Cancer Survival in Africa, Asia, the Caribbean and Central America

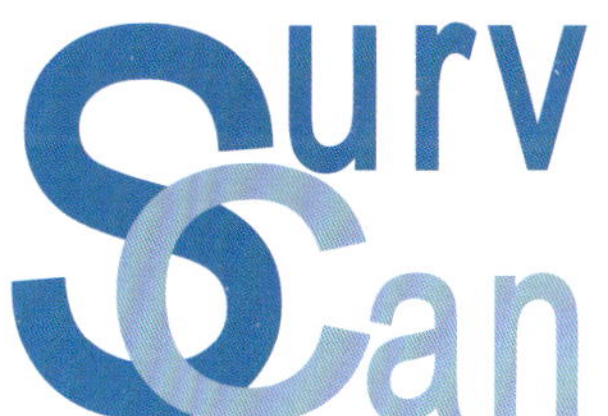

Also available online at http://survcan.iarc.fr

INTERNATIONAL AGENCY FOR RESEARCH ON CANCER

The International Agency for Research on Cancer (IARC) was established in 1965 by the World Health Assembly, as an independently financed organization within the framework of the World Health Organization. The headquarters of the Agency are at Lyon, France.

The Agency conducts a programme of research concentrating particularly on the epidemiology of cancer and the study of potential carcinogens in the human environment. Its epidemiological studies are supplemented by studies of the mechanisms of carcinogenesis carried out in the Agency's laboratories in Lyon. The promotion of collaborative research among scientists worldwide is a strong feature of the Agency's activities. The Agency also conducts a programme for the education and training of personnel for cancer research.

The publications of the Agency are intended to contribute to the dissemination of authoritative information on different aspects of cancer research. Information about IARC publications and how to order them is also available via the Internet at: **http://www.iarc.fr/**

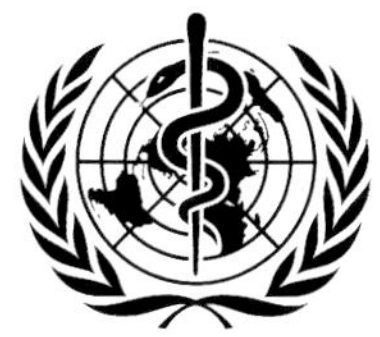

International Agency for Research on Cancer
World Health Organization

Cancer Survival in Africa, Asia, the Caribbean and Central America

Edited by
R. Sankaranarayanan, MD
R. Swaminathan, MSc, PhD

IARC Scientific Publications No. 162

International Agency for Research on Cancer
Lyon, 2011

Foreword

The success of early detection and cancer treatment may be measured by improvements in survival from cancer. Long-term survival reflects cure and is a positive measure that can be used by planners and health professionals to discuss the outcome of cancer diagnosis and treatment. It is also the result of most interest to patients, their families and the general public.

Cancer survival estimated from hospitals and clinical trial settings at best reflects the selective experience of groups of patients in specific settings, and cannot be generalized as reflecting the overall efficiency of the cancer health services in a given region or country. On the other hand, estimates of population-based survival based on all cancer patients diagnosed by all means in a given geographical region or country incorporate the influence of different socio-economic factors, natural histories, health-seeking behaviours, awareness, early detection practices and treatment availability and accessibility. Therefore, such estimates reflect the general efficiency of cancer health services and provide a key indicator of progress in cancer control in a given region. Such estimates can be derived from studying the survival experience of cancer patients registered in population-based cancer registries.

Comparative data on cancer survival from different regions could serve as the baseline for future improvement, through adequate and determined investments in improving awareness, health services infrastructure and accessibility. Population-based survival studies that have systematically analysed the survival outcomes of cancer patients are readily available in Europe, North America and other more-developed regions. However, they are relatively rare from countries in Africa, Asia and Central America. This gap was offset to an extent by the appearance, in 1999, of the first volume of the International Agency for Research on Cancer (IARC) scientific publication on *Cancer Survival in Developing Countries*.

The Agency presents here the second volume in the series, which includes survival data from 27 cancer registries in 14 countries from Africa, Asia, the Caribbean and Central America. This study would not have been possible without the availability of population-based cancer registries, thus underscoring the urgent need for organizing such information systems in sentinel populations in the least-represented areas of sub-Saharan Africa, central Asia and the Middle East.

For this volume, the response from registries has been overwhelming: the geographic coverage has a wider representation, the number of registries participating increased nearly threefold, and the number of cancer sites and incident cases analysed has increased manifold compared to the first volume. This provides a unique example of cooperation at the international level for improvement in cancer control, and the Agency is proud to play its part in this collaborative effort.

Considerable emphasis has been placed on improving follow-up for vital status of cancer patients by instituting a variety of innovative active and passive follow-up methods and on improving overall data quality by appropriate validation studies, although some level of overestimation of survival cannot be ruled out. The understanding and applicability of cancer survival estimates can be further improved by better collection of data for clinical stage and treatment of cancer as well as for vital status by the population-based cancer registries.

The striking inequalities in cancer survival between countries and within countries described in this volume are largely related to the differences in general awareness, availability of early detection practices, trained human resources, diagnosis and treatment and the development and accessibility to cancer services, as well as, to a lesser extent, to issues of data quality and reliability. The findings described in this scientific publication emphasize the need for urgent and adequate investments in comprehensive cancer control, including improving public and professional awareness, early detection, prompt treatment using locally feasible yet effective regimens, health services infrastructure and human resources development, as well as ensuring referral pathways and improved and equitable accessibility to health services.

The differences in cancer survival reported in populations observed between and within countries studied in this volume provide valuable insights for future planning and investment by governments in primary prevention activities, early detection initiatives and tertiary care to achieve meaningful cancer control. They should also prove a stimulus to those involved in cancer prevention and control to redouble their efforts to ensure that all cancer patients have the best possible chance to survive their own experience of this disease.

Christopher P. Wild
Director

Acknowledgements

The authors gratefully acknowledge the generous support of the following organizations for this cancer survival study:

- Association for International Cancer Research (AICR), St. Andrews, UK
- Association pour la Recherche sur le Cancer (ARC) Villejuif, France
- The Bill & Melinda Gates Foundation, Seattle, USA

We are thankful to all the personnel and agencies involved in data acquisition for this multinational study.

We are grateful to Ms. Evelyn Bayle, Ms. Odile Bouvy, Mr John Daniel, Ms. Krittika Guinot, Dr. Richard Muwonge and Dr. Catherine Sauvaget for their assistance in the preparation of this publication.

Final analysis was carried out during the post-doctoral fellowship awarded by the International Agency for Research on Cancer (IARC) to Dr. Rajaraman Swaminathan.

List of contributors

Introductory chapters

Brenner H
Division of Clinical Epidemiology and Aging Research
German Cancer Research Centre
69115 Heidelberg
GERMANY
E-mail: h.brenner@Dkfz-Heidelberg.de

Ganesh B
Division of Hospital Cancer Registry
and Biostatistics
Tata Memorial Centre
E.Borges Road
Mumbai 400012
INDIA
E-mail: b_ganeshbala@rediffmail.com

Hakama M
Finnish Cancer Registry
Institute for Statistical and Epidemiological Cancer Research
FI-00130 Helsinki
FINLAND
E-mail: Matti.Hakama@cancer.fi

Jayant K
Barshi Cancer Registry
Nargis Dutt Memorial Cancer Hospital
Agalgaon Road, Barshi 413401
Solapur District. Maharashtra
INDIA
E-mail: kasturijayant2010@gmail.com

Lucas E
Screening Group
Early Detection and Prevention Section
International Agency for Research on Cancer
69008 Lyon
FRANCE
E-mail: lucas@iarc.fr

Mathew A
Department of Clinical Research and Epidemiology
Regional Cancer Centre
Medical College Campus
Thiruvananthapuram 695011
INDIA
E-mail: amathew@rcctvm.org

Sankaranarayanan R
Screening Group
Early Detection and Prevention Section
International Agency for Research on Cancer
69008 Lyon
FRANCE
E-mail: sankar@iarc.fr

Swaminathan R
Division of Epidemiology and Cancer Registry
Cancer Institute (W.I.A)
Chennai 600036
Tamil Nadu
INDIA
E-mail: iarcsurvival@yahoo.co.uk

List of contributors

Registry chapters

CHINA, Hong Kong SAR

Hong Kong Cancer Registry
c/o Department of Clinical Oncology
Queen Elizabeth Hospital
30 Gascoigne Road, Kowloon
Hong Kong SAR
CHINA
Tel: (852) 2958-6021
Fax: (852) 2958-5559
E-mail: lawck@ha.org.hk

Law SC
Mang OW

CHINA, Qidong

Qidong Cancer Registry
Department of Epidemiology
Qidong Liver Cancer Institute
785 Jianghai Zhong Road
Qidong 226200 Jiangsu
CHINA
Tel: (86) 513-833-46201
Fax: (86) 513-830-86803
E-mail: chenjg@vip.sina.com

Chen JG
Zhu J
Zhang YH
Lu JH

CHINA, Shanghai

Shanghai Cancer Registry
Shanghai Cancer Institute
2200 Xie Tu Road
Shanghai 200032
CHINA
Tel: (86) 21-6404-3057
Fax: (86) 21-6404-1428
E-mail: ybxiang@online.sh.cn

Xiang YB
Jin F
Gao YT

CHINA, Tianjin

Tianjin Cancer Registry
Department of Epidemiology
Tianjin Cancer Institute & Hospital
Huanhu Xi Road
Tiyuan Bei, Hexi district,
Tianjin 300060
CHINA
Tel: (86) 22-23340123 Ext 5226
Fax: (86) 22-23359984
E-mail: chenkexin1963@yahoo.com

Xishan H
Chen K
Min H
Shufen D
Jifang W

COSTA RICA

Universidad de Costa Rica
Sede Rodrigo Facio
Escuela de Salud Pública
San Predro Montes de Oca
San José
COSTA RICA
Tel: (506) 351-7760
Fax: (506) 221-1167
E-mail: adolfo.ortiz@ucr.ac.cr

Ortiz-Barboza A
Gómez L
Cubero C
Bonilla G
Mena H

CUBA

Registro Nacional de Cancer de Cuba
Instituto Nacional Oncologia y Radiobiologia
29 y F Vedado
CP 10 400
La Habana
CUBA
Tel: (53) 7-552584
Fax: (53) 7-552593
E-mail: leticiaf@infomed.sld.cu

Garrote LF
Alvarez YG
Babie PT
Yi MG
Alvarez MG
Cecili ML

THE GAMBIA

National Cancer Registry, The Gambia
c/o IARC-Gambia Hepatitis Intervention Study
MRC Laboratories, Fajara
P.O.Box 273,
Banjul
THE GAMBIA
Tel: (220) 495229
Fax: (220) 496117
E-mail: ebah@iarc.fr

Bah E
Sam O
Whittle H
Ramanakumar A
Sankaranarayanan R

INDIA, Barshi

Barshi Cancer Registry
Nargis Dutt Memorial Cancer Hospital
Agalgaon Road
Barshi 413401
Solapur District
Maharashtra
INDIA
*Tata Memorial Hospital
Dr. E.Borges Road, Parel, Mumbai 400012
INDIA
Tel: (91) 2184-222699
Fax: (91) 2184-226657
E-mail: spr_bmnene@sancharnet.in

Jayant K
Nene BM
*Dinshaw KA**
*Badwe RA**
Panse NS
Thorat RV

INDIA, Bhopal

Bhopal Cancer Registry
Department of Pathology
Gandhi Medical College
Bhopal
INDIA
*Tata Memorial Hospital
Dr. E.Borges Road, Parel, Mumbai 400012
INDIA
Tel: (91) 22-2413 9318
Fax: (91) 22-2416 8440
E-mail: dixr24@hotmail.com

*Dikshit R**
Kanhere S
Surange S

INDIA, Chennai

Madras Metropolitan Tumour Registry
Cancer Institute (WIA)
38 Sardar Patel Road
Chennai 600036
INDIA
Tel: (91) 44-22350131
Fax: (91) 44-24912085
E-mail: iarcsurvival@yahoo.co.uk

Swaminathan R
Rama R
Nalini S
Shanta V

INDIA, Karunagappally

Natural Background Radiation Registry
Vavvakkavu P.O.
Karunagappally 690528
Kollam District Kerala
INDIA
Tel: (91) 476-620609
E-mail: nbrrkply@gmail.com

Jayalekshmi P
Gangadharan P

INDIA, Mumbai

Bombay Cancer Registry
Indian Cancer Society
74 Jerbai Wadia Road, Parel
Mumbai 400012
INDIA
Tel: (91) 22-4122351
Fax: (91) 22-4122351
E-mail: bcrics@vsnl.com

Yeole BB
Kurkure AP
Sunny L

PAKISTAN, South Karachi

Karachi Cancer Registry
Sindh Government Services Hospital (Premises)
M.A.Jinnah Road
Karachi 75600
PAKISTAN
Tel: (92) 21-5868421
Fax: (92) 21-21-5868421
E-mail: yasmin.bhurgri@gmail.com

Bhurgri Y

PHILIPPINES, Manila

Manila Cancer Registry
Philippine Cancer Society Inc.
P.O.Box 3066
310 San Rafael St., San Miguel
1005 Manila
PHILIPPINES
Tel: (63) 2-734-2114
Fax: (63) 2-734-2128
E-mail: yago_md@yahoo.com

Laudico A
Mapua C

PHILIPPINES, Rizal

Rizal Cancer Registry
Department of Health
Rizal Medical Center
Pasig Boulevard, Pasig City
1600 Metro Manila
PHILIPPINES
Tel: (63) 2-532-1879
Fax: (63) 2-532-1879
E-mail: dbesteban@yahoo.com

Esteban DB
Lumague RM
Laudico A

REPUBLIC OF KOREA, Busan

Busan Cancer Registry
Division of Cancer Control and Epidemiology
National Cancer Center Research Institute
809 Madu-Dong, Ilsan-Gu
Koyang
Kyonggi 411-764
REPUBLIC OF KOREA
Tel: (82) 31-920-2003
Fax: (82) 31-920-1520
E-mail: shinhr@wpro.who.int

Shin HR
Lee DH
Lee SY
Lee JT
Park HK
Rha SH
Whang IK
Jung KW
Won YJ
Kong HJ

REPUBLIC OF KOREA, Incheon

Incheon Cancer Registry
The College of Medicine,
Inha University
Incheon
REPUBLIC OF KOREA
Tel: 82-2-740-8394
Fax: 82-2-747-4830
Email: ychong1@snu.ac.kr

Woo ZH
Hong YC
Kim WC
Pu YK

REPUBLIC OF KOREA, Seoul

Seoul Cancer Registry
Department of Preventive Medicine
Seoul National University College of Medicine
Seoul
REPUBLIC OF KOREA
Tel: (82) 2-740-8322
Fax: (82) 2-764-9416
E-mail: yoahn@snu.ac.kr

Ahn YO
Shin MH

SAUDI ARABIA, Riyadh

King Faisal Specialist Hospital & Research Centre
Non-Communicable Diseases
Ministry of Health
Riyadh
SAUDI ARABIA
Tel: (966) 505482874
E-mail: nalhamdan@kfmc.med.sa

Hamdan NA
Ravichandran K
Dyab AR

SINGAPORE

Singapore Cancer Registry
Centre for Molecular Epidemiology
c/o Department of Community, Occupational and
Family Medicine, National University of Singapore
MD3, 16 Medical Drive
SINGAPORE 117597
Tel: (65) 68744977
Fax: (65) 67791489
Email: cofcks@nus.edu.sg

Chia KS

THAILAND, Chiang Mai

Chiang Mai Tumour Registry
Maharaj Nakorn Chiang Mai Hospital
Faculty of Medicine
Chiang Mai University
Chiang Mai 50200
THAILAND
Tel: (66) 53-947730
Fax: (66) 53-217144
E-mail: ssrisukh@mail.med.cmu.ac.th

Sumitsawan Y
Srisukho S
Sastraruji A
Chaisaengkhum U
Maneesai P
Waisri N

THAILAND, Khon Kaen

Khon Kaen Provincial Cancer Registry
Cancer Unit, Srinagarind Hospital
Faculty of Medicine
Khon Kaen University
Khon Kaen, 40002
THAILAND
Tel: (66) 43-202485
Fax: (66) 43-202485
E-mail: krisuw@kku.ac.th

Suwanrungruang K
Vatanasapt P
Kamsa-ard S
Sriamporn S
Wiangnon S

THAILAND, Lampang

Lampang Cancer Registry
Lampang Cancer Center,
Lampang 52000
THAILAND
Tel.: (66) 5433-5262 Ext.168
Fax : (66) 5433-5273
Email: tarathornmartin169@hotmail.com

Martin N
Pongnikorn S
Patel N
Daoprasert K

THAILAND, Songkhla

Songkhla Cancer Registry
Faculty of Medicine
Prince of Songkhla University
Hat Yai, Songkhla 90110
THAILAND
Tel: (66) 19901340
Fax: (66) 74212900
E-mail: hutcha.s@psu.ac.th

Sriplung H
Prechavittayakul P

TURKEY, Izmir

Izmir Cancer Registry
Izmir Provincial Health Directorate
KIDEM, Il Saglik Mudurlugu
35210 Alsancak
Izmir
TURKEY
Tel: (90) 232 4410571
Fax: (90) 232 4418111
E-mail: sultan.eser@gmail.com

Eser S

UGANDA, Kampala

Kampala Cancer Registry
Department of Pathology
Makerere University Faculty of Medicine
P.O.Box 7072 Kampala
UGANDA
Tel: (256) 41-531730
Fax: (256) 41-245580
E-mail: hwabinga@med.mak.ac.ug

Wabinga H
Parkin DM
Nambooze S
Amero J

ZIMBABWE, Harare

Zimbabwe National Cancer Registry
Parirenyatwa Hospital
P.O.Box A 449
Avondale, Harare
ZIMBABWE
Tel: (263) 4-791631 Ext 152
Fax: (263) 4-794445
E-mail: cancer@ecoweb.co.zw

Chokunonga E
Brook MZ
Chirenje ZM
Nyabakau AM
Parkin DM

Chapter 1

Introduction

Sankaranarayanan R

Abstract

The dearth of reliable survival statistics from developing countries was very evident until the mid-1990s. This prompted the International Agency for Research on Cancer (IARC) to undertake a project that facilitated hands-on-training and thereby transfer of knowledge and technology on cancer survival analysis to a majority of researchers from the participating population-based cancer registries, which culminated in the publication of the first volume of the IARC scientific publication on Cancer Survival in Developing Countries in 1998. The present study is the second in the series with wider geographical coverage and is based on data from 27 registries in 14 countries in Africa, Asia, the Caribbean and Central America. The calendar period of registration of incident cases for the present study ranges between 1990 and 2001. Data on 564 606 cases of 1–56 cancer sites from different registries are reported. Data from eleven registries were utilized for eliciting survival trend and seventeen registries for reporting survival by clinical extent of disease. Besides chapters on every registry and general chapters on methodology, database and overview, the availability of online comparative statistics on cancer survival data by participating registries or cancer site in the form of tables or graphs is an added feature (available online at http://survcan.iarc.fr).

Reliable data on the magnitude of the cancer problem are essential for monitoring the health of the community, assessing the performance of the health care system and allowing authorities to make informed decisions. The International Agency for Research on Cancer (IARC) has been collating data on cancer incidence and mortality worldwide, including from developing countries, for five decades now [1]. This is complemented by collaborative survival studies that are systematically analysed involving cancer patients in Europe [2], the United States of America [3] and other developed countries [4,5].

The dearth of reliable survival statistics from developing countries was very evident until the mid-1990s. Until then, a few isolated reports on survival using standard methods and based on the hospital-based series of selected cancer cases were available [6,7,8,9]. However, there were no population-based incident cancer case series from population-based cancer registries, which include all the cases diagnosed in a given population. The population-based cancer survival estimates are unbiased by selection, as they reflect the mixture of different socio-economic factors, health care seeking behaviours, natural histories, and the efficiency of the health care services in responding to the needs of early diagnosis, prompt treatment and follow-up care. Population-based survival represents the average prognosis of a given cancer in a given setting and is a very useful summary measure to evaluate progress in cancer control and to advocate for improved and equitable cancer care. Hence, several interested researchers from the well-laid network of population-based cancer registries in the developing countries with cooperation from all quarters, realized the urgent need of a comprehensive study on cancer survival.

This prompted the start of the collaborative survival project along these lines at the IARC in Lyon, France in 1994. The uniqueness of this study was that all the data submitted were subjected to central scrutiny and analysis, based on established and evolved norms, in a uniform manner. Furthermore, this project facilitated hands-on-training and thereby transfer of knowledge and technology on cancer survival analysis to a majority of researchers from the participating registries, which equipped the institutions with the required expertise to conduct such studies independently in future. All of these culminated in the publication of the first volume of the IARC scientific publication on Cancer Survival in Developing Countries in 1998 [10]. The major outcome of this study was that reliable cancer survival statistics from the developing countries were made available for the first time for comparison with the developed countries. Apart from that, the single most positive thing to happen was the overwhelming response it generated among other researchers, with more registries showing their willingness to take part in such collaborative survival studies. This led to the conception of the present study with the aim of increased coverage, utilisation of the recent methods in the estimation of survival, analysis of survival trend and wider implications aided by central data scrutiny and analysis at IARC.

Table 1 gives the coverage of the previous volume of Cancer Survival in Developing Countries and the present scientific publication in terms of geography, cancer sites/types reported and cases included for study for every country and registry that participated. Table 2 summarizes the coverage of all participating registries in terms of cases and analysis. The contributing registries present are mapped in Figure 1. The geographic coverage is seen to have a wider representation in the present volume with the inclusion of the continent of Africa joining Asia, the Caribbean and Central America as data providers. The total number of participating countries and registries also witnessed a nearly three-fold increase in the present volume: from ten registries in five countries in the first volume to 27 registries in 14 countries in this second volume. Nine out of ten registries that contributed data to the first volume continued to do so for the second volume. The other eighteen registries are new entrants to the scientific publication series on cancer survival.

The calendar period of registration of incident cases for the present study ranges from 1990 to 2001. It ranged between 1982 and 1992 in the earlier study. Thus, the most needed continuity in calendar time for the comparison of observations from the two studies and their meaningful interpretations has been preserved. Furthermore, six of the nine registries, which provided data for both volumes, have reported cases without discontinuity in calendar period.

The number of cancer sites or types for which the data on survival has been reported in the present study has also seen a substantial increase from the previous one. Three of ten registries had reported data for 20 or more cancers in the previous volume, while the corresponding figures in this volume are 14 of 27. All registries except two that contributed data for both volumes have reported either the same number or increased the number of cancers. The number of cancers reported in the present study ranges from a solitary cancer site to 56.

The increase in the number of registries and cancer sites or types in the present study has resulted in a significant increase in the number of cases reported. It ranges between a low of 300 and a high of >110 000. The corresponding figures were <300 and >65 000 in the previous volume.

The total cases submitted for central scrutiny at IARC for this study exceeded 630 000 cases, compared to about 169 000 in the previous volume, a 4-fold increase. The main analysis involved the cohort of cases from the latest calendar period and comprised the ascertainment of data quality, absolute and relative survival up to 5 years for all ages together, for both sexes and for classified age-groups. The trend analysis focussed on observations of the current period compared to the immediate preceding one. In selected instances, wherein data on incidence and follow-up was available for a very long period, as well as for recent years, the trend was analysed using the novel period approach of estimating survival and compared with the traditional cohort approach. The ratio of the number of cases included in this volume compared to the previous one was 4:1 for the main analysis; additional cases used was 9:1 for the trend analysis. Eleven registries contributed data for the trend analysis and there were seventeen for estimating survival by clinical extent of disease in this study; the corresponding figures for the previous study were one and eight respectively.

Chapter 2 deals with the statistical methods for cancer survival analysis discussing the basic entities, methods utilized in the estimation of absolute and relative survival and the most recent approach of age standardization.

Chapter 3 deals with loss-adjusted methods for estimating survival in the presence of substantial loss to follow-up with empirical examples.

Chapter 4 is the database chapter, giving details of the variables submitted for scrutiny, validation checks, data quality indices and types of analysis performed as a lead to the subsequent chapters on individual registries.

The subsequent chapters are dedicated to the observations on individual registries, with a concise write-up and standard sets of tables.

The final chapter gives an overview of cancer survival in participating countries, deals with discussion on the observed inter- and intra-country differences and the implications of the findings for cancer control, and makes a case for investing in the improvement of cancer health care services in low- and medium-resource countries.

Online dynamic functions are available at http://survcan.iarc.fr, to generate tables and figures giving comparative statistics by registry and by cancer site.

Table 1. Coverage of the previous and present volumes by country/registry/geographical area, number of cancer sites/types and cases

	Volume I			Volume II		
	Calendar peroid of registration	No. of cancer sites	No. of cases included	Calendar peroid of registration	No. of cancer sites	No. of cases included
CHINA				**1991–2001**	**33–52**	**270 468**
Hong Kong SAR				1996–2001	45	110 190
Qidong+	1982–1991	16	16 922	1992–2000	33	20 167
Shanghai+	1988–1991	39	66 449	1992–1995	52	70 006
Tianjin+				1991–1999	51	70 005
COSTA RICA$				1995–2000	2	6297
CUBA+	1988–1989	17	12 796	1994–1995	13	8150
THE GAMBIA*				1993–1997	6	505
INDIA				**1990–2000**	**15–28**	**73 432**
Bangalore	1982–1989	8	4781			
Barshi+	1988–1992	1	247	1993–2000	15	1188
Bhopal				1991–1995	16	1863
Chennai+	1984–1989	18	11 246	1990–1999	20	22 618
Karunagappally				1991–1997	22	1601
Mumbai+	1882–1986	2	5226	1992–1999	28	46 162
PAKISTAN						
South Karachi				1995–1999	4	677
PHILIPPINES				**1994–1997**	**1–4**	**2339**
Manila*				1994–1995	4	1040
Rizal+	1987	12	1400	1996–1997	1	1299
REPUBLIC OF KOREA				**1993–2001**	**42–56**	**139 824**
Busan				1996–2001	48	41 434
Incheon				1997–2001	42	20 563
Seoul				1993–1997	56	77 827
SAUDI ARABIA						
Riyadh				1994–1996	1	298
SINGAPORE+				1993–1997	45	27 016
THAILAND				**1990–2000**	**13–40**	**27 313**
Chiang Mai+	1983–1992	39	14 582	1993–1997	36	7276
Khon Kaen+	1985–1992	35	10 338	1993–1997	13	2253
Lampang				1990–2000	40	11 195
Songkhla				1990–1999	36	6589
TURKEY						
Izmir				1995–1997	12	4381
UGANDA						
Kampala*				1993–1997	15	1916
ZIMBABWE						
Harare*				1993–1997	17	1990

+ Data on previous calendar periods used for trend analysis;
$ Includes in-situ cancers of the cervix analysed separately;
** Random sample of cases for selected sites.*

Table 2. Summary of coverage in the two volumes: cases and analysis *(all registries together)*

	Volume I Cancer survival in developing countries	Volume II Cancer survival in Africa, Asia, the Caribbean and Central America
Total cases submitted for scrutiny among included registries (*all sites*)	168 869	632 361
Number of cases reported		
(selected sites and with at least 25 cases)		
Registered cases	144 268	610 938
Included for main analysis	143 987	564 606
Additional for trend analysis	18 171	168 181
No. of countries providing data	5	14
Number of registries included		
Main analysis	10	27
Trend analysis	1	11
Survival by clinical extent of disease	8	17
Calendar period of case registration*		
Main analysis	1982–1992	1990–2001
Trend analysis	1972–1991	1968–2000

** Period varies for individual registries*

Figure 1. Notional world map showing study locations

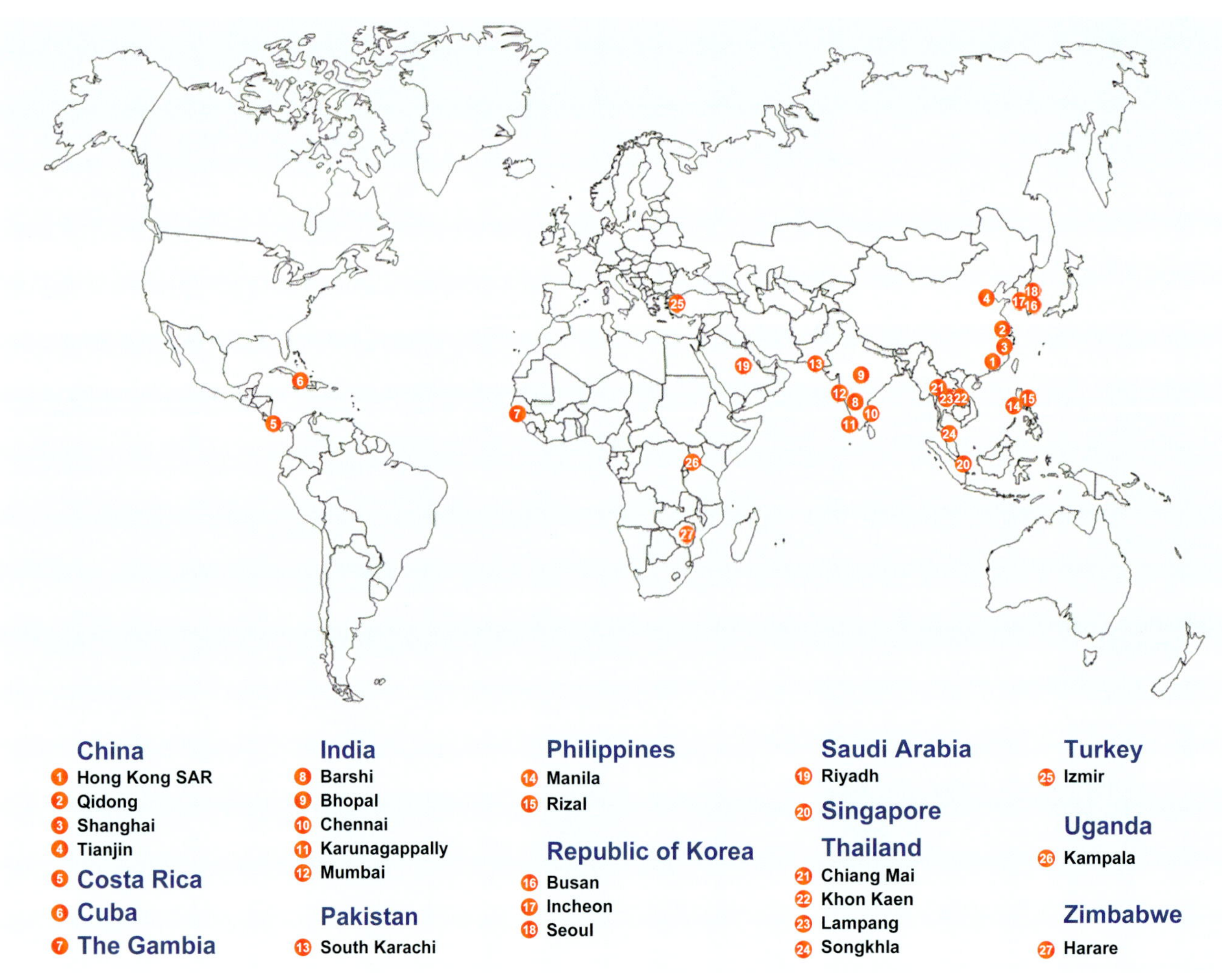

References

1. Parkin DM, Whelan SL, Ferlay J and Storm H. *Cancer Incidence in Five Continents, Vol I to VIII. IARC Cancerbase No. 7*. IARCPress, Lyon, 2005.

2. Sant M, Allemani C, Santaquilani M, *et al*. EUROCARE-4. Survival of cancer patients diagnosed in 1995–1999. Results and commentary. *Eur J Cancer* 2009;45: 931–991.

3. Ries LAG, Harkins D, Krapcho M, Mariotto A, Miller BA, Feuer EJ, Clegg L, Eisner MP, Horner MJ, Howlader N, Hayat M, Hankey BF and Edwards BK (eds). *SEER Cancer Statistics Review, 1975–2003*, National Cancer Institute. Bethesda, MD, 2006. http://seer.cancer.gov/csr/1975_2003/

4. Coleman MP, Quaresma M, Berrino F, et al. Cancer survival in five continents: a worldwide population-based study (CONCORD). *Lancet Oncol* 2008;9:730–756.

5. Tsukuma H, Ajiki W, Ioka A, Oshima A, Research Group of Population-Based Cancer Registries of Japan. Survival of cancer patients diagnosed between 1993 and 1996: a collaborative study of population-based cancer registries in Japan. *Jpn J Clin Oncol* 2006;36:602–607.

6. Lee AW, Poon YF, Foo W, Law SC, Cheung FK, Chan DK, Tung SY, Thaw M and Ho JH. Retrospective analysis of 5,037 patients with nasopharyngeal carcinoma treated during 1976–1985: Overall survival and patterns of failure. *Int J Radiat Oncol Biol Phys* 1992; 23(2): 261–270.

7. Nair MK, Sankaranarayanan R, Nair KS, Amma NS, Varghese C, Padmakumari G and Cherian T. Overall survival from breast cancer in Kerala, India, in relation to menstrual, reproductive and clinical factors. *Cancer* 1993; 71(5): 1791–1796.

8. Pavlovsky S, Sackmann MF, Santarelli MT, Svarch E, Jimenez E, Kohan R and Rosso A. An update of the results of intensive therapy in children with acute lymphoblastic leukaemia. *Leukemia* 1992; 6 (Suppl 2): 167–170.

9. Pengsaa P, Pesi M, Udomthavornsuk B, Tungvorapongchai V, Vatanasapt W and Shibata Y. *J Med Assoc Thai* 1989; 72(6): 346–350.

10. Sankaranarayanan R, Black RJ and Parkin DM. *Cancer Survival in Developing Countries. IARC Scientific Publications No. 145*. IARCPress, Lyon, 1998.

Chapter 2

Stastistical methods for cancer survival analysis

Swaminathan R and Brenner H

Abstract

Adequate and complete follow-up is a prerequisite for the conduct of any survival study. Passive follow-up relies on routine availability of mortality data through unique data linkage possibilities, while active follow-up supplements mortality ascertainment, for which there are a variety of methods. Cox proportional-hazard model was employed to test whether censoring was random in presence of loss to follow-up. Absolute survival probability was estimated by the actuarial method following semi-complete approach for all registries, and the period approach was also used wherever possible. Expected survival probability for registries was estimated from the respective country-, age- and sex-specific abridged life tables. Relative survival, as the ratio of absolute to expected survival, was calculated to exclude the effect arising from different background mortalities. To account for the differences in the age structure of the cancer cases, relative survival was adjusted for age and reported as age-standardized relative survival. Estimated incident cancer cases from less-developed countries together for every classified cancer site served as the standard population. Weights were assigned to individual patients, depending on their age, and standardization was carried out using weighted individual data. Analyses were done using the publicly available macros in SAS software.

Introduction and background

The life table, one of the basic tools in the description of mortality experience of a population, was first developed as early as 1693 by E. Halley in England. It forms the basis for calculation of the life table estimate of the survivor function, which is still widely used today in the analysis of data from epidemiological studies. Information on survival has long been recognized as an important component in monitoring cancer control activities [1]. Like all other health indices, survival statistics are useful primarily as comparative measures. It is these comparisons that help us to suggest possible reasons for the variations and provide targets for improvement and a means of monitoring progress towards them [2]. Survival data obtained from a population-based cancer registry ideally portrays the average outcome of the disease in the pertaining region covered since it is based on an unselected series of incident cancer cases [3].

Follow-up

Adequate and complete follow-up is a prerequisite to conducting a survival study. Lengthy periods of time may be required until the event of interest (any death is the outcome studied in this publication) occurs in all cases studied and maintenance of surveillance on patients may be extremely difficult. Hence, a closing date for follow-up is typically imposed keeping in mind the adequacy of follow-up information needed to estimate the survival at a specified time. Complete follow-up is deemed to have been achieved when the vital status (alive/dead) at closing date is known for an individual. If not known, then the follow-up is incomplete.

With passive follow-up, information on deaths is routinely received either by-law or via an arrangement with the vital statistics division. Using this procedure, those patients for whom no information of death has been received may be considered to be "alive" until that point of time. The main requirement for this method to work efficiently is that there is a high quality of registration of mortality data and unique data linkage possibilities which ensure the follow-up of cases to be complete with the exception of migration or rare losses. A few of the registries contributing data to this scientific publication have relied almost entirely on this means of obtaining follow-up information.

Active follow-up is necessary in the absence of a reliable health information system, and it may supplement the latter in case of incomplete passive follow-up. Most registries that contributed data to

after diagnosis. For this purpose, only subjects potentially under observation for at least 5 years and having a potentially complete follow-up of five years are taken into consideration. This approach, which has been called cohort analysis [7] has the disadvantage that even the most recent survival estimates are exclusively based on patients diagnosed many years ago. For example, with a database that includes patients diagnosed between 1989 and 1999 with a closing date of follow-up at the end of 1999, a cohort estimate of 5-year survival could be obtained from patients diagnosed in 1994 at the latest, because patients diagnosed in later years could not possibly have 5-year follow-up by the end of 1999. This approach is illustrated by the solid black frame in Figure 1.

Complete analysis

This is the approach to be used when there is no restriction on the potential follow-up time to equal, e.g., five years from the index date for which the survival is estimated. Rather, all subjects who are diagnosed as incident cancers until the closing date of the follow-up period qualify for inclusion in the analysis. Apart from the subjects with a complete follow-up of five years, those under observation for a variable period of time and having an incomplete follow-up of less than five years are included [7]. In the example given above, all patients diagnosed in 1995–1999 could be included in addition to those diagnosed in earlier years for the derivation of a complete estimate of 5-year survival. This approach is illustrated by the dashed black frame in Figure 1.

Figure 1. Types of analysis to derive up-to-date 5-year survival estimates based on data of patients diagnosed in 1989–1999 and followed until the end of 1999

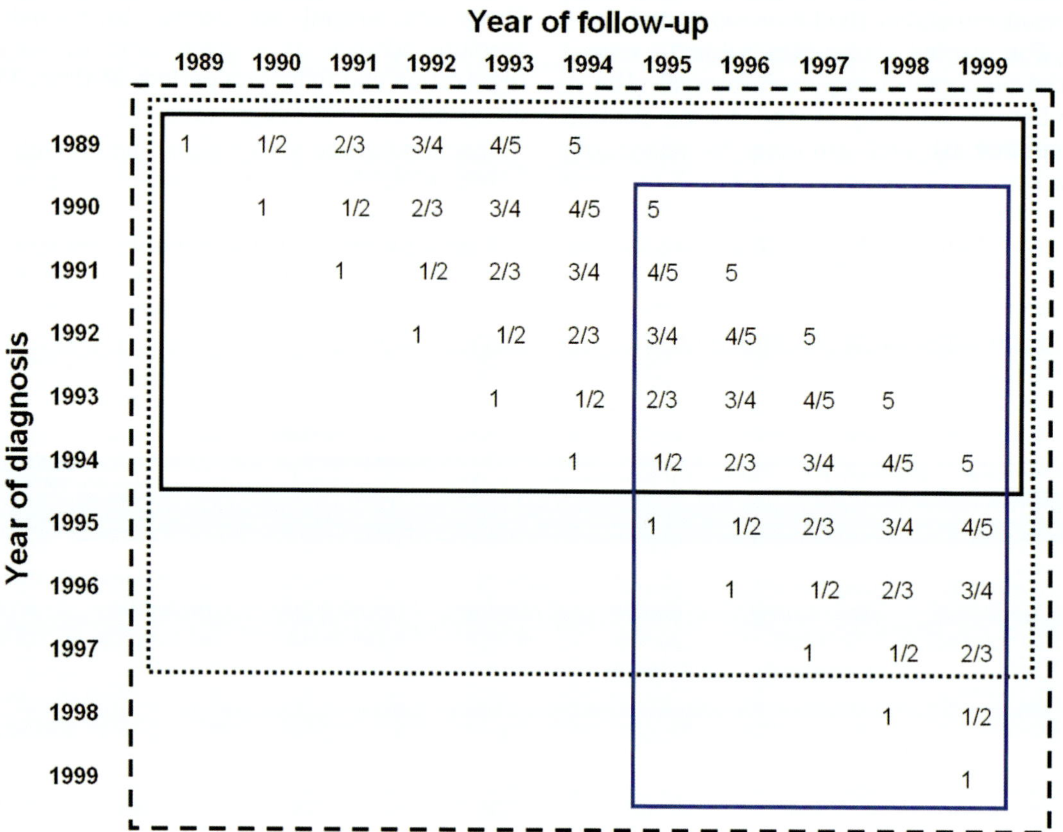

Cohort analysis: solid black frame;
Complete analysis: dashed black frame;
Semi or partially complete analysis: dotted black frame;
Period analysis: solid blue frame.
The numbers within the cells indicate the years since diagnosis.

Semi or partially complete analysis

This approach is widely practised in the estimation of survival by cancer registries. It was adopted in the previous publication on cancer survival [6], and is used for most analyses in this publication as well. Here, not all patients diagnosed until the closing date of follow-up are included. Rather, only patients who have had some minimum potential follow-up time at the closing date of follow-up, such as two or three years, are included. In our example, a partially complete estimate of 5-year survival may be obtained from patients diagnosed in or before 1997 and who have had a minimum of two potential years of follow-up at the end of 1999. This approach, which is in between the pure cohort and pure complete analysis, is illustrated by the dotted black frame in Figure 1.

Period analysis

This is an alternative approach [8] to deriving more up-to-date estimates of cancer patient survival by exclusively utilising the survival information pertaining to the most recent incidence and follow-up periods. The period of interest could be a single calendar year or more. Period analysis exclusively reflects the survival experience of subjects within the most recent calendar period for which the follow-up is available. This is achieved by left truncation of observations at the beginning of this period in addition to censoring at its end [9].

In our example, assume that a period estimate of 5-year survival is to be derived for the 1995–1999 period, the most recent period for which pertinent data are available, then all observations are left truncated at the beginning of 1995 in addition to being censored at the end of 1999. The 5-year period estimate of survival would be obtained from patients diagnosed in 1990–1999 for whom some proportion of 5-year follow-up might have fallen in the 1995–1999 period. With this approach, illustrated by the solid blue frame in Figure 1, different parts of the survival function would be derived from patients diagnosed in various calendar years. Survival during the first year following diagnosis would be estimated for patients diagnosed in 1994–1999, survival during the second year following diagnosis would be estimated for patients diagnosed in 1993–1998, and so on, until survival experience during the fifth year following diagnosis which would be obtained for patients diagnosed in 1990–1995. These conditional survival probabilities are then combined in the usual way to generate 5-year cumulative survival estimates for the 1995–1999 period. It has been shown that period analysis is the approach that clearly provides the most up-to-date estimates of cancer patient survival, and that period estimates of survival for some given period quite closely predict survival experience of patients diagnosed during that period [10]. In this publication, however, period analysis could not routinely be used because incidence data had not been collected up to the closing date of follow-up by most registries. That said, period analysis was used with data from registries in Qidong and Tianjin, China, and Singapore. A comparison of the survival estimates by cohort and period approaches has been done and the trends over calendar time were depicted.

Relative survival

Berkson [11] in 1942 introduced the concept of relative survival. The relative survival (R_i) for a group of patients at the end of an interval beginning at time t_i is defined as

$$R_i = \frac{S_i}{S_i^*}$$

where S_i is the absolute survival for subjects with a particular cancer and S_i^* is the expected survival of a group of individuals with the same demographic characteristics (age, sex, etc.) who are at risk of death only from causes other than the cancer under study [12]. Berkson and Gage [13] suggested that the observed proportion of survivors of cancer can be compared with an expected proportion of survivors derived from similar people from the general population, most of whom do not have the disease under study. The concept of relative survival methodology has primarily been designed for cancer survival studies to exclude the effect arising from different background mortalities.

Estimation of expected survival probabilities

Expected survival probabilities are usually estimated from age- and sex-specific (sometimes also race-specific) life tables of the general population for the registry area. At least three different methods have been proposed to estimate expected survival, the so-called Ederer I [12], Ederer II [14] and Hakulinen [15] methods. For follow-up times up to 5 years (as reported in this publication) they generally give very similar results. In this study, expected survival probabilities are estimated from country-, age- and sex-specific abridged life tables [16] according to the Ederer II method [14] (for 5-year survival) and the Hakulinen method [15] (for 10- and 15-year survival), the latter of which corrects for potential heterogeneity in patient withdrawal over long potential follow-up times. The estimation of expected survival for earlier calendar periods is done using the country-, age- and sex-specific life tables of the respective calendar periods.

Age-standardization of survival

Most biological phenomena are related to age; there is no reason to expect that survival is not. It is important to note that use of relative rather than absolute survival does not make age-standardization unnecessary. For many types of cancer, the risk of dying as a result of the cancer itself is clearly associated with a subject's age at diagnosis. The ages at diagnosis of cases of any cancer in the developing and developed countries are vastly different [17]. When comparing survival in different groups of patients from different regions, there is a definite need to standardize both absolute and relative survival estimates for age.

For this purpose, direct standardization of survival estimates has been advocated [18]. This is commonly done by using direct standardization of age-specific survival estimates to derive summary statistics called age-standardized absolute survival (ASAS) or age-standardized relative survival (ASRS). For example, ASAS at the end of some follow-up period i is given by

$$ASAS_i = \frac{\sum_x a_{ix} st_x}{\sum_x st_x}$$

where the a_{ix} are age-specific (x:0–4;5–9; etc.) absolute survival estimates at the end of follow-up period ti and stx are the age-specific proportions used as "standard or weight" for standardization. The st_x could be arbitrary. Traditionally, the weights have been chosen to reflect the age distribution at diagnosis of some standard cancer population, such as the world standard cancer population [19].

However, for relative survival, the traditional age-standardization, as outlined above, provides results that are conceptually different from crude survival data [20]. Furthermore, traditional age-standardization is often difficult if not impossible to carry out in the presence of sparse and censored data. Hence, in this publication, an alternative approach to age-standardization [21] has been adopted. In this approach, one first assigns the weights to the individual patients depending on their age and then carries out conventional survival analyses using the "weighted individual data". The weights are defined as the ratio of the proportion of patients in the respective age group (x) in the standard population (st) divided by the proportion of patients in the respective age group in the study population. Whereas in the unadjusted (crude analyses), each patient in the study population and her/his contributions to the numbers of persons at risk and deaths are (implicitly) entered with a weight of 1, the proposed form of age-adjustment gives weights higher (lower) than 1 to patients in age groups which are under-represented (over-represented) in the study population compared to the standard population. The advantages of doing this type of adjustment are: (i) it remains feasible with sparse data, even in situations where survival estimates cannot be derived for certain age groups, and (ii) it provides age-adjusted estimates of relative survival that are conceptually consistent with the crude estimates. In particular, age-adjustment to the study population's own age structure yields a standardized relative survival that is identical to the crude one.

In this study, the weights are defined as the ratio of the proportion of patients in the respective age group in the standard population as summarized in GLOBOCAN 2002 [22], divided by the proportion of patients in the respective age group in the study population registry for every classified cancer site/type.

Software used

While absolute survival can be estimated with any of a large number of commercially available statistical software packages, there are only few specialized programs for relative survival analysis. In this study, analyses are done using the publicly available SAS macros "period" or "periodh" (age-specific and crude analysis, [10]) or "adperiod" or "adperiodh" (age-adjusted analysis, [21]) , which can be used to calculate both absolute and relative survival (Ederer and Hakulinen methods) with either the cohort, semi-complete or period approach.

References

1. WHO/IARC. *Cancer Statistics: Report of a WHO/IARC Expert Committee, WHO Technical Report Series No. 632*. World Health Organization, Geneva, 1979.

2. Black RJ, Sankaranarayanan R and Parkin DM. Interpretation of population based cancer survival data. In: *Cancer Survival in Developing Countries*. (eds) R. Sankaranarayanan, RJ Black and DM Parkin. IARC Scientific Publications No. 145. IARCPress, Lyon, 1998, pp 13–17.

3. Sankaranarayanan R, Black RJ and Parkin DM. Eds. *Cancer Survival in Developing Countries*. IARC Scientific Publications No. 145. IARCPress, Lyon, 1998.

4. Cox DR. Regression models and life tables. *J R Statistic Soc (B)* 1972;34: 187–220.

5. Cutler SJ, Ederer F. Maximum utilization of the life table method in analysing survival. *J Chron Dis.* 1958;8: 699–712.

6. Black RJ and Swaminathan R. Statistical methods for the analysis of cancer survival data. In: *Cancer Survival in Developing Countries* (eds) Sankaranarayanan R, Black RJ and Parkin DM. IARC Scientific Publications No. 145. IARCPress, Lyon, 1998; pp 3–7.

7. Brenner H, Gefeller O. Deriving more up-to-date estimates of long term patient survival. *J Clin Epidemiol* 1997; 50: 211–216.

8. Brenner H, Gefeller O. An alternative approach to monitoring cancer patient survival. *Cancer* 1996; 78: 2004–2010.

9. Brenner H, Gefeller O, Hakulinen T. A computer program for period analysis of cancer patient survival. *Eur J Cancer* 2002; 38: 690–695.

10. Brenner H, Hakulinen T. Up-to-date long-term survival curves of patients with cancer by period analysis. *J Clin Oncol* 2002; 20: 826–832.

11. Berkson J. The calculation of survival rates. In: *Carcinoma and other malignant lesions of the stomach.* (eds) W. Wlaters, HK Gray and JT Priestly, 467–484. Philadelphia: Sanders, 1942.

12. Ederer F, Axtell LM and Cutler SJ. The relative survival rate: a statistical methodology. *Monogr Natl Cancer Inst* 1961; 6: 101–121.

13. Berkson J, Gage RP. Calculation of survival rates for cancer. *Proc Mayo Clinic* 1950; 25: 270–286.

14. Ederer F, Heise H. *Instructions to IBM 650 programmers in processing survival computations. Methodological note No. 10.* Bethesda, National Cancer Institute, 1959.

15. Hakulinen T. Cancer survival corrected for heterogeneity in patient withdrawal. *Biometrics* 1982; 38: 933–942.

16. Lopez AD, Ahmad OB, Guillot M, Inoue M, Ferguson BD, Salomon JA. *Life tables for 191 countries for 2000: data, methods, results (GPE discussion paper No. 40). Health Systems Performance Assessments Peer Review, Technical Documentation. IV Outcomes: Population Health. Evidence and information for Policy (EIP).* WHO, October 2001.

17. Parkin DM, Whelan SL, Ferlay J, Teppo L and Thomas DB. Eds. *Cancer Incidence in Five Continents, Vol VIII. IARC Scientific Publications No. 155.* IARCPress, Lyon, 2002.

18. Parkin DM and Hakulinen T. Analysis of survival. In: Jensen OM, Parkin DM, MacLennan R, Muir CS and Skeet RG (eds) *Cancer Registration, Principles and Methods. IARC Scientific Publications No. 95.* IARCPress, Lyon, 1991; pp 159–176.

19. Black RJ and Bashir SA. World standard cancer patient populations: A resource for comparative analysis of survival data. In: *Cancer Survival in Developing Countries.* (eds) Sankaranarayanan R, Black RJ and Parkin DM. IARC Scientific Publications No. 145. IARCPress, Lyon, 1998; pp 9–11.

20. Brenner H, Hakulinen T. On crude and age-adjusted relative survival rates. *J Clin Epidemiol* 2003; 56: 1185–1191.

21. Brenner H, Arndt V, Gefeller O, Hakulinen T. An alternative approach to age-adjustment of cancer survival rates. *Eur J Cancer* 2004; 40: 2317–2322.

22. Ferlay J, Bray F, Pisani P and Parkin DM. *GLOBOCAN 2002: Cancer Incidence, Mortality and Prevalence Worldwide. IARC CancerBase No. 5*, version 2.0. IARCPress, Lyon, 2004.

Chapter 3

Loss-adjusted hospital and population-based survival of cancer patients

Ganesh B, Swaminathan R, Mathew A, Sankaranarayanan R and Hakama M

Abstract

This chapter presents formulae that methodologically adjust for losses, and gives examples describing magnitude of bias in survival estimates without such adjustment. Loss-adjusted survival is estimated under the assumption that survival of patients lost to follow-up is the same as that for patients with known follow-up time and similar characteristics of different prognostic factors at first entry. The observed number of losses to follow-up is then relocated into expected numbers of death and survivors on this basis. Standard methods, such as the actuarial one, are then applied with the sum of observed and expected outcome events. A total of 336 hospital series of treated new breast cancer cases from Mumbai with 24% lost to follow-up revealed a substantial bias of 7 per cent units for 3-year survival estimated with (54%) and without (61%) loss-adjustment. Stepwise adjustment of losses established that increasing the number of prognostic factors explained the bias better. Population-based series comprising 13 371 cases of top ranking cancers from Chennai, with loss to follow-up ranging from 7–24%, revealed negligible bias, ranging from 0–2% in 5-year survival by the loss-adjusted approach for different cancers. Data source seems to affect the need for loss-adjustment, and the loss-adjusted approach is recommended when hospital-based cancer registry data of a low- or medium-resource country are used to evaluate the outcome of cancer patients.

Introduction

Cancer survival is the main indicator of outcome of cancer health services or treatment, and an important component in maintaining cancer control activities [1]. Cancer registries have long served as potential sources of data for estimating survival. Hospital-based cancer registries usually report survival of a selected series of treated patients that are registered in a hospital or group of hospitals without specific coverage of geographical area or background population. On the other hand, population-based cancer registries, which include all incident cases treated or not from a specific geographical area, usually report average survival in specific regions. Cancer survival reported from both settings may have different perspectives, but estimation of survival rates is routinely done using standard life table approaches such as the actuarial [2] or Kaplan-Meier [3] methods.

The actuarial method [2] of estimating survival by follow-up time allows utilization of all information independent of the length of follow-up of an individual patient, so that even recently diagnosed patients contribute to long-term survival. Patients who have a potential follow-up shorter than the time of the maximum estimated survival are "censored" cases. Censored cases are usually withdrawals, surviving at date of last follow-up: this date can be either individual for each patient or a common closing date for all patients. However, censorship in terms of losses to follow-up takes place if follow-up fails before this potential withdrawal. There is a qualitative difference between these two groups of censored cases.

Losses to follow-up may cause major bias. This holds true if the losses are common and correlated with the patient prognosis or survival. In most low- or medium-resource countries, such losses are common due to deficiencies in health infrastructure and recording of health statistics. The losses are also likely to be related to the patient's prognosis: low social status is related to lack of continuous patient surveillance; extent of disease is related to the motivation of follow-up, etc. Hence, this correlation, explained by information on prognostic factors, can be utilized to correct survival estimates.

A method to estimate loss-adjusted survival rates corrected, for possible bias due to losses to follow-up, is described here through two examples, one each from hospital-based and population-based registry settings. The loss-adjusted survival results are compared with the crude actuarial estimate to demonstrate the magnitude of bias.

Methods

Follow-up

Follow-up was carried out by passive and active methods. The passive approach was by data linkage either with patients' records on regular follow-up at the outpatient clinic and/or with mortality data from the vital statistics division. The active approach was by contacting the patients or their families directly by means of postal/telephone/e-mail/house visit enquiries for information on survival status.

Determinants of loss to follow-up or survival

Categorical factors (like age, sex, literacy status, tumour stage, treatment, etc.), each with reference and subcategory levels, that have the potential to influence either follow-up (complete or lost to follow-up) or survival (alive or dead) were first determined by using test of proportions (univariate only), logistic regression (unifactorial or multifactorial) or Cox proportional-hazard model (univariate or multi-factorial using survival time information). A differential pattern of follow-up or survival outcome, either between factors or within subcategories of factors, would indicate an association of non-random nature.

Estimation of loss-adjusted survival rate - stratified method

The life table method estimates annual survival during a given follow-up year by specifying four types of events including the outcome experienced by the patient: surviving throughout the year; dying (outcome) during the year; withdrawn alive, where patient was known to be alive at closing date of follow-up; and loss to follow-up, where the known survival time terminates during the follow-up year, but before closing date. Unlike traditional survival analysis, which grouped withdrawals and losses together, the proposed method for estimating loss-adjusted survival differentiated the two. For the time being, methods are developed for potential follow-up time of all subjects equalling the time for which survival is estimated. In other words, potential follow-up time for all cases would have to be five years to estimate 5-year loss-adjusted survival rate.

Every prognostic stratum is composed of a unique combination of subcategories of all identified determinants of follow-up or survival. In the estimation of loss-adjusted survival, it is assumed that those lost to follow-up in specific prognostic stratum have the same probability of death as others still remaining under observation and belonging to the same stratum. At any given follow-up time, the observed numbers of losses to follow-up in each stratum are relocated into expected numbers of deaths, withdrawals and survivors on the basis of observed survival in those without loss to follow-up in the same stratum. The actuarial method, or any other, is then applied to the sum of observed and expected events.

In the follow-up interval i in prognostic stratum j, there will be n_{ij} patients alive at beginning of interval, of whom d_{ij} will die, w_{ij} will be withdrawn alive and l_{ij} will be lost to follow-up during the interval. Since potential follow-up exceeds i intervals for all patients, w_{ij} = 0. The number with complete follow-up, n'_{ij} , is then given by:

$$n'_{ij} = n_{ij} - l_{ij}$$

The proportion dying with complete follow-up, q'_{ij} given the prognostic factors $x_i,\ldots..x_k$, is first estimated for patients not lost to follow-up, n'_{ij} , in the interval i:

$$q'_{ij} = \frac{d_{ij}}{n'_{ij}}\,.$$

The expected number of deaths in patients lost for follow-up in interval i is:

$$d'_{ij} = q'_{ij}\, l_{ij}$$

and the expected proportion of deaths in the n_{ij} cases is:

$$q_{ij} = \frac{(d_{ij} + d'_{ij})}{n_{ij}}$$

$$= \frac{D_{ij}}{n_{ij}}$$

The procedure is repeated for the next interval (i = i +1) as follows:

$$n'_{(i+1)j} = n_{ij} - D_{ij} - l_{(i+1)j} \quad \text{and with}$$

$$l'_{(i+1)j} = l_{(i+1)j} + l_{ij} - d'_{(i+1)j} \quad \text{with}$$

$$d'_{(i+1)j} = q'_{(i+1)j}\, l'_{(i+1)j} \quad \text{and for the other}$$

prognostic strata.

Accumulating over prognostic strata will result in an annual loss-adjusted rate:

$$q_i(Loss\ Adjusted) = \frac{\sum_j D_{ij}}{\sum_j n_{ij}}$$

and the cumulative loss-adjusted survival probability is:

$$P_i(Loss\ Adjusted) = (1-q_1)(1-q_2)......(1-q_i).$$

Logistic regression approach to estimate expected deaths among loss to follow-up

The correction of bias in survival estimation adjusted for loss to follow-up is optimal when it is determined by including as many factors as possible. An increase in number of determinants (factors with subcategories) of follow-up or survival would result in a corresponding increase in the number of prognostic strata. Cross-tabulation of all of these factors simultaneously would require adequate sample size to keep a majority of prognostic strata non-empty. Adjusting all factors simultaneously by logistic regression is a simplification of the computational procedure to estimate expected deaths among lost to follow-up and offers maximal effect in reducing the bias.

The proportion dying in the $\sum_j n'_{ij}$ patients followed completely during the interval is:

$$q'_i = \frac{\exp(\mu'_i)}{(1+\exp(\mu'_i))}$$

where

$$\mu'_i = \beta_{0i} + \beta_{1i}x_{1i} + \beta_{2i}x_{2i} + ... + \beta_{ki}x_{ki}$$

is a linear combination of the determinant or prognostic factors. The above methods are described in detail elsewhere [4,5].

Other approaches

Loss-adjusted survival can also be estimated using the Kaplan-Meier approach [6]. Stratum-specific expected deaths are estimated and the Kaplan-Meier curve is corrected at time points when the expected deaths occur.

Results

Example 1: Hospital-based cancer registry series

A total of 336 new cases of female breast cancer cases that were diagnosed and received complete treatment at Tata Memorial Hospital, Mumbai (Bombay), India, in 1985 and followed-up until 1988 formed the study population. These cases were allocated to 64 strata involving four factors associated with follow-up or prognosis: age (in completed years: <45, 45–54, 55–64, 65+ years); stage of disease (TNM staging classification: I, II, III, IV); type of treatment (chemotherapy: without, with); place of residence (Mumbai: residents, non-residents). Outcome event with respect to follow-up was loss to follow-up <3 years from diagnosis, and outcome event for loss-adjusted survival was death due to any cause.

Patients below 55 years of age comprised 65%, with an overall mean of 49 years (Table 1). There was an equal distribution of resident and non-resident patients from Mumbai city. A majority were diagnosed in stage II (48%) followed by stage III (37%) of the disease. About 58% of the patients were treated with either surgery or radiotherapy or in combination but not with chemotherapy, while the remaining 42% were treated with chemotherapy either alone or in combination with other modalities. Differential pattern of proportion (%) or risk (odds ratio) of loss to follow-up by different prognostic factor categories was forthcoming. The proportion of patients lost to follow-up was not very different between subcategories of age and type of treatment, with 0 to 30% increased risk over corresponding reference categories that was statistically not significant. The proportion lost to follow-up was doubled among non-residents versus residents of Mumbai, with two- to three-fold increased risk that was statistically significant. The risk was two to three times higher among stage III or IV patients and 50% higher among stage II compared to stage I patients, but not statistically significant (Table 1). The findings suggest an association between these prognostic factors and loss to follow-up.

The data was further analysed to estimate loss-adjusted survival by stratification of two or three factors at a time and by logistic regression approaches. Survival was estimated at the end of 3-year follow-up by actuarial method without and with adjustment for loss to follow-up (Table 2). The 3-year survival obtained by loss-adjustment showed lower survival compared to rates obtained by standard actuarial assumption without specific adjustment for loss to follow-up. The bias in survival estimation is represented as the difference in per cent units of survival rates (%) without and with loss-adjustment for each factor. This varied from 5.4 for patients aged 55 to 64 years to 8.6 for those aged <45 years. The bias was lesser among Mumbai residents (3.2) than non-residents (8.8). Three-year loss-adjusted survival was higher among residents (56.2%) than non-residents (54.4%), but this was the opposite for corresponding survival figures without loss-adjustment (59.4% and 63.2%), respectively. A decrease in survival (Table 2) and increase in proportion of lost to follow-up (Table 1) with severity of disease was forthcoming, which indicated a positive association between risk of dying and loss to follow-up in all disease stages. Loss-adjusted survival was greater in stage I patients, but lesser in other stages, compared to respective survival estimates without loss-adjustment. Following the elimination of bias by loss-adjustment, the difference in loss-adjusted survival between stages I and III patients increased from 51 per cent units to 61 per cent units (Table 2). The proportion of deaths in the chemotherapy group was twofold more than in the non-chemotherapy group. The comparison between actuarial and loss-adjusted survival showed that the adjusted unbiased difference between the two groups was bigger (43 per cent units) than the unadjusted ones (38 per cent units).

The variable extent of bias in survival estimation that could be elicited in the presence of loss to follow-up by utilizing information from one to four prognostic factors is shown stepwise for all cases in Table 3. The unadjusted actuarial 3-year survival was 61%. The loss-adjustment yielded a decrease of 7 per cent units in survival when all four prognostic factors were considered simultaneously by logistic regression method. The stepwise introduction of each of the prognostic factors into the adjustment procedure, by stratified method of estimating loss-adjusted survival, increased the correction of bias as follows: 1.7 per cent units when adjusted only for residential status; 2 per cent units when age was added; 3.8 per cent units when stage was added to the previous two factors; and 4.7 per cent units when all factors were adjusted.

Example 2: Case series from Chennai population-based cancer registry

A total of 13 371 cases comprising cancers of the uterine cervix (3134), female breast (1923), stomach (1845), oesophagus (1403), lung (1237), mouth (1202), lymphomas (768), tongue (670), leukaemias (668), and of ovary (521) ranked within the top ten in

Table 1. Number and proportion (%) of patients and losses at 3 years and risk (odds ratio) of loss to follow-up with 95% confidence interval by patient characteristics among female breast cancer patients diagnosed in Tata Memorial Hospital, Mumbai, India, in 1985 and followed through 1988

Patient characteristics	Patients (n=336)		Lost to follow-up (n=80; 24%)		Odds ratio (95% CI)
	Number	%[a]	Number	%[b]	
Age at diagnosis					
≤ 44 years	101	30	22	22	1.0*
45–54	117	35	29	25	1.2 (0.6–2.3)
55–64	77	23	19	25	1.2 (0.6–2.5)
65+ years	41	12	10	24	(0.5–2.9)
Residential status (Mumbai city)					
Residents	169	50	26	15	1.0*
Non-residents	167	50	54	32	2.6 (1.5–4.6)[$]
Stage of disease (TNM summary)					
I	29	9	4	14	1.0*
II	160	48	30	19	1.5 (0.5–5.6)
III	126	37	40	32	2.9 (0.9–10.6)
IV	21	6	6	29	2.5 (0.5–12.9)
Treatment					
With chemotherapy	194	58	42	22	1.0*
Without chemotherapy	142	42	38	27	1.3 (0.8–2.3)

[a] *Percentage of total breast cancer cases;*
[b] *Percentage of total cases in respective categories;*
CI: Confidence interval;
** Reference category;*
[$] *p=0.05.*

Table 2. Number and proportion (%) of patients and deaths and comparison of 3-year survival with and without adjustment for loss to follow-up by patient characteristics among female breast cancer patients diagnosed in Tata Memorial Hospital, Mumbai, India, in 1985 and followed through 1988

Patient characteristics	Number of patients	Deaths		3-year survival %	
		Number	%[a]	Actuarial assumption	Loss-adjusted by logistic regression*
Age at diagnosis					
≤ 44 years	101	34	34	60.1	51.5
45–54	117	42	36	56.7	48.7
55–64	77	20	26	67.7	62.3
65+ years	41	12	29	65.4	58.5
Residential status (Mumbai city)					
Residents	169	60	35	59.4	56.2
Non-residents	167	48	29	63.2	54.4
Stage of disease (TNM summary)					
I	29	2	9	92.2	93.2
II	160	36	22	74.4	71.2
III	126	55	44	41.2	31.8
IV	21	15	71	0.0	0.0
Treatment					
With chemotherapy	194	39	20	76.6	71.2
Without chemotherapy	142	69	48	38.1	28.2

[a] *Percentage of total cases in respective categories;*
* *Adjusted for other factors in the table.*

Table 3. Comparison of 3-year survival without loss-adjustment by actuarial assumption, stepwise loss- adjustment of factors using stratified method and loss-adjustment using all factors together by logistic regression for all female breast cancer patients diagnosed in Tata Memorial Hospital, Mumbai, India, in 1985 and followed through 1988

Loss-adjustedment of factors	3-year survival %
Without loss-adjustment and using actuarial assumption only	61.2
Loss-adjustment done by stratification	
Residential status	59.5
Residential status and age at diagnosis	59.2
Residential status, age at diagnosis and stage of disease	57.4
Residential status, age at diagnosis, stage of disease and treatment	56.5
Loss-adjustment done by logistic regression	
Residential status, age at diagnosis, stage of disease and treatment	54.5

the Population-Based Cancer Registry, Chennai, India, during 1990–1996 and followed-up until 2001 formed the study population.

The determinants of loss to follow-up at less than 5 years from diagnosis for each site were identified using Cox proportional-hazard model by following the method outlined in Chapter 2 of this publication. Five-year loss-adjusted absolute survival of patients through stratified method was estimated by allocating cases to 128 strata defined by 4 factors (with reference and subcategories): age at diagnosis (<45, 45–54, 55–64 and 65+ years); literacy status based on years of education (Nil, ≤ 5, 6–12 and ≥ 12 years); clinical extent of disease as a surrogate for tumour stage (localized, regional, distant metastasis and unknown); treatment status (no or unknown and yes). Outcome event was death due to any cause.

Table 4 gives the proportion of cases lost to follow-up and comparison of 5-year absolute survival estimated with and without adjustment for loss to follow-up for each cancer site. The losses ranged between 7% (oesophagus) and 24% (ovary) for different sites. Loss-adjusted survival was consistently lesser than the corresponding unadjusted estimate for all sites. Bias in survival estimation in the presence of non-random loss to follow-up, expressed in terms of absolute difference between survival (%) estimates obtained with and without loss-adjustment was minimal, ranging between 0.2 to 1.7 per cent units for different cancer sites.

Discussion

The success of cancer treatment is, as a rule, measured by survival. Population-based survival reflects the availability, development of and accessibility to cancer health services in a region. Survival based on hospital series reflects the impact of clinical services specific to the hospital. In both instances, high-level completeness of ascertainment of mortality data is an important prerequisite, and when such completeness cannot be assured, survival rates should be carefully interpreted [7,8].

Conventionally, estimation of survival was done using life table approaches by either actuarial [2] or Kaplan-Meier [3] methods. Both methods utilize observed survival time independently of whether it ends at the death of a patient. Patients withdrawn alive at closing date provide censored information that is unbiased, since closing date is independent from probability of death. If this is not true, Hakulinen [9] and Brenner [10] give means to adjust for withdrawal pattern and to correct for effects of improvement of survival by time.

Losses to follow-up because of reasons other than closing date (e.g., migration) are often few in developed countries and are dealt with identically as withdrawals. This is not justified if the losses are many and are correlated with risk of death. Distance from clinical care facility increases the likelihood of not undergoing a follow-up examination, as does serious morbidity and poverty. The factors in failure to obtain follow-up data are the same. Therefore, it is likely that patients lost to follow-up have poor prognosis and could not be compared with those under follow-up and surveillance. The direction in bias may also be the other way: those lost to follow-up have a better survival than those under follow-up, as was shown in our example on stage I breast cancer hospital series patients.

Our example from a hospital series shows that the bias due to losses may be substantial. Mathew[6] showed similar differences by applying loss-adjustment in the Kaplan-Meier survival method for hospital series ovarian cancer patients. Much of the original deficiencies in the hospital data were, however, removed by active follow-up using a postcard enquiring the vital status of patient. Only marginal adjustment effect appeared after the enquiry. However, in the example involving breast cancer hospital series, a large bias still existed after such attempts of active follow-up. On the other hand, the example involving population-based series of several cancers revealed negligible bias. In both

Table 4. Number of incident cases, proportion (%) lost to follow-up and comparison of 5-year absolute survival with and without loss-adjustment for top-ranking cancers in a population-based cancer registry, Chennai, during 1990–1996 and followed through 2001

Cancer site/type	Number of incident cases	Lost to follow-up %	5-year survival % No loss-adjustment	5-year survival % With loss-adjustment	Absolute difference in survival
Cervix	3134	21.8	52.1	50.4	1.7
Breast	1923	20.7	39.5	39.1	0.4
Stomach	1845	8.0	9.4	8.7	0.7
Oesophagus	1403	6.7	7.7	7.5	0.2
Lung	1237	7.8	8.2	8.1	0.1
Mouth	1202	11.6	30.1	29.1	1.0
Lymphomas	768	11.5	26.5	25.6	0.9
Tongue	670	13.0	20.2	18.9	1.3
Leukaemias	668	8.2	19.8	19.2	0.6
Ovary	521	24.0	25.7	24.2	1.5

instances, loss-adjusted survival was lesser than the actuarial estimate without adjustment indicating that under-ascertainment of deaths among loss to follow-up cases may be the problem. Most population-based cancer registries are based on systems that integrate linkage or collection of mortality data as a routine and hence result in small differential bias only [5]. Hence, the data source seems to affect the need for loss-adjustment, and the problem may be more substantial in hospital-based cancer registries and clinical series. The loss-adjusted approach is likely to be useful especially when hospital-based cancer registry data of a low- or medium-resource country are used to evaluate the outcomes of cancer patients.

One may conclude that if routine follow-up is poor, the first priority is to increase the actual follow-up visits on humanitarian and scientific grounds. The second is to improve the data by instituting rigorous active follow-up measures. The improvement of data by these means may indirectly improve routine follow-up activity. Analytical methods to correct the survival data with adjusting for losses are to be used in surveillance and evaluation and in scientific comparisons. However, such means do not directly improve human health, but have the potential to improve the organization itself.

References

1. WHO/IARC. *Cancer Statistics: Report of a WHO/IARC Expert Committee. WHO Technical Report Series No. 632*. World Health Organization, Geneva, 1979.

2. Cutler SJ, Ederer F. Maximum utilization of the life table method in analysing survival. *J Chron Dis* 1958;8: 699–712.

3. Kaplan EL and Meier P. Non parametric estimation from incomplete observation. *J Amer Stat Assoc* 1958;53:457–481.

4. Ganesh B. *Effect of loss to follow-up in estimating survival rates. Acta Universitatis Tamperensis, Ser A, Vol 440*. University of Tampere, Tampere, 1995.

5. Sriamporn S, Swaminathan R, Parkin DM, Kamsa-Ard S, Hakama M. Loss-adjusted survival of cervix cancer in Khon Kaen, Northeast Thailand. *B J Cancer* 2004;91(1):106–110.

6. Mathew A. Removing bias in cancer survival estimates by active follow-up and information on determinants of loss to follow-up. Acta Universitatis Tamperensis, Ser A, vol 525. University of Tampere, Tampere, 1996.

7. Brenner H, Hakulinen T. Implications of incomplete registration of deaths on long-term survival estimates from population-based cancer registries. *Int J Cancer 2009*;125:432–437.

8. Swaminathan R, Rama R, Shanta V. Lack of active follow-up of cancer patients in Chennai, India: implications for population-based survival estimates. *Bull World Health Organ*. 2008;86:509–515.

9. Hakulinen T. Cancer survival corrected for heterogeneity in patient withdrawal. *Biometrics*. 1982;38: 933–942.

10. Brenner H, Gefeller O. An alternative approach to monitoring cancer patient survival. *Cancer*. 1996;78: 2004–2010.

Chapter 4

Cancer survival in Africa, Asia, the Caribbean and Central America: Database and attributes

Swaminathan R, Lucas E and Sankaranarayanan R

Abstract

Thirty-one registries in 17 countries submitted data for systematic and centralized scrutiny. Data on 564 606 cases of different cancers ranging 1–56 sites/types from 27 registries in 14 low-/medium-resource countries in Eastern and Western Africa, the Caribbean, Central America and four regions of Asia, registered during 1990–2001 (period varying for individual registries) were reported. The database for this survival study comprised data that were classified as mandatory and optional. Mandatory variables provided by all registries included case-ID, age at diagnosis, sex, incidence date, most valid basis of diagnosis, cancer site/type (ICD-10 codes C00-96), vital status at follow-up and corresponding date. Clinical extent of disease was prominent among the optional variables provided by 17 registries and analysed. The grouping of cancer sites for analysis was based on standard norms, and only categories with at least 25 cases were reported. Cases registered based on a death certificate only, cases lacking any follow-up after initial registration, or cases rejected based on validation checks were excluded from the survival analysis. An easy guide to contents in subsequent chapters, especially tables and graphs describing data quality indices, survival statistics and online dynamic functions, is provided.

Introduction

The database for the survival study was conceived on the basis of data routinely collected in population-based cancer registries in most countries. Accordingly, the variables needed were classified under three major headings: the person, the disease and the follow-up. Under each heading the variables were classified as either mandatory or optional. The variables are summarized in Table 1.

The choice of registries for participation in this study was mainly those whose data on cancer incidence and mortality were published in any volume of *Cancer Incidence in Five Continents* [1]. The response was overwhelming: thirty-one registries in 17 countries submitted data for centralized scrutiny. One or some of the mandatory data variables required were not provided by two of the registries and in four there was a significant incompleteness in follow-up. Hence the data from these four registries were rejected after cursory introspection. Thus data submitted by 27 registries from 14 countries were included for further systematic scrutiny.

Inclusion and exclusion criteria

The broad inclusion and exclusion criteria fixed for this study are given in Table 2. The processing of data for individual registries with a pre-specified set of minimal checks for validity and consistency of data revealed the different procedures followed by some of the registries [2]. The first step undertaken was to standardize the norms to facilitate an unambiguous exclusion of cases from the study. The distinction between a Death Certificate initiated cases (DCN) for further trace-back of information and cases finally registered based on a Death Certificate Only (DCO) without any additional information was established after several exchanges of correspondence with the concerned registries. Such DCO cases with the incidence date the same as the date of death were excluded from survival analysis. In rare instances, the date of follow-up was mistaken to be the date of follow-up attempt rather than the date corresponding to the vital status. Such cases were mostly notified by a code for loss to follow-up or not coded for vital status in the data. These discrepancies were addressed diligently and resolved in consultation with the respective registries to classify them as having incomplete or no follow-up. Cases with lack of any follow-up were then excluded from the analysis. Cases with multiple primaries were identified both by the registry and by routine checks, and were excluded from survival analysis. Thus, a compact set of validation checks for mandatory and optional data variables, as described in Table 3, was evolved and carried out systematically for all the registries. Cases rejected on the basis of these checks were then excluded from the survival analysis.

Data processing

The data sent by the registries were not in a uniform format. These were all converted as database files (dbf) for uniformity.

Registry code & name

A two-digit code based on the ascending alphabetical order of the participating countries was assigned.

Cancer site or type

The data submitted by the registries did not have a uniform coding format, even for mandatory variables. The most prominent among these was the coding for the primary site and/or histology type of cancer. The calendar period of case registration for this study coincided with the smooth transition in coding practices that most registries were undergoing: from one version of ICD-O to another and thereby to

Table 1. Summary of data variables requested from the registries for the survival study

Person-realated data		Disease-realated data		Follow-up realated data	
Mandatory	**Optional**	**Mandatory**	**Optional**	**Mandatory**	**Optional**
• Case ID • Age at diagnosis • Sex	• Socio-demographic • Socioeconomic	• Incidence date • If ICD-O codes used - Site of primary - Histology type - Behaviour • If ICD-10 codes used - Cancer diagnosis • Basis of diagnosis	• If ICD-10 codes used - Histology type • Tumour grade • Clinical extent of disease • Tumour stage	• Vitas status • Date corresponding to vital status	• None

Note: For analysis of survival trend, mandatory data on person, disease and follow-up related variables for preceding years were requested.

Table 2. Inclusion and exclusion criteria for the survival study

Inclusion criteria	:	A cohort of single primary, incident, invasive cancers diagnosed within a specified consecutive calendar period from 1st January to 31st December with a potential follow-up period of five years or more for a sizeable number of cases
Exclusion criteria	:	Cases registered on the basis of a death certificate notification and continuing to remain as a case of Death Certificate Only (DCO) - Incidence date same as the date of death
		Cases without any follow-up information after the first registration - Lack of any follow-up
		Cases rejected on validation checks of submitted variables to the survival database - Details of checks listed separately

Table 3. Details of validation checks carried out and the decision made

Validation checks carried out		Decision made
Age at diagnosis, sex, incidence date and follow-up date unknown	:	Reject case
Multiple cancers signified by duplicate case ID or otherwise	:	Reject case
Duplicate registry ID numbers signifying same case with one cancer	:	Include one case only
<u>Out of range codes</u>		
Age at diagnosis (0–98 years)	:	Reject case
Sex (1–2)	:	Reject case
Incidence and follow-up months (1–12)	:	Reject case
Incidence and follow-up years (as applicable)	:	Reject case
Vital status (1–2)	:	Reject case
ICD-O and ICD-10 codes	:	Reject case
<u>Inconsistent data</u>		
Incidence date > Follow-up date	:	Reject case
Age, site and histology combination (based on IARC CHECK program)	:	Include case if listed as a warning Reject case if listed as invalid
Other logical checks on optional variables submitted for scrutiny	:	As appropriate

ICD-10. Some of them remained with ICD-9 coding even after having changed to higher versions of ICD-O [3–7]. These prompted to have the cancer diagnosis converted into a uniform format and codes of four digits following ICD-10 [8]. The case listings of warnings and invalid conversions were sent to the respective registries, and the queries were resolved by mutual consent. The classification of cancer sites or types was based on the same lines as in *Cancer Incidence in Five Continents*, Volume VIII [9] and is described in Table 4. Only categories with at least 25 cases were considered for analysis and reporting.

Age at diagnosis

This refers to the age in completed years on the incidence date. This was verified with the date of birth when provided. Age unknown cases were excluded, and age above 97 years was coded as 98.

Clinical extent of disease

Though this is an optional variable in this study, it has the greatest significance in correlating local factors with the estimated survival. This data is routinely available or collected by most registries, and in this study seventeen registries submitted this information. The broad norms adopted in classifying this variable into four categories are as follows:

- Localized: Tumour confined to the organ of origin without invasion into the surrounding tissue/organ and without involvement of any regional or distant lymph nodes or organs;
- Regional: Tumour not confined to the organ of origin with invasion into the surrounding tissue/organ, with or without the involvement of the regional lymph nodes and not involving or spread to the non-regional lymph nodes or organs;
- Distant metastasis: Tumour involving or spread to the non-regional lymph nodes or distant organs;
- Unknown: The above information is unknown.

Index date

The starting date for calculating survival in this study is the incidence date. The definition of incidence date did not reveal any substantial variation between registries. Most of the registries resorted to the first date of unequivocal diagnosis of cancer, by any means, as the incidence date. Other alternatives encountered were hospital admission date or the date of histological verification. Such a variation might result in minimal differences in short-term survival (say <2 years) and negligent differences for long-term survival [10]. Data on the incidence date was submitted as exact dates or to the level of the month and year of diagnosis. In this study, the index date varied between 1st January 1990 and 31st December 2001, with the period varying for individual registries.

Closing date or date of last follow-up

This date varied between registries and ranged between 31st December 1999 and 31st December 2003. The vital status of each patient was classified as dead, alive or lost to follow-up corresponding to this date. This information was submitted as exact dates or to the level of month and year of follow-up by the registries. To measure extent of incompleteness in follow-up, especially for registries that employed active methods of follow-up, a variable called 'Follow-up' was created, and the extent of loss to follow-up in years from index date was classified as <1 year, 1–3 years, 3–5 years and >5 years on survival time.

Survival time

This was calculated as the time (in months) between the index date and the date of death from any cause, date of loss to follow-up or the closing date, whichever was earliest.

Most valid basis of diagnosis

The codes for the most valid basis of diagnosis were also different among registries. Based on the key to these codes, a new variable, 'Histological verification', was created for unambiguity and uniformity.

Inclusion status

Systematic validation of the data was undertaken for the registries by performing the checks listed in Table 3. More customized checks were performed depending on the data type on optional variables provided by each registry. A list of potential errors was returned to the registries for clarification. Registries undertaking follow-up predominantly by passive methods were urged to improve follow-up by resorting to feasible active methods like repeated scrutiny of medical records and linkage of data at sources of registration of cases. After the rectification of errors, if any, the checks were repeated on the revised data. The inclusion status was then classified as follows: Included (I) or excluded for reasons of being a DCO case (D), with lack of any follow-up (F) or due to any other reasons (O) on validation checks.

Data quality indicators

The indices that would determine the data quality can be summarized as follows:

- The frequency of cases, expressed as number and percentage, that were registered as a DCO;
- The frequency of cases, expressed as percentage, that had a histologically confirmed cancer diagnosis;
- The frequency of cases, expressed as number and percentage, that were excluded from survival analysis including those with lack of any follow-up or other errors;
- The frequency of cases, expressed as number and percentage, with incomplete follow-up.

All of the above, by classified cancer site or type, are included as standard tables in the chapters dealing with individual registry data.

Study database

Two databases were created for analysis and reporting of results:

- The file SURVDB.DBF deals with all cases submitted for scrutiny and includes 16 variables. This file is essentially for eliciting the data quality.
- The file SURVDB2.DBF deals with cases included for analysis and comprises 10 variables. This file is essentially for eliciting data on survival.

The description of the variables is given in Table 5.

A lead to the chapters on individual registries

An overview of the issues in the background of the survival data and the analysis carried out for each registry is given in Table 6, as a lead to the forthcoming chapters on individual registries. The cancer registration and follow-up are seen to be completely carried out by active methods in eleven registries (all five from India, two from Thailand, one

Table 4. Details of validation checks carried out and the decision made

ICD-10 code	ICD-10 title	ICD-10 description
C00	Lip	Lip
C01–02	Tongue	Base, other and unspecified tongue
C03–06	Oral cavity	Gum, floor of mouth, palate, buccal mucosa and other mouth
C07–08	Salivary gland	Major salivary glands
C09	Tonsil	Tonsil
C10	Other oropharynx	Vallecula, anterior surface of epiglottis and other oropharynx
C11	Nasopharynx	Nasopharynx
C12–13	Hypopharynx	Pyriform fossa, post cricoid and other hypopharynx
C15	Oesophagus	Oesophagus
C16	Stomach	Stomach
C17	Small intestine	Small intestine
C18	Colon	Colon
C19–20	Rectum	Rectosigmoid junction and rectum
C21	Anus	Anal canal and anus
C22	Liver	Liver
C23–24	Gallbladder	Gallbladder and unspecified biliary tract
C25	Pancreas	Pancreas
C26	Gastrointestinal tract unspecified	Other unspecified gastrointestinal tract
C30–31	Nose/Sinuses	Nasal cavity, middle ear and other accessory sinuses
C32	Larynx	Larynx
C33–34	Lung	Trachea, bronchus and lung
C37–38	Other thoracic organs	Thymus, mediastinum, pleura and heart
C40–41	Bone	Bone, joints and articular cartilage
C43	Melanoma skin	Melanoma of skin
C44	Other skin	Non-melanoma of skin
C45	Mesothelioma	Mesothelioma
C46	Kaposi sarcoma	Kaposi sarcoma
C47;C49	Connective tissue	Peripheral, connective and other soft tissues
C48	Peritoneum	Retroperitoneum and peritoneum
C50	Breast	Male and female breast
C51	Vulva	Vulva
C52	Vagina	Vagina
C53	Cervix	Cervix uteri
C54	Corpus uteri	Endometrium and corpus uteri
C55	Uterus unspecified	Unspecified uterus
C56	Ovary	Ovary
C57	Other female genital	Other and unspecified female genital organs
C58	Placenta	Placenta
C60	Penis	Penis
C61	Prostate	Prostate
C62	Testis	Testis
C63	Other male genital organs	Other and unspecified male genital organs
C64	Kidney	Kidney
C65	Renal pelvis	Renal pelvis
C66	Ureter	Ureter
C67	Urinary bladder	Urinary bladder
C68	Other urinary organs	Other urinary organs
C69	Eye	Eye and adnexa
C70–72	Brain & nervous system	Meninges, brain and other parts of central nervous system
C73	Thyroid	Thyroid gland
C74	Adrenal gland	Adrenal gland
C75	Other endocrine	Other endocrine glands and related structures
C81	Hodgkin lymphoma	Hodgkin lymphoma
C82–85;C96	Non-Hodgkin lymphoma	Non-Hodgkin lymphoma
C90	Multiple myeloma	Multiple myeloma
C91	Lymphoid leukaemia	Lymphoid leukaemia
C92–94	Myeloid leukaemia	Myeloid, monocytic and myeloblastic leukaemia
C95	Leukaemia unspecified	Unspecifed leukaemia

Table 5. Cancer Survival in Africa, Asia, the Caribbean and Central America, database

Database format for all cases submitted (SURVDB.DBF)

Variable name	Codes/Description	Field length
Registry code	Codes to identify the registry	2
Registry name	Name of the registry & country	25
Cancer diagnosis	4 digit ICD-10 codes	4
Age at diagnosis	00–98 in completed years 98 for 98+ years of age	2
Sex	1: Male; 2: Female	1
Clinical extent of disease	1: Localized; 2: Regional; 3: Distant metastasis; 4: Unknown	1
Histology	ICD-O codes including type, behaviour and grade of tumour	6
Year of diagnosis	As applicable	4
Month of diagnosis	01–12	2
Year of follow-up	As applicable	4
Month of follow-up	01–12	2
Vital status	1: Alive; 2: Dead	1
Inclusion status	I: Included; D: DCO; F: Lack of follow-up; O: Excluded for other invalid reasons	1
Histological verification	0: No; 1: yes	1
Type of follow-up	C: Complete follow-up at 5-years; 1: Lost to follow-up (LFU) within 1-year; 3: LFU between 1-3 years; 5: LFU between 3-5 years; 6: LFU after 5 years	1
Survival time	In months	3.1

Database format for all cases included for survival analysis (SURVDB2.DBF)

Variable name	Codes/ Description	Field length
Registry code	Codes to identify the registry	2
Cancer diagnosis	2 digit ICD-10 codes (numeric only)	2
Age at diagnosis	00–98 in completed years 98 for 98+ years of age	2
Sex	1: Male; 2: Female	1
Clinical extent of disease	1: Localized; 2: Regional; 3: Distant metastasis; 4: Unknown	1
Year of diagnosis	As applicable	4
Month of diagnosis	01–12	2
Year of follow-up	As applicable	4
Month of follow-up	01–12	2
Vital status	1: Alive; 2: Dead	1

each from Pakistan, Turkey, Uganda and Zimbabwe). Among the remaining four registries wherein cancer registration is carried out entirely by active methods, the follow-up methods are done in a mixed manner: predominantly by active methods with a minimal passive component in Manila and Rizal, Philippines, and predominantly by passive methods in Tianjin, China and Incheon, South Korea. Cancer registration and follow-up are entirely done by passive methods in only Singapore. In Hong Kong, the cancer registration

Table 6. An overview of basic characteristics of survival data and analysis done by registry

Cancer Survival in Africa, Asia, the Caribbean and Central America

Country/registry	Method adopted for		Estimation of survival probability by			Analysis of survival	
	Cancer registration	Follow-up	Cohort analysis	Semi complete analysis	Period analysis	Trend	Extent disease
CHINA							
Hong Kong SAR	P + A	P		Y			Y[$]
Qidong	P + A	A + P	Y	Y*	Y	Y	
Shanghai	P	P + A		Y		Y	
Tianjin	A	P + A	Y	Y	Y	Y	
COSTA RICA	P	P + A		Y			Y
CUBA	P	P + A		Y		Y	Y
The GAMBIA	P + A	A		Y			
INDIA							
Barshi	A	A		Y		Y	
Bhopal	A	A		Y			Y
Chennai	A	A		Y		Y	Y
Karunagappally	A	A		Y			Y
Mumbai	A	A		Y		Y	Y
PAKISTAN							
South Karachi	A	A		Y			Y
PHILIPPINES							
Manila*	A	A+ P		Y			Y
Rizal	A	A + P		Y		Y	Y
REPUBLIC OF KOREA							
Busan	P + A	P + A		Y			
Incheon	A	P + A		Y			
Seoul	P + A	P + A		Y			
SAUDI ARABIA							
Riyadh	P + A	P + A		Y			Y
SINGAPORE	P	P	Y	Y	Y	Y	Y
THAILAND							
Chiang Mai	A	A		Y		Y	Y
Khon Kaen	A + P	A + P		Y		Y	Y
Lampang	P	P + A		Y			Y
Songkhla	A	A		Y			Y
TURKEY							
Izmir	A	A		Y			Y
UGANDA							
Kampala	A	A		Y			
ZIMBABWE							
Harare	A	A		Y			

A: Active; P: Passive; A + P: Predominantly active; P + A; Predominantly passive; Y: Yes
** Complete analysis; [$] for breast cancer only*

is mixed while the follow-up is entirely by passive methods. The cancer registration and follow-up are both carried out by a mixture of active and passive methods in all the other registries.

The various approaches to estimating survival probability are illustrated in Chapter 2. The analysis by the semi-complete approach has been done for all the registries excepting Qidong, for which the analysis was done by the complete approach. The analysis of survival trend by the semi-complete approach involving two calendar periods was done for eleven registries, while a comparative analysis of survival trend by cohort and period approaches for several calendar periods was possible in Qidong and Tianjin, China and Singapore. Analysis of survival by clinical extent of disease for selected cancer sites was possible in 17 registries.

A guide to the tables and graphs in the individual registry chapters

A chapter is dedicated to each participating registry. It comprises a concise summary describing the background and salient features of the results combined with standard/optional tables and figures.

Table 1 deals with the main data quality indices prior to and after the commencement of follow-up. It gives the total number of cases registered, proportion (%) of histologically verified diagnosis, frequency of type of exclusions from study like DCOs, lack of follow-up and others, and the total number of excluded and included cases for the study for each classified cancer site/type category.

Table 2 refers to the data quality index on completeness of follow-up. For registries that resorted to passive means of follow-up entirely, this table gives the distribution of vital status (alive/dead) by classified cancer site/type. For others, this table gives the frequency of cases with complete follow-up at the closing date, as well as at 5 years from the index date, and the extent of incompleteness in follow-up by duration (classified years from diagnosis) of loss to follow-up for every classified cancer site/type. The non-randomness of loss to follow-up or informative censoring is indicated wherever encountered. The median follow-up (in months) is given for every registry and classified cancer site/type.

Table 3 gives the crude and age-adjusted survival statistics. Absolute and relative survival (%) at one, three and five years from index date and 5-year age-standardized relative survival for all ages together and for the age interval 0-74 years are given for every classified cancer site/type.

Table 4 deals with survival statistics by sex and classified age groups. The frequency of cases and five-year absolute and relative survival (%) by sex and the frequency of cases and five-year relative survival (%) by the age groups 0–44, 45–54, 55–64, 65–74 and 75+ years are given for every classified cancer site/type.

Figure 1a portrays the top five or ten cancers ranked by 5-year relative survival for those registries that contributed data on sufficient number of cancer sites/types.

Figure 1b displays the top five cancers ranked by 5-year relative survival among males.

Figure 1c represents the top five cancers ranked by 5-year relative survival among females.

Analysis of survival by clinical extent of disease (Table 5)

This is carried out for selected cancer sites only: cancers of the head and neck, female breast, cervix and ovary. The frequency (%) of cases by classified clinical extent of disease categories and the corresponding 5-year absolute survival are presented as a table.

Figure 2 either depicts the absolute survival by clinical extent of disease for available cancer sites and registries or trend of survival by cohort and period approaches as appropriate.

Analysis of trend of survival (Table 6)

This is done in two ways:

For registries that provided data for any one preceding calendar period of time, the 5-year absolute and relative survival were estimated by semi-complete approach for the two periods for the available cancer sites/types and presented as a table.

For registries that provided data for more than two 5-year calendar periods preceding the latest one, the 5-year absolute and relative survival were estimated for the latest two calendar periods for the available cancer sites/types and presented as a table. Additionally, the frequency of cases by 5-year calendar periods by cancer site/type is given in a table. Correspondingly, the five-, ten- and fifteen-year relative survival were estimated by cohort and period approaches for available cancer site/type depending on the availability of data and presented as one or two tables, as necessary. These are depicted as figures also.

Online features of the publication

A dedicated website has been designed to host the new version of Cancer Survival in Africa, Asia, the Caribbean and Central America (SurvCan), available at http://survcan.iarc.fr. Users will be able to access all the chapters of the publication, including abstracts, tables and figures, and will be able to export each chapter in full or part in PDF format. Users will also be able to access the previous volume of the publication (1998) if available. References cited in the chapters are directly linked to PubMed or to the specific website of the publication as appropriate. Online dynamic functions are also supplied to let users generate comparative statistics: users will be able to list all the available tables/figures for a registry, compare values between registries for a specific cancer site, based on ICD-10 codes, and generate specific dynamic figures on survival statistics (5-year absolute survival or 5-year relative survival, etc.) according to the sex, age group and extent of disease. An online help tool is available to facilitate the use of the online statistical functions.

References

1. Parkin DM, Whelan SL, Ferlay J and Storm H. *Cancer Incidence in Five Continents, vol I to VIII. IARC Cancerbase No 7*. IARCPress, Lyon, 2005.

2. Swaminathan R, Black RJ and Sankaranarayanan R. Database on Cancer Survival from Developing Countries. In: *Cancer Survival in Developing Countries* (eds) R.Sankaranarayanan, RJ Black and DM Parkin. IARC Scientific Publications No. 145. IARCPress, Lyon, 1998.

3. *WHO. International Classification of Diseases for Oncology (ICD-O), First edition.* World Health Organization, Geneva, 1976.

4. *WHO. International Classification of Diseases for Oncology (ICD-O), Second edition.* World Health Organization, Geneva, 1990.

5. *WHO. International Classification of Diseases for Oncology (ICD-O), Third edition.* World Health Organization, Geneva, 2000.

6. *WHO. International Classification of Diseases, Ninth Revision* (ICD-9). World Health Organization, Geneva, 1976.

7. *WHO. International Statistical Classification of Diseases and Related Health Problems, Tenth Revision* (ICD-10), Volume 1. World Health Organization, Geneva, 1992.

8. Ferlay J. *IARCcrgTools, Version 1.01*. IARCPress, Lyon, 2003.

9. Parkin DM, Whelan SL, Ferlay J, Teppo L and Thomas DB. *Cancer Incidence in Five Continents, vol VIII*: IARC Scientific publications No 155. IARCPress, Lyon, 2002.

10. Berrino F, Sant M, Verdecchia A, Capocaccia R, Hakulinen T and Esteve J. (eds) *Survival of Cancer Patients in Europe: the EUROCARE Study. IARC Scientific Publications No. 132*. IARCPress, Lyon, 1995.

Chapter 5

Cancer survival in Hong Kong SAR, China, 1996–2001

Law SC and Mang OW

Abstract

The Hong Kong cancer registry was established in 1963, and cancer registration is done by passive and active methods. The registry contributed data on 45 cancer sites or types registered during 1996–2001 for this survival study. Follow-up has been carried out by passive methods with median follow-up ranging from 4–60 months. The proportion of cases with histologically verified cancer diagnosis ranged from 38–100%; death certificates only (DCOs) ranged from 0–11%; 83–99% of total registered cases were included for survival analysis. The 5-year age-standardized relative survival exceeded 100% for lip and non-melanoma skin followed by thyroid (94%) and testicular (92%) cancers. The corresponding survival for common cancers were breast (90%), colon (61%), liver and lung (22%), nasopharynx (70%), rectum (59%) and stomach (39%). The 5-year relative survival by age group showed a decreasing trend with increasing age groups for most cancers. A decreasing survival with increasing clinical extent of disease was noted.

Hong Kong cancer registry

The Hong Kong cancer registry was established in 1963 and is currently based at the clinical oncology department, Queen Elizabeth Hospital, Hospital Authority of Hong Kong. The registry has been contributing data to the quinquennial IARC publication *Cancer Incidence in Five Continents* since Vol IV [1]. Cancer notification is by an administrative order without a specific law. Hence, cancer registration is done by passive and active methods. The principal sources of information on cancer cases are the records in more than 50 institutions comprising the hospitals in public and private sectors, radiation centres and pathology laboratories as well as voluntary notifications from private practitioners. The registry covers the entire country (1104 km^2) and a population of about 6.9 million with a sex ratio of 1076 females to 1000 males in 2004. The average annual age-standardized incidence rate is 265 per 100 000 among males and 197 per 100 000 among females, with a lifetime cumulative risk of one in four of developing cancer in the period 1998–2002. The top ranking cancers among males are lung followed by liver and colon. Among females, the order is breast, lung and colon [2].

The registry contributed data on survival from 45 cancer sites or types for the first time in this volume of the IARC publication *Cancer survival in Africa, Asia, the Caribbean and Central America.*

Data quality indices (Table 1)

The proportion of cases with histologically verified cancer diagnosis in our series is 86%, varying from 38% (cancer of the pancreas) to 100% (melanoma of the skin and kidney, and mesothelioma). The proportion of cases registered as death certificates only (DCOs) is 1%, ranging between 0% for many cancers and 11% for unspecified leukaemia. Cases excluded without any follow-up are negligible. Thus, 83–99% of the total cases registered are included in the estimation of the survival probability (see note on next page).

Outcome of follow-up (Table 2)

Follow-up has been carried out by passive methods. This included obtaining cancer mortality information from the death certificates in births, deaths and marriages registry of the Government. The mortality data are periodically matched with the incident cancer database. Unmatched incident cases are then presumed to be alive on the last date of the year for which the mortality data is fully available.

The closing date of follow-up is 31st December 2003. The median follow-up ranged from four months in cancer of the pancreas and unspecified leukaemia to 60 months in lip cancer.

Survival statistics

All ages and both sexes together (Table 3)

The 5-year relative survival is the highest in non-melanoma skin and lip cancers (102%) followed by thyroid (94%), testis (90%) and breast (90%). The lowest survival is encountered with pancreatic cancer (17%) preceded by lung (21%), liver and gallbladder (22%) and unspecified leukaemia (25%). Salivary gland (83%) and nasopharynx (75%) among other head and neck cancers and colon and rectum (61%) among gastrointestinal cancers have higher survival rates than others. Survival from cancers of the urinary system is 76% for urinary bladder and 66% for kidney. Hodgkin lymphoma had a better survival (84%) than non-Hodgkin lymphoma (56%). The survival figures for leukaemias are lymphoid (60%) and myeloid (34%).

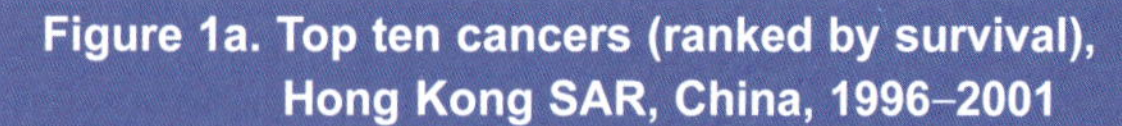

Figure 1a. Top ten cancers (ranked by survival), Hong Kong SAR, China, 1996–2001

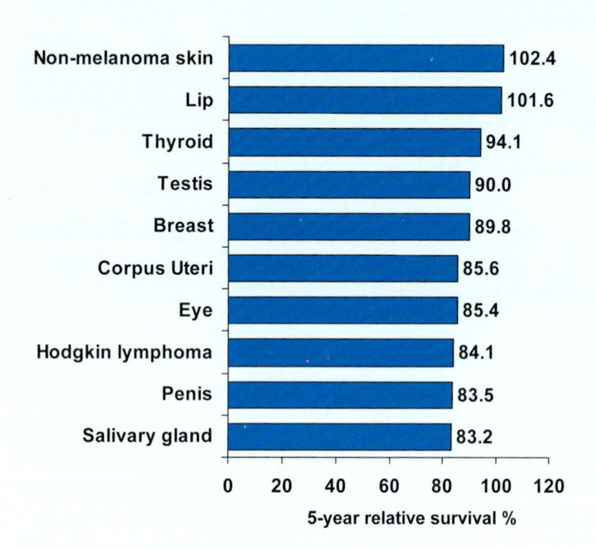

The 5-year age-standardized relative survival (ASRS) probability for all ages together is generally lesser than or similar to the corresponding unadjusted one for most cancers. Also, the 5-year ASRS (0–74 years of age) is generally higher than or similar to the corresponding ASRS (all ages) for a majority of cancers.

Sex

Male (Table 4a)

The top five cancers ranked on the 5-year relative survival probabilities are lip (102%), non-melanoma skin (101%), breast (100%), testis and thyroid (90%). Survival from breast cancer is noticeably higher among males than females.

Figure 1b. Top five cancers (ranked by survival), Male, Hong Kong SAR, China, 1996–2001

Site	5-year relative survival %
Lip	101.7
Non-melanoma skin	100.7
Male breast	99.8
Testis	90.0
Thyroid	89.6

Female (Table 4a)

The highest 5-year relative survival probability is observed for non-melanoma skin cancer (104%), followed by lip (102%), thyroid (95%), Hodgkin lymphoma (92%) and salivary gland (90%). The survival is distinctly higher among females than males in most of the head and neck cancers, oesophagus, nose and sinuses, mesothelioma, adrenal glands, Hodgkin lymphoma and unspecified leukaemia.

Figure 1c. Top five cancers (ranked by survival), Female, Hong Kong SAR, China, 1996–2001

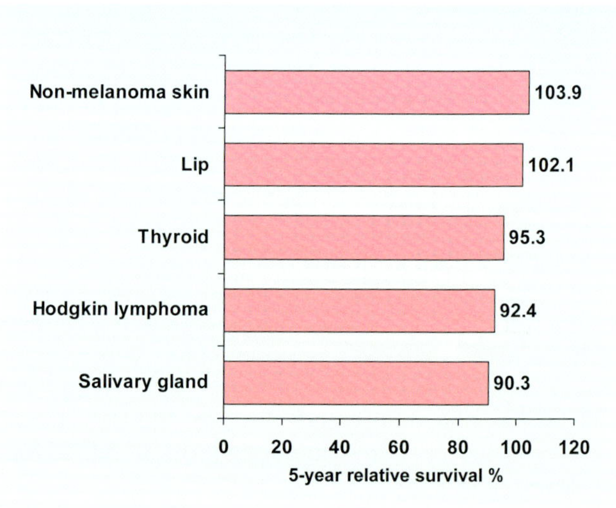

Age group (Table 4b)

The 5-year relative survival by age group reveals an inverse relationship: a decreasing survival with increasing age at diagnosis for cancers of the oral cavity, nasopharynx, liver, nose and sinuses, lung, melanoma skin, soft tissue, cervix, ovary, bladder, thyroid, non-Hodgkin lymphoma and myeloid leukaemia. In the rest, it is observed to be fluctuating.

Extent of disease (Table 5)

A high proportion of cases of breast cancer is classified under the regional category of extent of disease (35%) followed by 12% in localized and 1% in distant metastasis categories. However, the extent of disease is unknown in 52%. The 5-year absolute survival by extent of disease followed the expected pattern: highest for localized cases followed by regional and distant metastasis cases among known categories of extent of disease. It is 83% for unknown category.

Figure 2. Absolute survival by extent of disease, Hong Kong SAR, China, 1996–2001, cancer of the breast

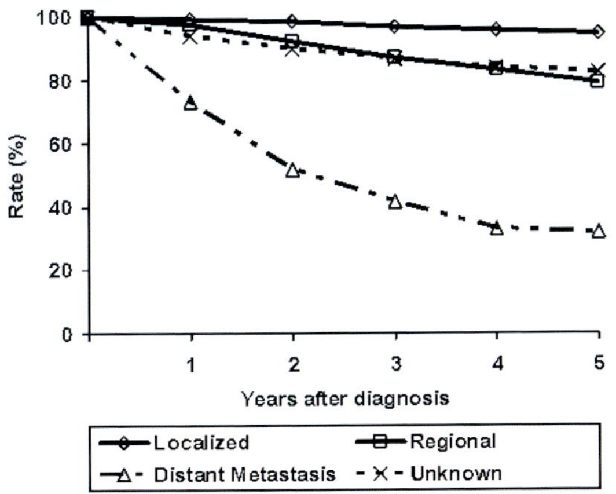

Note: The extent of disease of the breast cancer data presented here is a summary of a pilot study carried out retrospectively by the registry in 2003. The project was conducted on a cohort of breast cancer cases diagnosed between 1996 and 2001. Information on about 80% of cases was audited and updated. Follow-up was done passively by matching with the death register. Owing to technical difficulties, we made an assumption that each ever-registered case was alive if not known to be dead. The possibility exists that some patients (especially for distant-staged groups) seek more aggressive treatment outside Hong Kong and are eventually lost to follow-up or die in other regions without making death registration here. This may have inflated survival rates. The much lower proportion of patients with distant tumours may also lead to a higher overall relative survival in this category of extent of disease. Since information is not fully available on the variables influencing survival, this is of particular concern in the above survival comparisons. One should take account of these differences when comparing these results with other findings.

References

1. Parkin DM, Whelan SL, Ferlay J and Storm H. *Cancer Incidence in Five Continents, Vol I to VIII: IARC Cancerbase No. 7.* IARCPress, Lyon, 2005.

2. Curado MP, Edwards B, Shin HR, Storm H, Ferlay J, Heanue M and Boyle P. *Cancer Incidence in Five Continents, Vol. IX: IARC Scientific Publications No. 160.* IARCPress, Lyon, 2007.

Table 1. Data quality indices - Proportion of histologically verified and death certificate only cases, number and proportion of included and excluded cases by site: Hong Kong SAR, China, 1996–2001 cases followed-up until 2003

Site	ICD-10	Total registered	%		Excluded cases					Included cases	
			HV	DCO	DCO	Follow-up	Others	Total	%	No.	%
Lip	C00	47	85.1	2.1	1	0	4	5	10.6	42	89.4
Tongue	C01-02	737	92.8	0.3	2	0	58	60	8.1	677	91.9
Oral cavity	C03-06	605	94.0	0.5	3	0	41	44	7.3	561	92.7
Salivary gland	C07-08	347	91.1	0.0	0	0	17	17	4.9	330	95.1
Oropharynx	C09-10	237	92.8	0.4	1	0	17	18	7.6	219	92.4
Nasopharynx	C11	6 746	93.9	0.3	18	0	135	153	2.3	6 593	97.7
Hypopharynx	C12-13	402	94.8	0.5	2	0	40	42	10.4	360	89.6
Oesophagus	C15	3 054	92.8	1.0	32	3	187	222	7.3	2 832	92.7
Stomach	C16	6 209	92.4	1.0	63	2	265	330	5.3	5 879	94.7
Small intestine	C17	258	89.1	1.9	5	0	14	19	7.4	239	92.6
Colon	C18	11 685	90.4	1.1	134	7	519	660	5.6	11 025	94.4
Rectum, anus	C19-21	6 567	92.3	0.8	52	4	319	375	5.7	6 192	94.3
Liver	C22	9 920	60.3	4.0	392	10	262	664	6.7	9 256	93.3
Gall bladder	C23-24	1 702	61.7	2.3	39	0	62	101	5.9	1 601	94.1
Pancreas	C25	2 042	38.2	6.3	128	4	109	241	11.8	1 801	88.2
Nose/Sinuses	C30-31	309	90.0	0.6	2	0	19	21	6.8	288	93.2
Larynx	C32	1 284	92.3	0.5	6	0	68	74	5.8	1 210	94.2
Lung	C33-34	22 667	77.1	2.2	503	10	1023	1536	6.8	21 131	93.2
Other thoracic organs	C37-38	250	78.8	1.6	4	0	16	20	8.0	230	92.0
Bone	C40-41	280	80.0	2.1	6	0	18	24	8.6	256	91.4
Melanoma of skin	C43	276	100.0	0.0	0	0	15	15	5.4	261	94.6
Other skin	C44	2 719	97.1	0.1	2	0	131	133	4.9	2 586	95.1
Mesothelioma	C45	55	100.0	0.0	0	1	4	5	9.1	50	90.9
Connective tissue	C47+C49	1 025	95.1	0.7	7	1	47	55	5.4	970	94.6
Breast	C50	10 556	96.4	0.3	36	1	407	444	4.2	10 112	95.8
Vulva, vagina, other	C51-52+C57	256	91.4	0.0	0	0	24	24	9.4	232	90.6
Cervix	C53	2 727	95.8	0.2	5	0	98	103	3.8	2 624	96.2
Corpus uteri	C54	1 990	97.7	0.1	1	0	126	127	6.4	1 863	93.6
Ovary	C56	1 949	90.2	0.9	18	0	100	118	6.1	1 831	93.9
Penis	C60	163	95.7	0.0	0	0	2	2	1.2	161	98.8
Prostate	C61	3 441	90.7	0.5	17	1	217	235	6.8	3 206	93.2
Testis	C62	389	97.2	0.3	1	0	5	6	1.5	383	98.5
Kidney	C64	969	100.0	0.0	0	0	55	55	5.7	914	94.3
Urinary bladder	C67	3 750	92.3	0.4	15	0	261	276	7.4	3 474	92.6
Other urinary organs	C68	776	64.3	3.0	23	0	42	65	8.4	711	91.6
Eye	C69	66	92.4	1.5	1	0	0	1	1.5	65	98.5
Brain & nervous system	C70-72	1 349	82.1	3.6	49	0	31	80	5.9	1 269	94.1
Thyroid	C73	2 309	96.9	0.3	6	0	68	74	3.2	2 235	96.8
Adrenal gland, other	C74-75	173	67.6	8.1	14	0	0	14	8.1	159	91.9
Hodgkin lymphoma	C81	268	97.8	0.4	1	0	10	11	4.1	257	95.9
Non-Hodgkin lymphoma	C82-85+C96	3 516	95.3	0.9	32	3	163	198	5.6	3 318	94.4
Multiple myeloma	C90	857	90.4	2.5	21	0	40	61	7.1	796	92.9
Lymphoid leukaemia	C91	596	94.8	0.5	3	0	32	35	5.9	561	94.1
Myeloid leukaemia	C92-94	1 470	87.5	1.8	26	0	55	81	5.5	1 389	94.5
Leukaemia unspecified	C95	170	73.5	10.6	18	1	10	29	17.1	141	82.9

HV: histologically verified; DCO: death certificate only

Table 2. Number and proportion of cases by vital status and median follow-up (in months) by site: Hong Kong SAR, China, 1996–2001 cases followed-up until 2003

Site	ICD-10	Cases included	Dead		Alive		Complete FU		Median FU (in months)
			No.	%	No.	%	No.	%	
Lip	C00	42	6	14.3	36	85.7	42	100.0	59.6
Tongue	C01-02	677	288	42.5	389	57.5	677	100.0	41.6
Oral cavity	C03-06	561	278	49.6	283	50.4	561	100.0	34.5
Salivary gland	C07-08	330	83	25.2	247	74.8	330	100.0	54.8
Oropharynx	C09-10	219	130	59.4	89	40.6	219	100.0	27.0
Nasopharynx	C11	6 593	1 902	28.8	4 691	71.2	6 593	100.0	48.7
Hypopharynx	C12-13	360	268	74.4	92	25.6	360	100.0	16.4
Oesophagus	C15	2 832	2 216	78.2	616	21.8	2 832	100.0	9.7
Stomach	C16	5 879	4 009	68.2	1 870	31.8	5 879	100.0	15.6
Small intestine	C17	239	151	63.2	88	36.8	239	100.0	21.1
Colon	C18	11 025	5 506	49.9	5 519	50.1	11 025	100.0	35.2
Rectum, anus	C19-21	6 192	2 984	48.2	3 208	51.8	6 192	100.0	35.4
Liver	C22	9 256	7 445	80.4	1 811	19.6	9 256	100.0	5.6
Gall bladder	C23-24	1 601	1 303	81.4	298	18.6	1 601	100.0	7.0
Pancreas	C25	1 801	1 552	86.2	249	13.8	1 801	100.0	4.4
Nose/Sinuses	C30-31	288	119	41.3	169	58.7	288	100.0	41.6
Larynx	C32	1 210	507	41.9	703	58.1	1 210	100.0	41.6
Lung	C33-34	21 131	17 393	82.3	3 738	17.7	21 131	100.0	8.1
Other thoracic organs	C37-38	230	91	39.6	139	60.4	230	100.0	38.1
Bone	C40-41	256	77	30.1	179	69.9	256	100.0	49.7
Melanoma of skin	C43	261	124	47.5	137	52.5	261	100.0	33.5
Other skin	C44	2 586	519	20.1	2 067	79.9	2 586	100.0	50.7
Mesothelioma	C45	50	40	80.0	10	20.0	50	100.0	11.0
Connective tissue	C47+C49	970	341	35.2	629	64.8	970	100.0	42.6
Breast	C50	10 112	1 649	16.3	8 463	83.7	10 112	100.0	50.7
Cervix	C53	2 624	756	28.8	1 868	71.2	2 624	100.0	48.7
Corpus uteri	C54	1 863	372	20.0	1 491	80.0	1 863	100.0	48.7
Ovary	C56	1 831	653	35.7	1 178	64.3	1 831	100.0	42.6
Vulva/vagina, etc.	C57;C51-52	232	96	41.4	136	58.6	232	100.0	37.8
Penis	C60	161	60	37.3	101	62.7	161	100.0	44.6
Prostate	C61	3 206	1 271	39.6	1 935	60.4	3 206	100.0	38.2
Testis	C62	383	71	18.5	312	81.5	383	100.0	54.8
Kidney	C64	914	378	41.4	536	58.6	914	100.0	37.5
Urinary bladder	C67	3 474	1 438	41.4	2 036	58.6	3 474	100.0	40.5
Other urinary organs	C68	711	407	57.2	304	42.8	711	100.0	26.3
Eye	C69	65	12	18.5	53	81.5	65	100.0	49.7
Brain & nervous system	C70-72	1 269	709	55.9	560	44.1	1 269	100.0	27.4
Thyroid	C73	2 235	240	10.7	1 995	89.3	2 235	100.0	58.9
Adrenal gland, other	C74-75	159	51	32.1	108	67.9	159	100.0	49.7
Hodgkin lymphoma	C81	257	50	19.5	207	80.5	257	100.0	48.7
Non-Hodgkin lymphoma	C82-85+C96	3 318	1 672	50.4	1 646	49.6	3 318	100.0	32.5
Multiple myeloma	C90	796	571	71.7	225	28.3	796	100.0	20.4
Lymphoid leukaemia	C91	561	242	43.1	319	56.9	561	100.0	36.5
Myeloid leukaemia	C92-94	1 389	935	67.3	454	32.7	1 389	100.0	15.1
Leukaemia unspecified	C95	141	109	77.3	32	22.7	141	100.0	4.5

FU: follow-up

Table 3. Comparison of 1-, 3- and 5-year absolute and relative survival and 5-year age-standardized relative survival by site: Hong Kong SAR, China, 1996–2001 cases followed-up until 2003

Site	ICD-10	Cases included	% Absolute survival			% Relative survival			% ASRS at 5-years	
			1-year	3-year	5-year	1-year	3-year	5-year	all ages	0-74 years
Lip	C00	42	97.6	92.6	84.9	100.6	102.0	101.6	103.6	100.3
Tongue	C01-02	677	80.9	61.7	56.8	83.0	66.5	64.6	63.7	64.0
Oral cavity	C03-06	561	70.9	57.8	50.2	73.7	64.3	60.2	62.8	64.5
Salivary gland	C07-08	330	90.6	81.3	75.5	92.5	86.1	83.2	80.3	81.8
Oropharynx	C09-10	219	68.5	46.6	40.1	70.3	50.1	45.1	45.9	47.8
Nasopharynx	C11	6 593	92.1	78.5	70.2	93.2	81.4	74.6	69.6	74.0
Hypopharynx	C12-13	360	60.8	31.7	22.5	63.0	35.4	27.1	25.5	24.1
Oesophagus	C15	2 832	43.9	25.3	20.9	45.6	28.4	25.6	26.1	26.4
Stomach	C16	5 879	54.5	35.9	30.8	57.0	40.8	38.2	38.7	41.5
Small intestine	C17	239	57.7	40.4	35.7	59.8	44.4	41.7	41.4	48.5
Colon	C18	11 025	74.8	57.2	48.9	78.2	65.2	61.3	61.0	63.2
Rectum, anus	C19-21	6 192	79.2	59.3	49.9	82.4	66.4	60.6	59.2	63.4
Liver	C22	9 256	36.9	23.0	18.9	38.0	24.9	21.6	22.4	24.6
Gall bladder	C23-24	1 601	38.0	21.7	17.8	40.1	25.0	22.4	26.1	29.7
Pancreas	C25	1 801	27.3	15.2	13.7	28.4	17.0	16.5	17.2	19.9
Nose/Sinuses	C30-31	288	78.5	63.5	58.6	80.8	69.0	67.7	66.5	70.2
Larynx	C32	1 210	84.5	66.0	57.9	88.0	74.7	71.9	72.4	73.4
Lung	C33-34	21 131	39.6	20.8	17.0	41.4	23.6	21.1	22.1	25.1
Other thoracic organs	C37-38	230	75.2	63.0	60.2	76.6	65.7	64.7	54.9	72.2
Bone	C40-41	256	87.9	73.8	69.3	88.9	76.0	72.7	68.8	70.1
Melanoma of skin	C43	261	83.5	56.8	49.5	86.5	63.1	59.2	60.1	61.7
Other skin	C44	2 586	94.7	86.0	79.1	99.6	100.3	102.4	101.1	100.1
Mesothelioma	C45	50	48.0	28.0	23.6	49.6	30.1	26.2	28.0	38.1
Connective tissue	C47	970	82.0	69.4	63.6	83.6	73.3	69.4	62.8	66.5
Breast	C50	10 112	95.6	87.4	82.4	97.1	91.8	89.8	90.0	89.6
Vulva, vagina, other	C51-52+C57	232	84.1	62.4	57.6	87.2	69.6	69.5	71.0	73.4
Cervix	C53	2 624	88.8	76.1	70.4	90.3	80.0	76.8	77.3	79.5
Corpus uteri	C54	1 863	91.4	82.3	79.4	92.7	86.0	85.6	84.1	85.1
Ovary	C56	1 831	83.0	69.0	63.5	84.2	71.7	67.6	63.6	67.3
Penis	C60	161	87.6	72.9	64.1	92.0	85.1	83.5	83.9	86.8
Prostate	C61	3 206	87.8	69.2	55.6	93.8	85.2	79.9	79.3	78.2
Testis	C62	383	94.8	86.9	80.8	96.8	92.6	90.0	91.9	92.1
Kidney	C64	914	77.8	64.4	57.8	80.0	69.8	66.3	65.5	70.5
Urinary bladder	C67	3 474	81.3	65.7	57.8	85.7	76.9	75.5	75.9	81.2
Other urinary organs	C68	711	62.9	47.1	42.5	65.6	52.9	51.6	54.0	61.0
Eye	C69	65	93.8	85.9	78.6	96.0	90.8	85.4	59.4	51.9
Brain & nervous system	C70-72	1 269	65.7	49.0	43.9	66.8	50.7	46.4	46.7	48.7
Thyroid	C73	2 235	93.5	91.3	89.0	94.6	94.3	94.1	93.7	95.1
Adrenal gland, other	C74-75	159	81.8	71.5	68.0	82.8	73.5	71.1	57.8	71.2
Hodgkin lymphoma	C81	257	89.1	82.6	79.8	90.3	85.2	84.1	85.6	87.4
Non-Hodgkin lymphoma	C82-85+C96	3 318	67.4	54.1	48.9	69.5	58.8	56.1	61.6	64.7
Multiple myeloma	C90	796	62.4	37.6	25.1	65.1	42.4	31.0	34.8	37.8
Lymphoid leukaemia	C91	561	77.7	60.9	54.9	79.3	64.3	60.0	56.7	59.1
Myeloid leukaemia	C92-94	1 389	55.0	36.9	31.4	56.4	38.8	33.9	36.0	42.3
Leukaemia unspecified	C95	141	32.6	23.3	23.3	33.9	25.0	25.4	31.4	36.8

ASRS: age-standardized relative survival

Table 4a. Site-wise number of cases, 5-year absolute and relative survival by sex: Hong Kong SAR, China, 1996–2001 cases followed-up until 2003

Site	ICD-10	Cases included	Male	% 5-year survival		Female	% 5-year survival	
			No.	Abs	Rel	No.	Abs	Rel
Lip	C00	42	25	84.0	101.7	17	87.1	102.1
Tongue	C01-02	677	438	50.1	57.6	239	69.3	77.5
Oral cavity	C03-06	561	378	45.9	55.9	183	59.5	69.0
Salivary gland	C07-08	330	180	68.2	77.0	150	83.9	90.3
Oropharynx	C09-10	219	180	33.1	37.8	39	71.0	77.0
Nasopharynx	C11	6 593	4 751	67.6	72.2	1 842	77.0	80.7
Hypopharynx	C12-13	360	335	20.4	24.7	25	50.3	57.8
Oesophagus	C15	2 832	2 290	18.9	23.2	542	29.3	35.7
Stomach	C16	5 879	3 709	31.3	39.2	2 170	30.0	36.4
Small intestine	C17	239	126	34.8	41.6	113	36.8	41.7
Colon	C18	11 025	5 819	47.6	60.7	5 206	50.3	61.8
Rectum, anus	C19-21	6 192	3 638	48.2	59.2	2 554	52.5	62.6
Liver	C22	9 256	7 223	18.9	21.5	2 033	19.1	21.8
Gall bladder	C23-24	1 601	758	17.5	22.5	843	18.0	22.4
Pancreas	C25	1 801	989	14.9	17.9	812	12.2	14.7
Nose/Sinuses	C30-31	288	178	56.2	63.9	110	62.6	74.1
Larynx	C32	1 210	1 130	57.7	71.7	80	61.7	75.1
Lung	C33-34	21 131	14 375	16.8	21.0	6 756	17.5	21.2
Other thoracic organs	C37-38	230	134	59.8	64.4	96	60.4	64.8
Bone	C40-41	256	140	66.7	70.2	116	72.5	75.8
Melanoma of skin	C43	261	141	45.3	55.7	120	54.4	63.2
Other skin	C44	2 586	1 207	78.7	100.7	1 379	79.4	103.9
Mesothelioma	C45	50	30	16.0	18.5	20	35.0	37.6
Connective tissue	C47	970	511	58.2	65.1	459	69.7	74.2
Breast	C50	10 112	63	77.3	99.8	10 049	82.4	89.7
Vulva, vagina, other	C51-52+C57	232				232	57.6	69.5
Cervix	C53	2 624				2 624	70.4	76.8
Corpus uteri	C54	1 863				1 863	79.4	85.6
Ovary	C56	1 831				1 831	63.5	67.6
Penis	C60	161	161	64.1	83.5			
Prostate	C61	3 206	3 206	55.6	79.9			
Testis	C62	383	383	80.8	90.0			
Kidney	C64	914	592	56.0	64.9	322	61.0	68.8
Urinary bladder	C67	3 474	2 620	58.4	76.5	854	55.8	72.4
Other urinary organs	C68	711	440	43.5	53.8	271	40.9	48.3
Eye	C69	65	33	76.0	85.3	32	82.3	87.0
Brain & nervous system	C70-72	1 269	765	40.2	42.9	504	49.4	51.7
Thyroid	C73	2 235	488	82.2	89.6	1 747	91.0	95.3
Adrenal gland, other	C74-75	159	97	64.0	67.0	62	74.4	77.7
Hodgkin lymphoma	C81	257	153	74.2	78.3	104	87.9	92.4
Non-Hodgkin lymphoma	C82-85+C96	3 318	1 900	47.2	54.9	1 418	51.3	57.7
Multiple myeloma	C90	796	439	25.3	31.7	357	25.0	30.4
Lymphoid leukaemia	C91	561	310	54.6	60.7	251	55.2	58.9
Myeloid leukaemia	C92-94	1 389	766	30.0	32.7	623	33.2	35.2
Leukaemia unspecified	C95	141	70	15.6	17.2	71	31.0	33.6

Abs: absolute survival; Rel: relative survival

Table 4b. Site-wise number of cases and relative survival by age group: Hong Kong SAR, China, 1996–2001 cases followed-up until 2003

Site	ICD-10	Cases included	Number of cases by age group					Relative survival by age group % 5-year survival				
			< 45	45-54	55-64	65-74	> 75	< 45	45-54	55-64	65-74	> 75
Lip	C00	42	8	6	6	12	10	101.1	102.8	110.3	71.8	119.7
Tongue	C01-02	677	139	119	151	170	98	76.8	63.7	58.0	67.1	63.2
Oral cavity	C03-06	561	50	75	127	171	138	84.8	61.8	59.2	58.7	52.8
Salivary gland	C07-08	330	118	63	55	55	39	90.4	88.2	74.7	76.4	73.0
Oropharynx	C09-10	219	30	45	61	58	25	70.2	61.2	32.4	35.6	38.2
Nasopharynx	C11	6 593	2 726	1 744	1 094	759	270	80.8	76.1	67.5	64.0	57.1
Hypopharynx	C12-13	360	20	69	94	107	70	15.2	25.5	25.2	29.5	35.6
Oesophagus	C15	2 832	100	364	696	995	677	33.5	26.1	23.0	26.8	26.0
Stomach	C16	5 879	530	640	1 021	1 733	1 955	43.0	43.0	41.9	39.3	32.2
Small intestine	C17	239	36	42	41	57	63	44.5	47.5	53.3	47.4	21.5
Colon	C18	11 025	754	1 047	1 889	3 636	3 699	64.3	63.3	64.0	62.3	58.1
Rectum, anus	C19-21	6 192	508	718	1 238	2 076	1 652	62.5	65.5	64.7	61.8	53.1
Liver	C22	9 256	1 163	1 720	2 243	2 605	1 525	33.8	25.8	20.6	18.5	13.1
Gall bladder	C23-24	1 601	59	110	210	520	702	35.1	35.7	26.6	24.4	16.1
Pancreas	C25	1 801	93	187	348	600	573	25.1	22.6	23.1	13.0	12.5
Nose/Sinuses	C30-31	288	50	55	57	69	57	82.3	76.8	67.1	58.6	56.8
Larynx	C32	1 210	34	141	309	445	281	73.7	70.6	78.5	69.0	69.2
Lung	C33-34	21 131	904	1 834	4 063	7 490	6 840	30.4	28.9	25.9	20.2	15.5
Other thoracic organs	C37-38	230	90	38	31	50	21	63.0	83.9	74.2	71.4	6.6
Bone	C40-41	256	153	36	27	25	15	75.9	68.4	74.7	62.1	72.8
Melanoma of skin	C43	261	55	38	41	60	67	68.2	60.4	58.2	55.5	51.2
Other skin	C44	2 586	212	250	371	730	1 023	96.0	99.8	100.8	103.7	105.6
Mesothelioma	C45	50	5	6	12	16	11	80.7	17.0	27.1	29.4	0.0
Connective tissue	C47	970	415	146	127	160	122	80.4	68.8	61.0	58.8	51.7
Breast	C50	10 112	3 226	2 689	1 508	1 399	1 290	88.5	90.5	89.1	90.4	93.6
Vulva, vagina, other	C51-52+C57	232	35	23	25	74	75	71.6	65.7	84.6	69.3	64.8
Cervix	C53	2 624	758	563	420	508	375	83.6	80.1	77.4	73.4	60.6
Corpus uteri	C54	1 863	334	631	400	321	177	93.4	87.1	85.9	76.1	83.5
Ovary	C56	1 831	649	422	277	287	196	84.1	67.8	60.6	50.7	45.8
Penis	C60	161	16	11	28	54	52	75.4	94.7	90.6	87.2	72.6
Prostate	C61	3 206	3	36	352	1 329	1 486	68.0	70.2	71.0	82.9	80.2
Testis	C62	383	237	41	18	33	54	94.2	92.1	56.7	93.8	75.9
Kidney	C64	914	128	193	180	261	152	81.8	64.4	65.6	68.4	50.0
Urinary bladder	C67	3 474	141	252	568	1 195	1 318	92.9	85.1	79.4	77.3	67.7
Other urinary organs	C68	711	53	80	126	224	228	61.2	65.8	68.2	50.8	34.4
Eye	C69	65	43	1	4	9	8	96.8	0.0	81.9	43.6	97.3
Brain & nervous system	C70-72	1 269	585	198	175	203	108	66.4	37.9	31.8	20.7	21.1
Thyroid	C73	2 235	1 102	419	302	258	154	99.7	98.9	90.5	83.8	60.8
Adrenal gland, other	C74-75	159	97	25	17	14	6	71.1	90.5	66.6	62.2	22.5
Hodgkin lymphoma	C81	257	157	27	24	31	18	95.2	80.2	76.1	50.5	57.2
Non-Hodgkin lymphoma	C82-85+C96	3 318	714	457	585	821	741	70.0	69.1	60.5	49.3	36.0
Multiple myeloma	C90	796	35	92	137	279	253	46.7	53.1	29.9	30.4	21.4
Lymphoid leukaemia	C91	561	329	37	51	68	76	69.8	46.5	39.2	44.5	46.0
Myeloid leukaemia	C92-94	1 389	536	159	166	288	240	52.9	42.6	30.4	14.7	7.4
Leukaemia unspecified	C95	141	40	19	11	31	40	47.9	37.8	19.3	11.2	

Table 5. Proportion of cases and 5-year absolute survival by extent of disease of breast cancer: Hong Kong SAR, China, 1996–2001

Site	ICD-10	Cases included	% of cases by extent of disease				% 5-year absolute survival			
			Localized	Regional	Dist. met.	Unknown	Localized	Regional	Dist. met.	Unknown
Breast	C50	10 112	12.2	34.6	1.5	51.7	94.9	79.1	31.8	82.7

Chapter 6

Cancer survival in Qidong, China, 1992–2000

Chen JG, Zhu J, Zhang YH and Lu JH

Abstract

The Qidong cancer registry was established in 1972, and registration of cases is done by active and passive methods. The registry contributed data on 33 cancer sites or types registered during 1992–2000 for this survival study. Data on 22 cancers registered during 1972–2000 were utilized to elicit the survival trend by period and cohort approaches. Follow-up was done by a mixture of active and passive methods, with median follow-up ranging from 2–25 months. The proportion of cases with histologically verified cancer diagnosis ranged from 9–100%, and 87–100% of total registered cases were included for survival analysis. The top-ranking cancers on 5-year age-standardized relative survival (%) were thyroid (78%), breast (58%), corpus uteri (54%), larynx (51%) and urinary bladder (42%). The corresponding survival rates for common cancers were liver (6%), lung (7%) and stomach (18%). The 5-year relative survival by age group fluctuated and showed no distinct pattern or trend. The comparison of 5-year relative survival trend by cohort and period approaches revealed that period survival closely predicted the survival experience of cancer cases diagnosed in that period for most cancers.

Qidong cancer registry

The Qidong cancer registry was established in 1972 at the Qidong Liver Cancer Institute, Qidong. The registry has been contributing data to the quinquennial IARC publication *Cancer Incidence in Five Continents* since Vol VI [1]. Cancer registration is done by active and passive methods. The principal source of information on incident cancer cases is the data file received from lower-level registries managed by a physician or a health worker. The registry checks these files with cancer report lists to find missing and/or duplicate cases. The registry caters to a mixed rural and urban population about 1.2 million with a sex ratio of 1016 females to 1000 males in 1999. The average annual age-standardized incidence rate is 242 per 100 000 among males and 111 per 100 000 among females with a lifetime cumulative risk of one in 4 of developing cancer in the period 1993–1997. The common cancers among males are liver, lung and stomach. The rank order among females is liver, stomach, lung and breast [1].

The registry contributed data on survival to the first volume of the IARC publication on *Cancer Survival in Developing Countries* [2]. In the present volume, the main tables pertain to the period 1992–2000. The data on survival for the years 1972–1991 are also utilized to elicit the trend in cancer survival.

Data quality indices (Table 1)

The proportion of cases with histologically verified cancer diagnosis in the series is 35%, varying from 9% (liver cancer) to 100% (all leukaemias). The proportion of cases registered based on a death certificate only (DCO) is negligible. Cases excluded from the study without any follow-up information is the highest for thyroid cancers (13%). Thus, 87–100% of the total cases registered are included in the estimation of the survival probability.

Outcome of follow-up (Table 2)

The methods of follow-up have been a mixture of both active and passive ones. These included receiving mortality information from all causes of death and periodically matching with the incident cancer database. The vital status of the unmatched incident cases is then collected by scrutiny of medical reports and house visits.

The closing date of follow-up is 31st December 2000. The median follow-up ranged from 2 months for lymphoid and myeloid leukaemias to 25 months for breast cancer. The completeness of follow-up at 5 years from the incidence date is 100%, as there are no losses to follow-up.

Survival statistics

All ages and both sexes together (Table 3)

The top-ranking cancers on 5-year relative survival are thyroid (78%), breast and corpus uteri (59%), larynx (53%) and urinary bladder (43%). The lowest survival is encountered with lymphoid leukaemia and oesophagus (5%), preceded by liver and myeloid leukaemia (6%) and lung (7%). Colon (39%) and rectum (31%) cancers have a higher survival among gastrointestinal cancers. The figure for Non-Hodgkin lymphoma is 14%, and that for multiple myeloma is 11%.

Figure 1a. Top ten cancers (ranked by survival), Qidong, China, 1992–2000

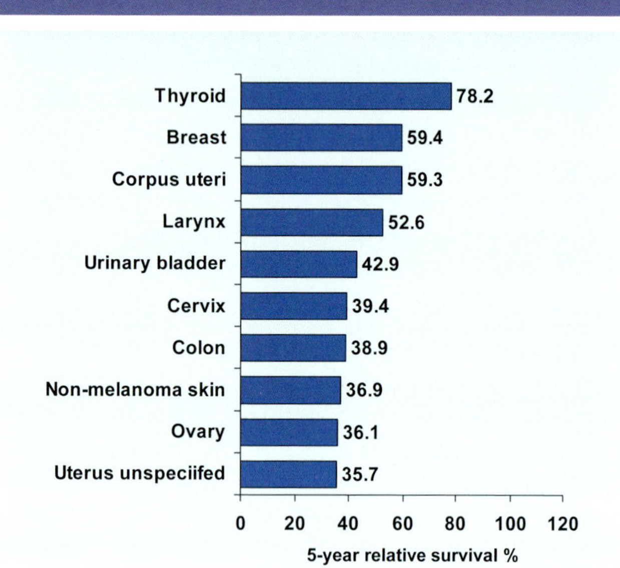

The 5-year age-standardized relative survival (ASRS) probability for all ages together is observed to be lesser than or similar to the corresponding unadjusted one for a majority of cancers. Also, the 5-year ASRS (0–74 years of age) is generally higher than or similar to the corresponding ASRS (all ages) for a majority of cancers.

Sex

Male (Table 4a)

Cancers of the breast (114%), larynx (60%), urinary bladder (43%), thyroid (42%) and soft tissue (39%) form the order when ranked on 5-year relative survival. Survival from prostate cancer is 32%. Cancers of the larynx, soft tissue and melanoma skin have a notably higher survival among males than females.

Figure 1b. Top five cancers (ranked by survival), Male, Qidong, China, 1992–2000

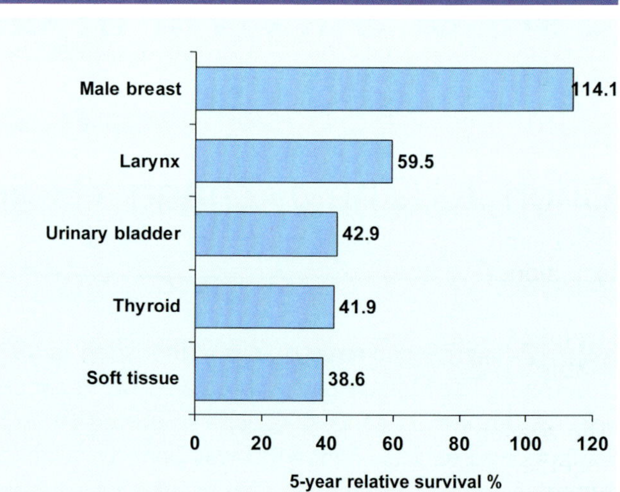

Female (Table 4a)

The rank order based on 5-year relative survival is cancer of the thyroid (93%), nose/sinuses (64%), corpus uteri and breast (59%) and non-melanoma skin (44%). Survival from cancers of the cervix and ovary are 39% and 36%, respectively. Survival is markedly higher among females than males in cancers of the nasopharynx, nose/sinuses, non-melanoma skin, kidney and thyroid.

Figure 1c. Top five cancers (ranked by survival), Female, Qidong, China, 1992–2000

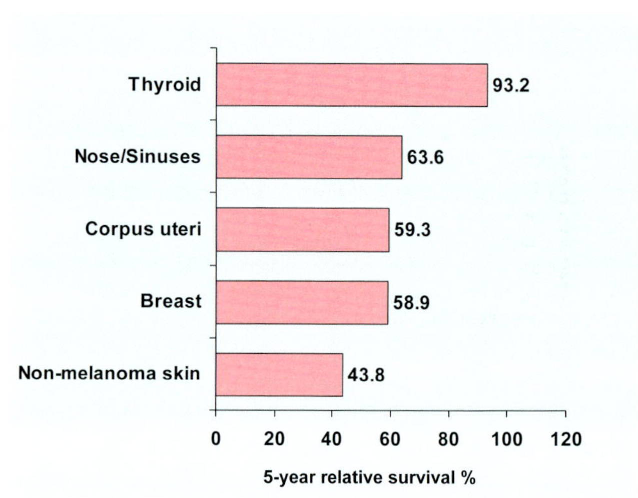

Age group (Table 4b)

The 5-year relative survival by age group reveals no distinct pattern or trend and is seen to fluctuate with increasing age groups.

Survival trend (Table 5)

The trend of survival data, estimated by the same method of semi-complete analytic approach, is available for 15 cancer sites or types spanning 19 years in the two time periods 1982–1991 and 1992–2000. An increasing trend in the 5-year relative survival with an absolute difference of 10% and more between 1982–1991 and 1992–2000 is observed only in cancer of the nose/sinuses. A decreasing survival of similar magnitude is forthcoming for cancers of skin melanoma and non-melanoma, soft tissue, prostate and kidney.

Trend of survival by period and cohort approaches (Tables 6 & 7; Figure 2)

The availability of data on registration and follow-up together for both a long (from the calendar year 1972) and a more recent period (year 2000) of calendar time led to the possibility of estimating up-to-date survival and trend by period approach. Survival is also estimated by cohort approach for comparison.

The 5-year relative survival by cohort and period approaches are estimated for the five calendar periods 1977–1981, 1982–1986, 1987–1991, 1992–1996 and 1997–2000. The period survival estimates in a calendar period are seen to resemble the cohort survival estimates of the succeeding calendar period for most cancers. Thus, period survival closely predicts the survival experience of cancer cases diagnosed in that period. However, this seems to vary for some calendar periods in a few cancers, indicating some limiting factor either in the ascertainment of follow-up information or some changes in the registration process in those periods.

References

1. Parkin DM, Whelan SL, Ferlay J and Storm H. *Cancer Incidence in Five Continents, Vol I to VIII: IARC Cancerbase No. 7*. IARCPress, Lyon, 2005.

2. Swaminathan R, Black RJ and Sankaranarayanan R. Database on Cancer Survival from Developing Countries. In: *Cancer Survival in Developing Countries* (eds) R Sankaranarayanan, RJ Black and DM Parkin. IARC Scientific Publications No. 145. IARCPress, Lyon, 1998.

Figure 2. Up-to-date 5-year relative survival estimates over the calendar periods by period and cohort approaches for selected cancers, Qidong, China, 1972–2000 cases followed through 2000

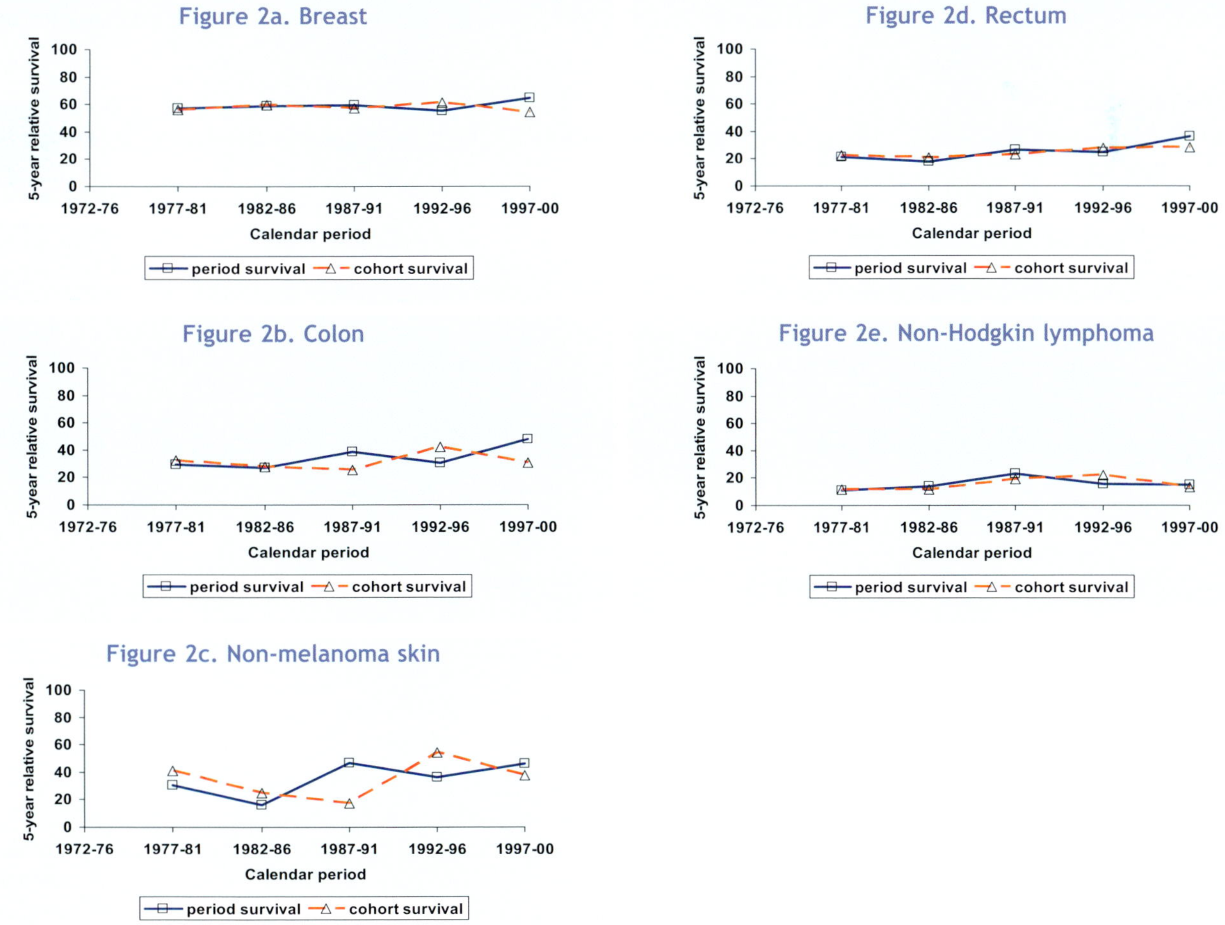

Figure 2a. Breast

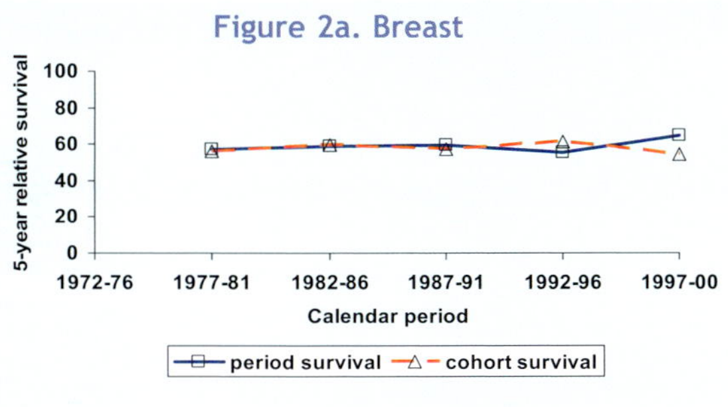

Figure 2b. Colon

Figure 2c. Non-melanoma skin

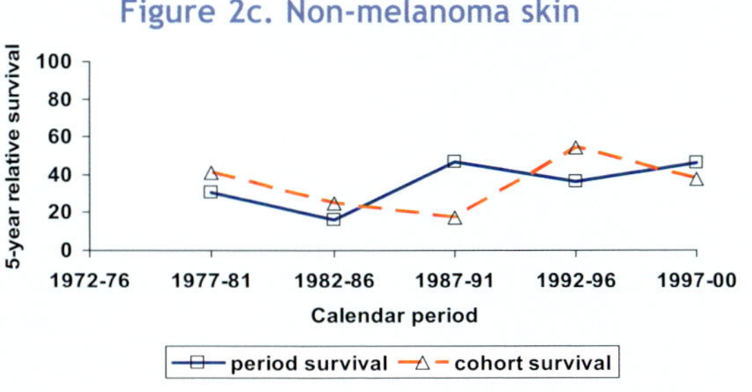

Figure 2d. Rectum

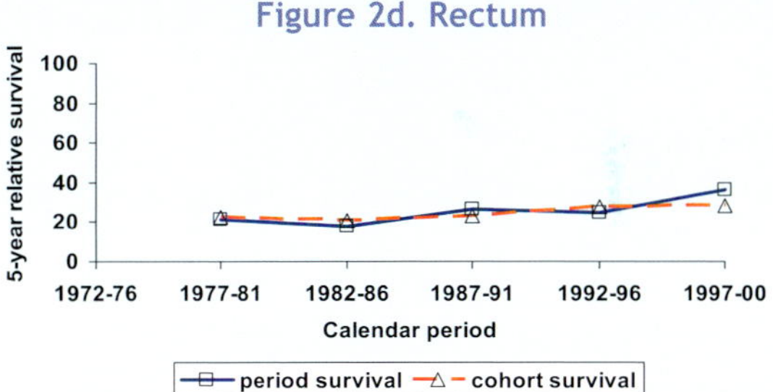

Figure 2e. Non-Hodgkin lymphoma

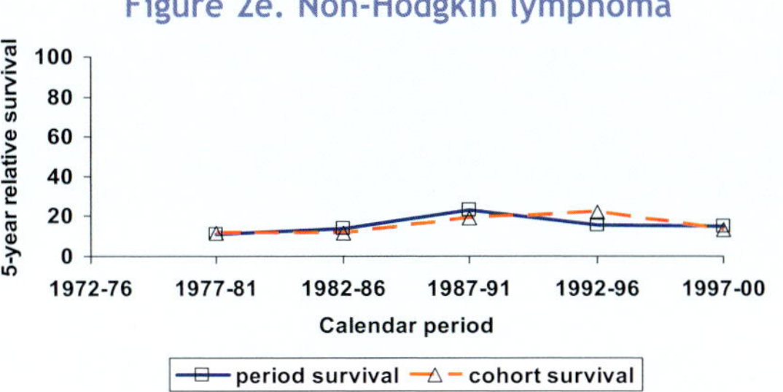

Table 1. Data quality indices - Proportion of histologically verified and death certificate only cases, number and proportion of included and excluded cases by site: Qidong, China, 1992–2000 cases followed-up until 2000

Site	ICD-10	Total registered	%		Excluded cases					Included cases	
			HV	DCO	DCO	Follow-up	Others	Total	%	No.	%
Oral cavity	C03-06	37	89.2	2.7	1	1	0	2	5.4	35	94.6
Nasopharynx	C11	166	77.7	0.6	1	1	0	2	1.2	164	98.8
Oesophagus	C15	948	30.5	0.2	2	4	0	6	0.6	942	99.4
Stomach	C16	3 289	54.8	0.2	5	30	0	35	1.1	3 254	98.9
Small intestine	C17	37	56.8	0.0	0	2	0	2	5.4	35	94.6
Colon	C18	326	73.6	0.3	1	10	0	11	3.4	315	96.6
Rectum	C19-20	1 026	77.4	0.4	4	12	0	16	1.6	1 010	98.4
Liver	C22	7 138	9.0	0.2	15	33	0	48	0.7	7 090	99.3
Gall bladder	C23-24	102	41.2	0.0	0	2	0	2	2.0	100	98.0
Pancreas	C25	672	25.4	0.6	4	7	0	11	1.6	661	98.4
Nose/Sinuses	C30-31	45	77.8	0.0	0	0	0	0	0.0	45	100.0
Larynx	C32	49	85.7	0.0	0	2	0	2	4.1	47	95.9
Lung	C33-34	3 303	10.4	0.3	11	11	0	22	0.7	3 281	99.3
Other thoracic organs	C37-38	38	36.8	0.0	0	0	0	0	0.0	38	100.0
Bone	C40-41	150	45.3	0.7	1	0	0	1	0.7	149	99.3
Melanoma of skin	C43	36	94.4	0.0	0	0	0	0	0.0	36	100.0
Other skin	C44	122	92.6	0.0	0	2	0	2	1.6	120	98.4
Connective tissue	C47+C49	34	91.2	0.0	0	2	0	2	5.9	32	94.1
Breast	C50	669	93.6	0.3	2	16	0	18	2.7	651	97.3
Cervix	C53	146	87.7	0.0	0	2	0	2	1.4	144	98.6
Corpus uteri	C54	72	93.1	0.0	0	3	0	3	4.2	69	95.8
Uterus unspecified	C55	42	73.8	0.0	0	1	0	1	2.4	41	97.6
Ovary	C56	105	78.1	0.0	0	4	0	4	3.8	101	96.2
Prostate	C61	55	67.3	0.0	0	0	0	0	0.0	55	100.0
Kidney	C64	72	55.6	0.0	0	0	0	0	0.0	72	100.0
Urinary bladder	C67	373	66.5	0.5	2	5	0	7	1.9	366	98.1
Brain & nervous system	C70-72	414	21.3	0.0	0	1	0	1	0.2	413	99.8
Thyroid	C73	55	94.5	0.0	0	7	0	7	12.7	48	87.3
Non-Hodgkin lymphoma	C82-85+C96	316	91.1	0.6	2	2	0	4	1.3	312	98.7
Multiple myeloma	C90	137	85.4	0.0	0	0	0	0	0.0	137	100.0
Lymphoid leukaemia	C91	83	100.0	1.2	1	1	0	2	2.4	81	97.6
Myeloid leukaemia	C92-94	217	100.0	0.5	1	0	0	1	0.5	216	99.5
Leukaemia unspecified	C95	107	100.0	0.0	0	0	0	0	0.0	107	100.0

HV: histologically verified; DCO: death certificate only

Table 2. Number and proportion of cases by vital status and median follow-up (in months) by site: Qidong, China, 1992–2000 cases followed-up until 2000

Site	ICD-10	Cases included	Dead		Alive		Complete FU		Median FU (in months)
			No.	%	No.	%	No.	%	
Oral cavity	C03-06	35	22	62.9	13	37.1	35	100.0	6.1
Nasopharynx	C11	164	106	64.6	58	35.4	164	100.0	8.2
Oesophagus	C15	942	871	92.5	71	7.5	942	100.0	3.6
Stomach	C16	3 254	2 625	80.7	629	19.3	3 254	100.0	4.5
Small intestine	C17	35	29	82.9	6	17.1	35	100.0	4.3
Colon	C18	315	184	58.4	131	41.6	315	100.0	7.4
Rectum	C19-20	1 010	696	68.9	314	31.1	1 010	100.0	7.8
Liver	C22	7 090	6 424	90.6	666	9.4	7 090	100.0	2.7
Gall bladder	C23-24	100	87	87.0	13	13.0	100	100.0	2.8
Pancreas	C25	661	595	90.0	66	10.0	661	100.0	2.8
Nose/Sinuses	C30-31	45	30	66.7	15	33.3	45	100.0	14.6
Larynx	C32	47	26	55.3	21	44.7	47	100.0	10.7
Lung	C33-34	3 281	2 940	89.6	341	10.4	3 281	100.0	3.4
Other thoracic organs	C37-38	38	32	84.2	6	15.8	38	100.0	4.9
Bone	C40-41	149	126	84.6	23	15.4	149	100.0	4.3
Melanoma of skin	C43	36	27	75.0	9	25.0	36	100.0	9.4
Other skin	C44	120	89	74.2	31	25.8	120	100.0	7.2
Connective tissue	C47+C49	32	21	65.6	11	34.4	32	100.0	9.8
Breast	C50	651	239	36.7	412	63.3	651	100.0	25.5
Cervix	C53	144	86	59.7	58	40.3	144	100.0	7.9
Corpus uteri	C54	69	27	39.1	42	60.9	69	100.0	21.1
Uterus unspecified	C55	41	25	61.0	16	39.0	41	100.0	8.1
Ovary	C56	101	61	60.4	40	39.6	101	100.0	9.7
Prostate	C61	55	39	70.9	16	29.1	55	100.0	5.3
Kidney	C64	72	50	69.4	22	30.6	72	100.0	3.8
Urinary bladder	C67	366	222	60.7	144	39.3	366	100.0	9.1
Brain & nervous system	C70-72	413	357	86.4	56	13.6	413	100.0	3.0
Thyroid	C73	48	12	25.0	36	75.0	48	100.0	20.3
Non-Hodgkin lymphoma	C82-85+C96	312	259	83.0	53	17.0	312	100.0	4.8
Multiple myeloma	C90	137	118	86.1	19	13.9	137	100.0	3.3
Lymphoid leukaemia	C91	81	70	86.4	11	13.6	81	100.0	2.4
Myeloid leukaemia	C92-94	216	197	91.2	19	8.8	216	100.0	2.4
Leukaemia unspecified	C95	107	99	92.5	8	7.5	107	100.0	3.6

FU: follow-up

Table 3. Comparison of 1-, 3- and 5-year absolute and relative survival and 5-year age-standardized relative survival by site: Qidong, China, 1992–2000 cases followed-up until 2000

Site	ICD-10	Cases included	% Absolute survival			% Relative survival			% ASRS at 5-years	
			1-year	3-year	5-year	1-year	3-year	5-year	all ages	0-74 years
Oral cavity	C03-06	35	44.6	32.2	32.2	46.0	35.5	36.2	40.3	43.8
Nasopharynx	C11	164	47.1	31.6	29.3	48.1	33.1	31.2	29.1	36.4
Oesophagus	C15	942	14.7	4.6	4.0	15.5	5.2	4.9	5.3	6.1
Stomach	C16	3 254	28.0	16.6	15.4	29.2	18.3	18.0	17.9	20.1
Small intestine	C17	35	36.4	14.5	6.2	37.6	16.4	7.7	5.5	6.3
Colon	C18	315	49.5	34.6	32.9	51.5	38.0	38.9	36.7	42.1
Rectum	C19-20	1 010	44.0	29.9	26.9	45.8	33.0	31.4	29.6	34.5
Liver	C22	7 090	13.3	6.5	5.2	13.5	6.8	5.6	5.6	5.4
Gall bladder	C23-24	100	20.8	12.5	12.5	21.5	13.5	14.4	15.2	17.5
Pancreas	C25	661	11.9	6.8	6.5	12.4	7.6	8.0	8.6	6.7
Nose/Sinuses	C30-31	45	57.8	34.5	24.6	59.1	37.4	29.9	44.1	22.3
Larynx	C32	47	55.1	41.3	41.3	57.2	46.8	52.6	50.5	48.7
Lung	C33-34	3 281	15.2	6.5	5.6	15.8	7.2	6.8	6.6	6.4
Other thoracic organs	C37-38	38	23.3	10.0	10.0	24.1	10.5	10.8	14.2	19.3
Bone	C40-41	149	27.5	14.3	13.0	28.2	15.6	14.8	13.7	15.2
Melanoma of skin	C43	36	46.3	30.8	15.4	48.0	33.9	18.1	22.2	26.6
Other skin	C44	120	39.2	27.3	26.0	42.1	33.2	36.9	38.5	37.3
Connective tissue	C47+C49	32	50.8	27.8	27.8	51.8	30.0	30.9	26.8	36.2
Breast	C50	651	77.7	63.0	56.0	78.6	65.0	59.4	57.6	58.3
Cervix	C53	144	45.8	39.0	36.5	47.1	40.8	39.4	43.8	47.9
Corpus uteri	C54	69	76.9	62.6	54.9	78.5	66.0	59.3	53.8	62.2
Uterus unspecified	C55	41	46.2	33.6	33.6	47.7	35.3	35.7	28.6	34.9
Ovary	C56	101	51.3	34.7	32.7	52.1	36.2	36.1	41.0	35.1
Prostate	C61	55	37.7	25.1	25.1	40.2	29.2	32.5	31.1	36.3
Kidney	C64	72	36.7	31.0	24.5	37.4	32.7	26.8	28.9	26.7
Urinary bladder	C67	366	51.5	38.7	32.9	54.3	45.3	42.9	42.1	47.3
Brain & nervous system	C70-72	413	18.0	11.2	8.8	18.3	11.6	9.2	10.7	11.1
Thyroid	C73	48	75.6	72.8	72.8	77.0	75.6	78.2	77.8	76.8
Non-Hodgkin lymphoma	C82-85+C96	312	26.3	16.8	12.3	27.0	18.0	13.9	13.1	13.4
Multiple myeloma	C90	137	14.7	9.1	9.1	15.1	10.1	11.1	11.1	10.9
Lymphoid leukaemia	C91	81	21.0	6.8	4.5	21.3	7.1	4.8	4.1	5.4
Myeloid leukaemia	C92-94	216	19.1	7.2	5.3	19.3	7.5	5.7	6.6	6.0
Leukaemia unspecified	C95	107	13.6	7.6	6.5	13.8	7.8	6.9	5.8	7.1

ASRS: age-standardized relative survival

Table 4a. Site-wise number of cases, 5-year absolute and relative survival by sex: Qidong, China, 1992–2000 cases followed-up until 2000

Site	ICD-10	Cases included	Male % 5-year survival			Female % 5-year survival		
			No.	Abs	Rel	No.	Abs	Rel
Oral cavity	C03-06	35	21	33.8	35.6	14	29.3	36.6
Nasopharynx	C11	164	114	24.4	26.0	50	40.2	42.6
Oesophagus	C15	942	645	4.0	4.9	297	3.9	4.9
Stomach	C16	3 254	2 038	16.0	19.0	1 216	14.4	16.3
Small intestine	C17	35	23	5.1	6.5	12		
Colon	C18	315	136	31.2	37.1	179	34.1	40.0
Rectum	C19-20	1 010	508	25.2	29.6	502	28.4	33.0
Liver	C22	7 090	5 338	5.1	5.5	1 752	5.3	5.7
Gall bladder	C23-24	100	54	10.5	11.5	46	15.0	18.1
Pancreas	C25	661	361	6.6	8.0	300	6.3	7.9
Nose/Sinuses	C30-31	45	35	16.4	21.1	10	58.5	63.6
Larynx	C32	47	42	46.5	59.5	5	0.0	0.0
Lung	C33-34	3 281	2 459	5.0	6.1	822	7.3	8.8
Other thoracic organs	C37-38	38	27	10.8	11.8	11		
Bone	C40-41	149	101	15.5	16.9	48	8.1	10.0
Melanoma of skin	C43	36	16	21.3	24.7	20	9.9	11.7
Other skin	C44	120	57	22.4	29.5	63	29.2	43.8
Connective tissue	C47+C49	32	15	35.2	38.6	17	20.8	23.5
Breast	C50	651	5	100.0	114.1	646	55.7	58.9
Cervix	C53	144				144	36.5	39.4
Corpus uteri	C54	69				69	54.9	59.3
Uterus unspecified	C55	41				41	33.6	35.7
Ovary	C56	101				101	32.7	36.1
Prostate	C61	55	55	25.1	32.5			
Kidney	C64	72	41	17.6	19.5	31	33.0	35.7
Urinary bladder	C67	366	287	32.5	42.9	79	33.8	42.7
Brain & nervous system	C70-72	413	237	6.4	6.7	176	12.3	12.7
Thyroid	C73	48	14	38.5	41.9	34	87.3	93.2
Non-Hodgkin lymphoma	C82-85+C96	312	179	13.2	14.9	133	11.0	12.5
Multiple myeloma	C90	137	72	10.7	14.1	65	7.6	8.4
Lymphoid leukaemia	C91	81	44	3.5	3.6	37	8.6	9.3
Myeloid leukaemia	C92-94	216	118	7.3	8.0	98	2.7	2.8
Leukaemia unspecified	C95	107	58	5.5	6.0	49	7.9	8.2

Abs: absolute survival; Rel: relative survival

Table 4b. Site-wise number of cases and relative survival by age group: Qidong, China, 1992–2000 cases followed-up until 2000

Site	ICD-10	Cases included	Number of cases by age group					Relative survival by age group % 5-year survival				
			< 45	45-54	55-64	65-74	> 75	< 45	45-54	55-64	65-74	> 75
Oral cavity	C03-06	35	5	5	9	11	5	34.2		42.8		0.0
Nasopharynx	C11	164	34	42	41	32	15	46.4	36.8	22.3	29.9	0.0
Oesophagus	C15	942	26	84	203	330	299	7.9	4.8	8.6	3.7	3.5
Stomach	C16	3 254	285	403	784	998	784	22.5	22.9	19.5	17.5	15.4
Small intestine	C17	35	6	1	10	9	9	0.0	0.0	28.2	0.0	0.0
Colon	C18	315	33	44	70	88	80	44.2	43.1	50.3	34.0	28.7
Rectum	C19-20	1 010	102	132	219	305	252	30.3	43.9	39.5	27.6	25.0
Liver	C22	7 090	2 458	1 812	1 380	946	494	5.5	6.1	5.2	5.0	7.8
Gall bladder	C23-24	100	11	15	22	27	25	32.9	20.4	4.9	16.9	8.9
Pancreas	C25	661	44	75	163	214	165	4.6	8.0	9.0	5.3	14.8
Nose/Sinuses	C30-31	45	5	5	12	20	3		0.0	20.7	29.6	79.5
Larynx	C32	47	2	2	12	20	11	51.4	51.9	32.4	59.7	66.8
Lung	C33-34	3 281	165	368	917	1 240	591	3.0	6.8	5.8	8.0	8.1
Other thoracic organs	C37-38	38	8	2	15	7	6		52.0	7.3	0.0	0.0
Bone	C40-41	149	38	21	34	31	25	22.0	24.8	10.0	8.5	10.1
Melanoma of skin	C43	36	7	4	7	11	7		68.9		14.0	0.0
Other skin	C44	120	16	5	21	28	50	45.4	61.7	20.5	28.4	50.6
Connective tissue	C47+C49	32	11	4	7	6	4	35.3	77.9		27.9	0.0
Breast	C50	651	205	200	119	85	42	60.5	66.4	49.1	56.5	57.7
Cervix	C53	144	36	25	27	31	25	61.2	67.4	24.1	31.1	15.1
Corpus uteri	C54	69	9	22	15	17	6	67.2	66.6	56.6	58.7	0.0
Uterus unspecified	C55	41	11	8	6	9	7	64.2	36.5	28.9	14.9	
Ovary	C56	101	27	30	26	11	7	32.8	43.5	9.3	55.3	90.0
Prostate	C61	55	3	3	11	19	19		0.0	30.2	45.4	31.8
Kidney	C64	72	12	8	21	23	8			26.7	24.1	36.0
Urinary bladder	C67	366	17	30	86	118	115	63.0	41.3	47.7	45.0	33.7
Brain & nervous system	C70-72	413	115	97	88	89	24	14.8	6.3	11.1		
Thyroid	C73	48	19	6	8	9	6	100.5	51.1	90.3	51.0	71.9
Non-Hodgkin lymphoma	C82-85+C96	312	76	32	78	79	47	10.5	15.4	19.3	15.1	10.8
Multiple myeloma	C90	137	19	12	37	52	17	21.4		0.0	10.7	14.3
Lymphoid leukaemia	C91	81	37	9	14	15	6	6.5	0.0	0.0	13.7	0.0
Myeloid leukaemia	C92-94	216	98	29	29	37	23	10.7	0.0	0.0	0.0	20.2
Leukaemia unspecified	C95	107	50	15	22	15	5	5.0	0.0	9.5	15.6	0.0

Table 5. Comparison of 5-year absolute and relative survival of cases diagnosed between 1982–1991 and 1992–2000, Qidong, China

Site	ICD-10	% 5-year absolute survival		% 5-year relative survival	
		1982–1991	1992–2000	1982–1991	1992–2000
Oral cavity	C03-06	28.2	32.2	34.0	36.2
Nasopharynx	C11	26.7	29.3	28.7	31.2
Oesophagus	C15	4.9	4.0	5.9	4.9
Stomach	C16	13.9	15.4	15.6	18.0
Small intestine	C17	14.9	6.2	17.5	7.7
Colon	C18	29.8	32.9	34.5	38.9
Rectum	C19-20	22.5	26.9	25.3	31.4
Liver	C22	3.0	5.2	3.2	5.6
Gall bladder	C23-24	16.2	12.5	19.1	14.4
Pancreas	C25	7.4	6.5	8.9	8.0
Nose/Sinuses	C30-31	13.6	24.6	16.3	29.9
Larynx	C32	48.0	41.3	54.5	52.6
Lung	C33-34	4.1	5.6	4.8	6.8
Other thoracic organs	C37-38	10.2	10.0	10.9	10.8
Bone	C40-41	19.9	13.0	22.7	14.8
Melanoma of skin	C43	51.9	15.4	54.5	18.1
Other skin	C44	51.9	26.0	54.5	36.9
Connective tissue	C47+C49	37.5	27.8	41.9	30.9
Breast	C50	56.5	56.0	59.5	59.4
Cervix	C53	33.5	36.5	37.2	39.4
Corpus uteri	C54	61.1	54.9	66.6	59.3
Uterus unspecified	C55	41.3	33.6	43.1	35.7
Ovary	C56	39.2	32.7	41.0	36.1
Prostate	C61	20.7	25.1	24.1	32.5
Kidney	C64	33.9	24.5	37.6	26.8
Urinary bladder	C67	34.4	32.9	40.1	42.9
Brain & nervous system	C70-72	8.8	8.8	9.0	9.2
Thyroid	C73	70.0	72.8	72.7	78.2
Non-Hodgkin lymphoma	C82-85+C96	18.7	12.3	20.0	13.9
Multiple myeloma	C90	3.5	9.1	4.6	11.1
Lymphoid leukaemia	C91	5.5	4.5	5.7	4.8
Myeloid leukaemia	C92-94	10.2	5.3	11.5	5.7
Leukaemia unspecified	C95	4.7	6.5	4.9	6.9

Table 6. Number of cases by cancer site and calendar period, Qidong, China, 1977–2000

Site	ICD-10	1977-81	1982-86	1987-91	1992-96	1997-2000	1977-2000
Nasopharynx	C11	92	81	91	95	69	428
Oesophagus	C15	479	476	510	550	392	2 407
Stomach	C16	1 708	1 774	2 082	1 935	1 319	8 818
Small intestine	C17	116	64	30	25	10	245
Colon	C18	90	109	146	148	167	660
Rectum	C19-20	275	381	465	581	429	2 131
Liver	C22	2 499	3 066	2 992	3 862	3 228	15 647
Pancreas	C25	264	323	392	356	305	1 640
Lung	C33-34	879	1 137	1 403	1 728	1 553	6 700
Bone	C40-41	61	68	73	88	61	351
Other skin	C44	55	60	74	77	43	309
Breast	C50	219	297	369	337	314	1 536
Cervix	C53	118	115	97	85	59	474
Ovary	C56	31	45	34	49	52	211
Prostate	C61	13	13	16	31	24	97
Kidney	C64	25	25	34	37	35	156
Urinary bladder	C67	84	113	140	205	161	703
Brain & nervous system	C70-72	116	118	167	214	199	814
Non-Hodgkin lymphoma	C82-85+C96	105	133	150	195	117	700
Multiple myeloma	C90	56	72	71	74	63	336
Myeloid leukaemia	C92-94	26	32	105	140	76	379
Leukaemia unspecified	C95	128	161	74	62	45	470

Table 7. Up-to-date 5-year relative survival estimates using cohort and period approaches by site and calendar period: Qidong, China, 1977–2000 cases followed-up until 2000

Site	ICD-10	Period approach					Cohort approach				
		1977–81	1982–86	1987–91	1992–96	1997–2000	1977–81	1982–86	1987–91	1992–96	1997–2000
Nasopharynx	C11	15.9	31.4	27.2	25.1	37.7	28.1	22.7	29.9	28.5	27.6
Oesophagus	C15	2.6	6.2	6.6	4.2	5.6	3.6	4.5	5.4	6.8	4.4
Stomach	C16	11.2	13.3	16.2	14.7	21.3	11.8	12.3	14.5	17.4	16.2
Small intestine	C17	8.0	11.9	23.3	13.2	8.6	12.2	8.9	16.5	20.7	5.9
Colon	C18	29.4	27.4	38.5	30.8	47.8	32.1	28.0	25.6	42.0	30.8
Rectum	C19-20	21.6	18.0	26.7	24.9	36.7	22.3	20.6	23.3	27.7	28.2
Liver	C22	2.3	1.2	3.8	4.8	5.6	2.4	1.8	2.4	4.0	5.0
Pancreas	C25	3.5	4.5	5.1	4.6	8.3	5.6	4.0	5.0	4.9	5.2
Lung	C33-34	3.3	4.5	5.1	4.6	8.3	5.6	4.0	5.0	4.9	5.2
Bone	C40-41	14.0	16.1	26.6	15.2	16.0	37.4	13.0	19.1	26.6	12.5
Other skin	C44	30.4	16.4	47.0	36.6	46.4	41.0	24.8	17.6	54.6	37.7
Breast	C50	57.1	58.9	59.7	55.4	64.8	56.2	59.4	57.3	61.4	54.2
Cervix	C53	39.1	32.1	40.8	30.6	41.9	56.7	28.7	39.0	35.1	39.8
Ovary	C56	25.9	48.1	34.8	33.8	36.3	30.3	27.5	48.6	31.0	24.2
Prostate	C61	4.5	28.1	22.4	31.2	29.2	14.3	11.4	19.6	29.7	35.0
Kidney	C64	13.9	40.2	40.6	31.5	27.3	31.4	13.9	45.0	34.6	26.7
Urinary bladder	C67	41.0	36.9	37.3	40.6	47.9	31.1	38.5	36.7	45.4	38.9
Brain & nervous system	C70-72	6.4	7.5	7.7	8.9	11.4	10.2	7.1	7.9	10.0	5.0
Non-Hodgkin lymphoma	C82-85+C9	10.8	13.9	23.1	15.7	14.9	11.8	11.3	19.1	21.7	13.5
Multiple myeloma	C90	1.2	3.0	8.8	4.0	13.6	7.9	0.0	7.3	2.1	11.7
Myeloid leukaemia	C92-94	0.0	17.8	7.3	7.6	8.4	4.4	3.9	12.9	11.2	5.3
Leukaemia unspecified	C95	1.1	2.6	12.0	7.6	2.9	2.6	1.6	3.4	8.5	12.1

Chapter 7

Cancer survival in Shanghai, China, 1992–1995

Xiang YB, Jin F and Gao YT

Abstract

The Shanghai cancer registry, established in 1963, is the oldest one in mainland China; cancer registration is entirely done by passive methods. The registry contributed data on 52 cancer sites or types registered during 1992–1995 for this survival study. The methods of follow-up have been a mixture of both active and passive ones, with median follow-up ranging 3–81 months. The proportion with histologically verified diagnosis for various cancers ranged from 14–95%; death certificates only (DCOs) ranged from 0–2% and 98–100% of total registered cases were included for survival analysis. The top ranking cancers on 5-year age-standardized relative survival (%) were thyroid (90%), non-melanoma skin (86%), penis (84%), corpus uteri (82%) and testis (80%). The corresponding survival rates for common cancers were lung (16%), stomach (30%), liver (9%), breast (78%) and colon (48%). The 5-year relative survival by age group reveals an inverse relationship for most cancers. An increasing trend in the 5-year absolute and relative survival was noted for all cancers registered in 1992–1995 compared to 1988–1991.

Shanghai cancer registry

The Shanghai cancer registry, established in 1963, is the oldest one in mainland China. It is based at the Shanghai Cancer Institute, Shanghai. The registry has been contributing data to the quinquennial IARC publication *Cancer Incidence in Five Continents* since Vol IV [1]. Cancer notification is by a regulation issued by the Shanghai Municipal Bureau of Public Health. Hence, cancer registration is entirely done by passive methods. The principal source of information on cancer cases is the notification card consisting of basic required information for cancer registration that is sent to the registry. The residential status of cancer cases is confirmed by house visit. The registry covers an area of 290 km^2 and caters to a population of about 6.4 million, with a sex ratio of 982 females to 1000 males in 1995. The average annual age-standardized incidence rate is 190 per 100 000 among males and 155 per 100 000 among females with a lifetime cumulative risk of one in 5 of developing cancer in the period 1993–1997. The common cancers among males are lung, stomach and liver. The rank order among females is breast, lung and stomach [1].

The registry contributed data on survival from 38 cancer sites or types registered during 1988–1991 to the first volume of IARC publication on *Cancer Survival in Developing Countries* [2]. In the present volume, data on survival from 52 cancers registered during 1992–1995 are reported.

Data quality indices (Table 1)

The proportion of cases with histologically verified cancer diagnosis in the series is 56%, varying from 14% (liver cancer) to 95% (corpus uteri cancer). The proportion of cases registered as death certificates only (DCOs) is the highest in lip cancer (2%), and cases without any follow-up are negligible. Thus, 98–100% of the total cases registered are included in the estimation of the survival probability.

Outcome of follow-up (Table 2)

The methods of follow-up have been a mixture of both active and passive ones. These included obtaining cancer mortality information from the death certificates in vital statistics section of Shanghai Hygiene and Anti-epidemic Centre. The mortality data are periodically matched with the incident cancer database. The vital status of the unmatched incident cases is then collected by house visits or postal/telephone enquiries.

The closing date of follow-up was 31st December 2000.

The median follow-up ranged from 3 months for cancers of the pancreas and liver to 81 months for cancer of the adrenal gland. The completeness of follow-up at 5 years from the incidence date is available in 95-100%.

Survival statistics

All ages and both sexes together (Table 3)

The top ranking cancers on 5-year relative survival are thyroid (90%), other male genital organ (89%), non-melanoma skin (86%), corpus uteri (86%) and penis (83%). The least survival is encountered with pancreatic cancer (8%), preceded by liver (9%), unspecified leukaemia (12%), lung and gallbladder (15%). Lip and salivary gland (73%) among other head and neck cancers and colon, rectum and anus (48–51%) among gastrointestinal cancers have higher survival than others. Survival from cancers of the urinary system is 65% for urinary bladder and 62% for renal pelvis. Hodgkin lymphoma had a better survival (66%) than non-Hodgkin lymphoma (39%). The survival figures for leukaemias are lymphoid (30%) and myeloid (27%).

Figure 1a. Top ten cancers (ranked by survival), Shanghai, China, 1992–1995

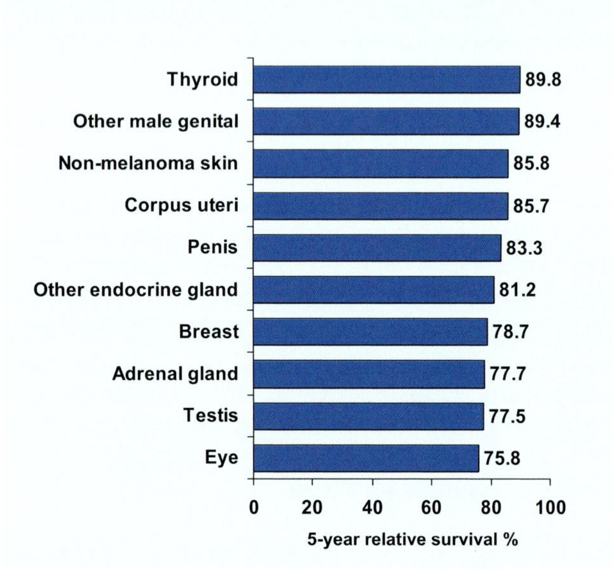

The 5-year age-standardized relative survival (ASRS) probability for all ages together is generally less than or similar to the corresponding unadjusted one for a majority of cancers. Also, the 5-year ASRS (0–74 years of age) is generally higher than or similar to the corresponding ASRS (all ages) for a majority of cancers.

Sex

Male (Table 4a)

The 5-year relative survival probabilities for lip, breast, renal pelvis, bladder, other urinary organ cancers and lymphoid leukaemia are noticeably higher among males than females.

Figure 1b. Top five cancers (ranked by survival), Male, Shanghai, China, 1992–1995

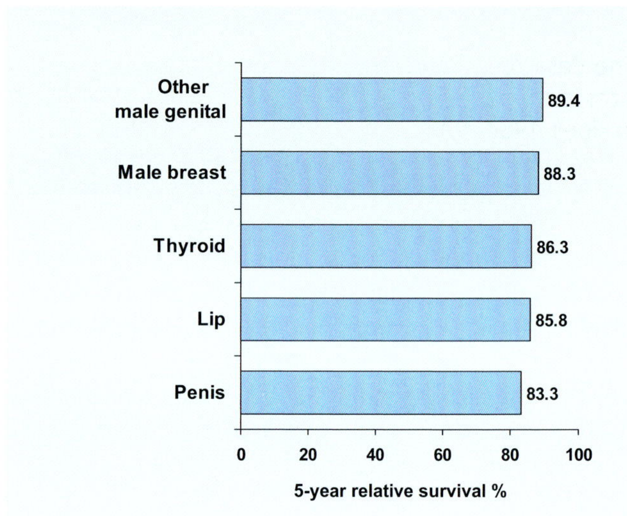

Female (Table 4a)

The 5-year relative survival is distinctly higher among females than males in cancers of the oral cavity, oropharynx, nasopharynx, nose/sinuses, ureter, brain and adrenal gland.

Figure 1c. Top five cancers (ranked by survival), Female, Shanghai, China, 1992–1995

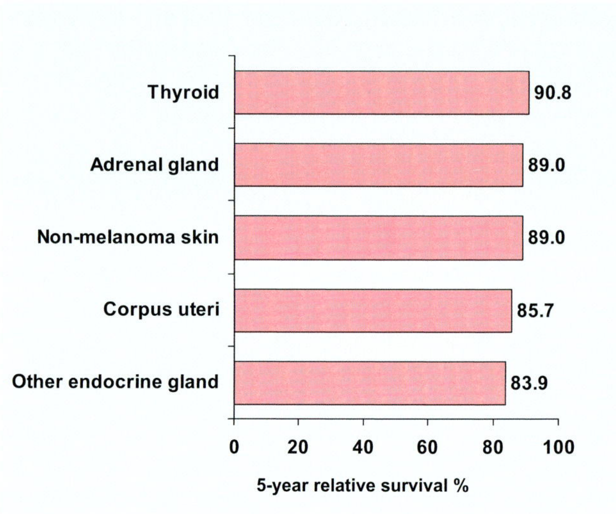

Age group (Table 4b)

The 5-year relative survival by age group reveals an inverse relationship: a decreasing survival with increasing age at diagnosis for many cancers such as tongue, salivary gland, nasopharynx, oesophagus, stomach, liver, pancreas, other thoracic organs, bone, uterus unspecified, ovary, bladder, thyroid and other endocrine glands. In the rest, it is observed to fluctuate.

Survival trend (Table 5)

The data on survival trend is available for 38 cancers sites or types spanning eight years in the two time periods 1988–1991 [2] and 1992–1995. An increasing trend in the 5-year absolute and relative survival probabilities is observed for most cancers registered in 1992–1995 compared to 1988–1991.

References

1. Parkin DM, Whelan SL, Ferlay J and Storm H. *Cancer Incidence in Five Continents, Vol. I to VIII: IARC Cancerbase No. 7*. IARCPress, Lyon, 2005.

2. Jin F, Xiang YB and Gao YT. Cancer survival in Shanghai, People's Republic of China. In: *Cancer Survival in Developing Countries* (eds) R Sankaranarayanan, RJ Black and DM Parkin. IARC Scientific Publications No. 145. IARCPress, Lyon, 1998, pp 37–50.

Table 1. Data quality indices - Proportion of histologically verified and death certificate only cases, number and proportion of included and excluded cases by site: Shanghai, China, 1992–1995 cases followed-up until 2000

Site	ICD-10	Total registered	%		Excluded cases					Included cases	
			HV	DCO	DCO	Follow-up	Others	Total	%	No.	%
Lip	C00	43	88.4	2.3	1	0	0	1	2.3	42	97.7
Tongue	C01-02	206	92.7	0.0	0	0	0	0	0.0	206	100.0
Oral cavity	C03-06	285	91.2	0.0	0	0	0	0	0.0	285	100.0
Salivary gland	C07-08	189	89.9	0.0	0	0	0	0	0.0	189	100.0
Tonsil	C09	59	89.8	0.0	0	0	0	0	0.0	59	100.0
Nasopharynx	C11	1 061	85.4	0.0	0	1	0	1	0.1	1 060	99.9
Hypopharynx	C12-13	37	94.6	0.0	0	0	0	0	0.0	37	100.0
Oesophagus	C15	2 990	47.5	0.1	2	0	0	2	0.1	2 988	99.9
Stomach	C16	11 741	59.7	0.0	2	4	0	6	0.1	11 735	99.9
Small intestine	C17	229	72.5	0.0	0	0	0	0	0.0	229	100.0
Colon	C18	4 785	70.2	0.0	1	2	0	3	0.1	4 782	99.9
Rectum	C19-20	3 285	74.9	0.0	0	1	0	1	0.0	3 284	100.0
Anus	C21	93	66.7	0.0	0	0	0	0	0.0	93	100.0
Liver	C22	6 959	13.9	0.0	3	2	0	5	0.1	6 954	99.9
Gall bladder	C23-24	1 383	41.9	0.0	0	0	0	0	0.0	1 383	100.0
Pancreas	C25	2 243	20.5	0.0	1	0	0	1	0.0	2 242	100.0
Nose/Sinuses	C30-31	200	79.5	0.0	0	0	0	0	0.0	200	100.0
Larynx	C32	625	86.2	0.2	1	0	0	1	0.2	624	99.8
Lung	C33-34	14 113	41.2	0.0	5	4	0	9	0.1	14 104	99.9
Other thoracic organs	C37-38	403	43.4	0.0	0	0	0	0	0.0	403	100.0
Bone	C40-41	523	40.9	0.0	0	0	0	0	0.0	523	100.0
Melanoma of skin	C43	110	86.4	0.0	0	0	0	0	0.0	110	100.0
Other skin	C44	473	88.8	0.0	0	1	0	1	0.2	472	99.8
Connective tissue	C47+C49	483	83.9	0.0	0	1	0	1	0.2	482	99.8
Breast	C50	5 184	86.3	0.0	0	0	0	0	0.0	5 184	100.0
Vulva	C51	54	85.2	0.0	0	0	0	0	0.0	54	100.0
Vagina	C52	45	91.1	0.0	0	0	0	0	0.0	45	100.0
Cervix	C53	548	85.4	0.0	0	0	0	0	0.0	548	100.0
Corpus uteri	C54	735	94.8	0.0	0	0	0	0	0.0	735	100.0
Uterus unspecified	C55	145	52.4	0.0	0	0	0	0	0.0	145	100.0
Ovary	C56	1 087	77.4	0.0	0	0	0	0	0.0	1 087	100.0
Other female genital org.	C57	35	94.3	0.0	0	0	0	0	0.0	35	100.0
Penis	C60	49	91.8	0.0	0	0	0	0	0.0	49	100.0
Prostate	C61	641	63.2	0.2	1	1	0	2	0.3	639	99.7
Testis	C62	113	85.8	0.0	0	0	0	0	0.0	113	100.0
Other male genital org.	C63	45	80.0	0.0	0	0	0	0	0.0	45	100.0
Kidney	C64	743	60.7	0.0	0	0	0	0	0.0	743	100.0
Renal pelvis	C65	67	79.1	0.0	0	0	0	0	0.0	67	100.0
Ureter	C66	68	82.4	0.0	0	0	0	0	0.0	68	100.0
Urinary bladder	C67	1 750	72.1	0.0	0	0	0	0	0.0	1 750	100.0
Other urinary organs	C68	26	65.4	0.0	0	0	0	0	0.0	26	100.0
Eye	C69	40	77.5	0.0	0	0	0	0	0.0	40	100.0
Brain & nervous system	C70-72	1 906	53.5	0.0	0	0	0	0	0.0	1 906	100.0
Thyroid	C73	868	88.0	0.0	0	0	0	0	0.0	868	100.0
Adrenal gland	C74	123	52.0	0.0	0	0	0	0	0.0	123	100.0
Other endocrine	C75	330	61.8	0.0	0	0	0	0	0.0	330	100.0
Hodgkin lymphoma	C81	99	80.8	0.0	0	0	0	0	0.0	99	100.0
Non-Hodgkin lymphoma	C82-85+C96	1 272	78.7	0.1	1	0	0	1	0.1	1 271	99.9

Table 1 (Continued).

Site	ICD-10	Total registered	%		Excluded cases					Included cases	
			HV	DCO	DCO	Follow-up	Others	Total	%	No.	%
Multiple myeloma	C90	233	70.0	0.9	2	1	0	3	1.3	230	98.7
Lymphoid leukaemia	C91	338	89.6	0.0	0	0	0	0	0.0	338	100.0
Myeloid leukaemia	C92-94	606	88.0	0.2	1	0	0	1	0.2	605	99.8
Leukaemia unspecified	C95	378	75.1	0.3	1	0	0	1	0.3	377	99.7

HV: histologically verified; DCO: death certificate only

Table 2. Number and proportion of cases with complete/incomplete follow-up (in years) and median follow-up (in months) by site: Shanghai, China, 1992–1995 cases followed-up until 2000

Site	ICD-10	Cases included	Complete FU Alive/dead at end of FU		Incomplete FU: lost to FU		% lost to FU: years from diagnosis				% with complete FU at 5 years	Median FU (in months)
			No.	%	No.	%	< 1	1-3	3-5	> 5		
Lip	C00	42	41	97.6	1	2.4	0.0	0.0	2.4	0.0	97.6	66.2
Tongue	C01-02	206	203	98.5	3	1.5	0.0	0.5	0.5	0.5	99.0	66.1
Oral cavity	C03-06	285	278	97.5	7	2.5	0.0	1.4	0.4	0.7	98.2	61.9
Salivary gland	C07-08	189	186	98.4	3	1.6	0.0	1.1	0.5	0.0	98.4	74.1
Tonsil	C09	59	56	94.9	3	5.1	3.4	1.7	0.0	0.0	94.9	47.8
Nasopharynx	C11	1 060	1 045	98.6	15	1.4	0.3	0.5	0.5	0.1	98.7	61.9
Hypopharynx	C12-13	37	37	100.0	0	0.0	0.0	0.0	0.0	0.0	100.0	11.8
Oesophagus	C15	2 988	2 980	99.7	8	0.3	0.1	0.1	0.1	0.0	99.8	6.8
Stomach	C16	11 735	11 656	99.3	79	0.7	0.2	0.2	0.2	0.1	99.4	9.3
Small intestine	C17	229	226	98.7	3	1.3	0.0	0.0	0.4	0.9	99.6	11.0
Colon	C18	4 782	4 734	99.0	48	1.0	0.1	0.3	0.4	0.2	99.2	31.4
Rectum	C19-20	3 284	3 249	98.9	35	1.1	0.1	0.3	0.4	0.3	99.2	32.5
Anus	C21	93	91	97.8	2	2.2	0.0	2.2	0.0	0.0	97.8	28.7
Liver	C22	6 954	6 942	99.8	12	0.2	0.1	0.1	0.0	0.0	99.8	3.0
Gall bladder	C23-24	1 383	1 378	99.6	5	0.4	0.2	0.1	0.1	0.0	99.6	3.8
Pancreas	C25	2 242	2 238	99.8	4	0.2	0.1	0.1	0.0	0.0	99.9	3.0
Nose/Sinuses	C30-31	200	195	97.5	5	2.5	0.5	0.5	1.0	0.5	98.0	31.4
Larynx	C32	624	621	99.5	3	0.5	0.0	0.2	0.1	0.2	99.7	56.5
Lung	C33-34	14 104	14 050	99.6	54	0.4	0.0	0.2	0.1	0.1	99.7	6.5
Other thoracic organs	C37-38	403	400	99.3	3	0.7	0.0	0.2	0.0	0.5	99.8	11.2
Bone	C40-41	523	520	99.4	3	0.6	0.0	0.2	0.2	0.2	99.6	8.2
Melanoma of skin	C43	110	109	99.1	1	0.9	0.9	0.0	0.0	0.0	99.1	40.9
Other skin	C44	472	459	97.2	13	2.8	0.0	1.3	1.5	0.0	97.2	74.1
Connective tissue	C47+C49	482	475	98.5	7	1.5	0.1	0.8	0.4	0.2	98.8	65.4
Breast	C50	5 184	5 094	98.3	90	1.7	0.3	0.6	0.5	0.3	98.6	73.5
Vulva	C51	54	54	100.0	0	0.0	0.0	0.0	0.0	0.0	100.0	49.8
Vagina	C52	45	44	97.8	1	2.2	0.0	2.2	0.0	0.0	97.8	29.1
Cervix	C53	548	541	98.7	7	1.3	0.2	0.3	0.4	0.4	99.1	62.1
Corpus uteri	C54	735	725	98.6	10	1.4	0.3	0.3	0.1	0.7	99.3	76.3
Uterus unspecified	C55	145	145	100.0	0	0.0	0.0	0.0	0.0	0.0	100.0	11.6
Ovary	C56	1 087	1 076	99.0	11	1.0	0.2	0.4	0.2	0.2	99.2	30.2
Other female genital org.	C57	35	34	97.1	1	2.9	2.9	0.0	0.0	0.0	97.1	56.1
Penis	C60	49	49	100.0	0	0.0	0.0	0.0	0.0	0.0	100.0	73.6
Prostate	C61	639	634	99.2	5	0.8	0.2	0.2	0.2	0.2	99.4	25.9
Testis	C62	113	112	99.1	1	0.9	0.0	0.9	0.0	0.0	99.1	78.4
Other male genital org.	C63	45	44	97.8	1	2.2	2.2	0.0	0.0	0.0	97.8	73.6
Kidney	C64	743	729	98.1	14	1.9	0.2	0.8	0.5	0.4	98.5	39.6
Renal pelvis	C65	67	67	100.0	0	0.0	0.0	0.0	0.0	0.0	100.0	61.4
Ureter	C66	68	66	97.1	2	2.9	0.0	0.0	2.9	0.0	97.1	47.3
Urinary bladder	C67	1 750	1 729	98.8	21	1.2	0.2	0.1	0.6	0.3	99.1	61.0
Other urinary organs	C68	26	26	100.0	0	0.0	0.0	0.0	0.0	0.0	100.0	31.6
Eye	C69	40	39	97.5	1	2.5	0.0	0.0	2.5	0.0	97.5	66.7
Brain & nervous system	C70-72	1 906	1 886	99.0	20	1.0	0.0	0.3	0.5	0.2	99.2	14.4
Thyroid	C73	868	841	96.9	27	3.1	0.3	1.1	1.2	0.5	97.4	77.9
Adrenal gland	C74	123	118	95.9	5	4.1	0.1	0.8	2.4	0.8	96.7	81.1
Other endocrine	C75	330	320	97.0	10	3.0	0.3	0.9	1.2	0.6	97.6	75.0

Table 2 (Continued).

Site	ICD-10	Cases included	Complete FU Alive/dead at end of FU		Incomplete FU: lost to FU		% lost to FU: years from diagnosis				% with complete FU at 5 years	Median FU (in months)
			No.	%	No.	%	< 1	1-3	3-5	> 5		
Hodgkin lymphoma	C81	99	97	98.0	2	2.0	1.0	0.0	0.0	1.0	99.0	65.5
Non-Hodgkin lymphoma	C82-85+C96	1 271	1 258	99.0	13	1.0	0.2	0.6	0.1	0.1	99.1	15.4
Multiple myeloma	C90	230	229	99.6	1	0.4	0.0	0.0	0.4	0.0	99.6	11.1
Lymphoid leukaemia	C91	338	338	100.0	0	0.0	0.0	0.0	0.0	0.0	100.0	13.9
Myeloid leukaemia	C92-94	605	601	99.3	4	0.7	0.0	0.2	0.3	0.2	99.5	12.4
Leukaemia unspecified	C95	377	377	100.0	0	0.0	0.0	0.0	0.0	0.0	100.0	3.6

FU: follow-up

Table 3. Comparison of 1-, 3- and 5-year absolute and relative survival and 5-year age-standardized relative survival by site: Shanghai, China, 1992–1995 cases followed-up until 2000

Site	ICD-10	Cases included	% Absolute survival			% Relative survival			% ASRS at 5-years	
			1-year	3-year	5-year	1-year	3-year	5-year	all ages	0-74 years
Lip	C00	42	83.3	71.4	59.5	86.8	80.9	73.9	78.8	84.1
Tongue	C01-02	206	72.3	59.7	54.8	74.3	64.0	61.5	64.1	66.9
Oral cavity	C03-06	285	75.1	60.6	53.4	77.7	67.0	63.4	68.5	70.9
Salivary gland	C07-08	189	87.8	74.0	65.9	89.7	78.7	73.4	71.0	73.7
Oropharynx	C09-10	59	72.4	56.2	52.6	74.6	60.9	60.4	61.0	62.1
Nasopharynx	C11	1 060	78.9	60.8	51.9	80.2	63.5	56.0	52.9	57.6
Hypopharynx	C12-13	37	51.4	29.7	24.3	53.4	33.2	29.7	31.2	31.0
Oesophagus	C15	2 988	34.7	15.9	13.1	36.3	17.9	16.0	18.0	20.6
Stomach	C16	11 735	45.8	28.7	24.8	47.6	31.7	29.3	30.4	36.0
Small intestine	C17	229	48.0	28.4	24.0	49.5	30.8	27.6	27.9	32.1
Colon	C18	4 782	66.3	48.6	43.0	68.4	53.4	50.6	48.2	54.0
Rectum	C19-20	3 284	70.5	48.6	40.8	72.7	53.2	47.7	44.1	51.0
Anus	C21	93	69.9	48.1	39.1	72.5	53.9	47.5	45.8	49.9
Liver	C22	6 954	18.4	8.9	7.5	19.0	9.6	8.6	8.9	9.8
Gall bladder	C23-24	1 383	24.1	14.4	12.7	25.0	16.0	15.2	19.2	21.0
Pancreas	C25	2 242	16.2	7.3	6.5	16.9	8.1	7.8	8.5	9.5
Nose/Sinuses	C30-31	200	67.9	48.7	43.6	69.9	52.7	49.8	48.5	52.4
Larynx	C32	624	74.8	56.7	49.9	77.8	63.5	60.6	61.7	67.2
Lung	C33-34	14 104	34.1	15.1	12.4	35.4	16.9	15.0	15.6	18.0
Other thoracic organs	C37-38	403	48.6	35.4	32.4	49.9	37.8	36.0	33.2	41.4
Bone	C40-41	523	42.8	29.6	27.3	44.2	31.6	30.1	27.8	34.0
Melanoma of skin	C43	110	74.4	55.1	44.1	77.0	60.5	51.5	55.4	61.7
Other skin	C44	472	84.5	74.5	69.5	88.0	84.2	85.8	86.0	85.9
Connective tissue	C47+C49	482	73.0	61.6	56.7	74.5	65.2	62.4	58.3	62.9
Breast	C50	5 184	90.8	79.2	73.1	92.0	82.6	78.7	77.8	79.4
Vulva	C51	54	68.5	51.9	48.1	71.2	57.5	57.7	55.9	56.5
Vagina	C52	45	71.1	48.8	41.8	73.0	52.9	47.9	42.8	49.5
Cervix	C53	548	77.0	57.8	52.4	79.0	62.5	60.1	61.6	63.5
Corpus uteri	C54	735	90.3	82.8	79.7	91.6	86.3	85.7	82.3	86.9
Uterus unspecified	C55	145	49.0	31.0	29.7	50.6	33.4	32.7	37.6	49.5
Ovary	C56	1 087	66.4	48.4	42.7	67.3	50.3	45.6	43.5	47.9
Other female genital org.	C57	35	91.3	67.7	47.1	92.9	71.2	51.6	55.6	50.1
Penis	C60	49	87.8	73.5	67.3	91.7	83.5	83.3	84.2	90.7
Prostate	C61	639	68.8	44.0	36.9	73.1	53.0	50.8	48.8	54.2
Testis	C62	113	82.3	77.0	74.3	83.2	79.0	77.5	80.1	81.7
Other male genital org.	C63	45	79.8	68.4	66.1	84.4	81.3	89.4	91.4	94.8
Kidney	C64	743	63.1	51.5	46.5	65.0	55.8	53.3	51.2	60.3
Renal pelvis	C65	67	74.6	55.2	50.7	77.2	61.6	61.6	70.7	71.2
Ureter	C66	68	85.3	54.4	48.4	87.8	59.3	56.1	65.6	73.0
Urinary bladder	C67	1 750	71.9	56.8	51.1	75.4	65.0	64.3	62.9	74.5
Other urinary organs	C68	26	84.6	46.2	42.3	88.9	53.0	54.0	62.1	64.3
Eye	C69	40	90.0	77.5	69.8	91.6	81.4	75.8	78.6	79.1
Brain & nervous system	C70-72	1 906	54.2	42.4	39.8	55.3	44.3	42.8	48.8	51.1
Thyroid	C73	868	90.5	87.2	85.6	91.5	89.6	89.8	89.7	91.2
Adrenal gland	C74	123	80.5	78.0	73.9	81.5	80.4	77.7	71.3	69.5
Other endocrine	C75	330	85.7	80.9	77.4	86.6	83.1	81.2	70.8	78.0
Hodgkin lymphoma	C81	99	80.7	67.4	62.3	81.8	69.9	66.0	75.1	77.6

Table 3 (Continued).

Site	ICD-10	Cases included	% Absolute survival			% Relative survival			% ASRS at 5-years	
			1-year	3-year	5-year	1-year	3-year	5-year	all ages	0-74 years
Non-Hodgkin lymphoma	C82-85+C96	1 271	56.3	39.2	35.1	57.7	41.9	39.2	43.3	45.6
Multiple myeloma	C90	230	49.1	28.3	19.5	50.6	30.6	22.3	25.1	28.1
Lymphoid leukaemia	C91	338	52.7	32.2	27.8	53.5	33.8	30.2	28.8	30.4
Myeloid leukaemia	C92-94	605	51.7	31.4	25.4	52.6	32.7	27.1	27.2	30.0
Leukaemia unspecified	C95	377	26.3	14.6	11.1	26.9	15.5	12.3	13.3	14.6

ASRS: age-standardized relative survival

Table 4a. Site-wise number of cases, 5-year absolute and relative survival by sex: Shanghai, China, 1992–1995 cases followed-up until 2000

Site	ICD-10	Cases included	Male % 5-year survival			Female % 5-year survival		
			No.	Abs	Rel	No.	Abs	Rel
Lip	C00	42	26	65.4	85.8	16	50.0	55.4
Tongue	C01-02	206	109	54.8	61.5	97	52.2	59.7
Oral cavity	C03-06	285	165	46.4	57.4	120	63.1	71.5
Salivary gland	C07-08	189	108	60.9	69.9	81	72.6	77.9
Tonsil	C09	59	38	42.6	51.1	21	70.6	76.7
Nasopharynx	C11	1 060	771	48.1	52.4	289	61.9	65.2
Hypopharynx	C12-13	37	28	25.0	31.4	9	22.2	24.8
Oesophagus	C15	2 988	2 001	13.2	16.6	987	12.8	15.0
Stomach	C16	11 735	7 670	25.2	30.6	4 065	24.1	27.1
Small intestine	C17	229	142	26.1	30.2	87	20.6	23.3
Colon	C18	4 782	2 404	41.5	50.6	2 378	44.5	50.6
Rectum	C19-20	3 284	1 838	40.1	48.4	1 446	41.6	46.8
Anus	C21	93	42	37.5	46.9	51	40.5	48.1
Liver	C22	6 954	4 952	7.9	9.1	2 002	6.4	7.3
Gall bladder	C23-24	1 383	510	12.5	15.7	873	12.8	14.9
Pancreas	C25	2 242	1 213	6.7	8.4	1 029	6.2	7.1
Nose/Sinuses	C30-31	200	128	40.1	46.4	72	49.6	55.8
Larynx	C32	624	555	50.1	61.2	69	48.8	56.1
Lung	C33-34	14 104	10 178	12.6	15.6	3 926	11.9	13.7
Other thoracic organs	C37-38	403	266	30.4	34.2	137	36.5	39.5
Bone	C40-41	523	268	27.9	31.1	255	26.7	29.0
Melanoma of skin	C43	110	52	46.2	54.9	58	42.2	48.4
Other skin	C44	472	257	66.3	83.0	215	73.3	89.0
Connective tissue	C47+C49	482	275	57.3	63.9	207	55.8	60.3
Breast	C50	5 184	58	72.1	88.3	5 126	73.1	78.6
Vulva	C51	54				54	48.1	57.7
Vagina	C52	45				45	41.8	47.9
Cervix	C53	548				548	52.4	60.1
Corpus uteri	C54	735				735	79.7	85.7
Uterus unspecified	C55	145				145	29.7	32.7
Ovary	C56	1 087				1 087	42.7	45.6
Other female genital org.	C57	35				35	47.1	51.6
Penis	C60	49	49	67.3	83.3			
Prostate	C61	639	639	36.9	50.8			
Testis	C62	113	113	74.3	77.5			
Other male genital org.	C63	45	45	66.1	89.4			
Kidney	C64	743	485	47.4	55.6	258	44.9	49.1
Renal pelvis	C65	67	42	54.8	70.2	25	44.0	48.2
Ureter	C66	68	48	43.7	51.8	20	60.0	66.1
Urinary bladder	C67	1 750	1 359	53.4	68.1	391	43.2	51.3
Other urinary organs	C68	26	19	57.9	73.9	7	0.0	0.0
Eye	C69	40	28	67.9	74.1	12	74.1	79.3
Brain & nervous system	C70-72	1 906	958	34.8	37.9	948	45.0	47.7
Thyroid	C73	868	192	78.9	86.3	676	87.5	90.8
Adrenal gland	C74	123	55	57.9	63.5	68	86.7	89.0
Other endocrine	C75	330	131	71.5	77.1	199	81.3	83.9

Table 4a (Continued).

Site	ICD-10	Cases included	Male % 5-year survival			Female % 5-year survival		
			No.	Abs	Rel	No.	Abs	Rel
Hodgkin lymphoma	C81	99	54	59.3	62.9	45	66.0	69.7
Non-Hodgkin lymphoma	C82-85+C96	1 271	758	32.2	36.7	513	39.4	42.8
Multiple myeloma	C90	230	136	19.8	23.1	94	19.1	21.2
Lymphoid leukaemia	C91	338	210	31.0	34.0	128	22.7	24.2
Myeloid leukaemia	C92-94	605	348	25.1	27.4	257	25.7	26.7
Leukaemia unspecified	C95	377	200	11.5	13.1	177	10.7	11.4

Abs: absolute survival; Rel: relative survival

Table 4b. Site-wise number of cases and relative survival by age group: Shanghai, China, 1992–1995 cases followed-up until 2000

Site	ICD-10	Cases included	Number of cases by age group					Relative survival by age group % 5-year survival				
			< 45	45-54	55-64	65-74	> 75	< 45	45-54	55-64	65-74	> 75
Lip	C00	42	5	4	7	12	14	81.0	77.6	92.8	82.2	48.5
Tongue	C01-02	206	37	28	49	62	30	82.1	80.7	59.8	48.9	46.6
Oral cavity	C03-06	285	30	19	71	101	64	77.4	81.7	63.9	62.5	50.7
Salivary gland	C07-08	189	50	31	39	49	20	92.9	76.4	69.1	58.9	55.6
Tonsil	C09	59	8	11	15	14	11	100.9	44.2	64.4	47.8	61.3
Nasopharynx	C11	1 060	331	209	277	189	54	64.1	60.0	55.4	41.6	40.1
Hypopharynx	C12-13	37	3	2	7	16	9	0.0	52.1	31.7	30.0	35.4
Oesophagus	C15	2 988	71	108	649	1 282	878	25.7	23.7	20.1	16.4	10.7
Stomach	C16	11 735	1 126	869	2 568	4 306	2 866	44.7	43.1	35.1	26.4	17.3
Small intestine	C17	229	28	25	58	80	38	35.9	45.7	26.8	24.4	16.8
Colon	C18	4 782	463	376	1 245	1 709	989	55.6	58.3	54.0	51.3	39.8
Rectum	C19-20	3 284	396	324	835	1 105	624	50.2	54.5	50.9	49.8	33.8
Anus	C21	93	6	9	22	32	24	50.7	45.9	60.3	44.2	39.5
Liver	C22	6 954	984	808	1 804	2 106	1 252	12.2	10.0	9.0	8.0	5.1
Gall bladder	C23-24	1 383	61	74	290	593	365	38.1	21.0	15.6	12.3	14.9
Pancreas	C25	2 242	95	147	500	892	608	17.1	9.3	7.8	7.3	6.9
Nose/Sinuses	C30-31	200	41	14	50	60	35	46.4	51.4	65.3	45.7	38.8
Larynx	C32	624	23	42	166	273	120	57.4	74.4	72.7	59.2	41.8
Lung	C33-34	14 104	534	756	3 341	6 073	3 400	19.7	21.7	19.4	13.9	10.2
Other thoracic organs	C37-38	403	100	39	78	125	61	52.6	49.7	42.0	25.7	10.4
Bone	C40-41	523	134	40	79	156	114	59.5	38.6	27.1	16.3	10.8
Melanoma of skin	C43	110	13	8	26	35	28	54.6	77.1	71.5	44.3	29.9
Other skin	C44	472	48	35	105	147	137	88.5	85.5	85.4	84.8	87.6
Connective tissue	C47+C49	482	165	60	102	100	55	71.1	75.5	61.5	48.4	45.8
Breast	C50	5 184	1 519	1 124	1 163	936	442	78.9	81.7	78.1	79.1	72.2
Vulva	C51	54	3	1	9	20	21	101.0	0.0	71.0	65.6	40.4
Vagina	C52	45	4	3	8	19	11	75.6	0.0	53.3	60.4	24.4
Cervix	C53	548	63	34	130	214	107	70.4	57.2	62.1	62.3	47.8
Corpus uteri	C54	735	99	172	257	167	40	91.8	95.4	83.4	80.2	65.0
Uterus unspecified	C55	145	23	12	29	30	51	87.9	77.0	32.9	15.4	2.9
Ovary	C56	1 087	308	192	256	236	95	59.4	47.4	42.2	38.5	22.1
Other female genital org.	C57	35	1	8	15	7	4		51.2	49.5	49.4	68.0
Penis	C60	49	8	4	10	12	15	88.9	104.0	67.1	106.8	64.9
Prostate	C61	639	2	4	91	268	274	50.9	52.3	54.3	54.5	46.2
Testis	C62	113	70	17	11	10	5	82.4	78.8	79.2	76.1	0.0
Other male genital org.	C63	45	2	0	12	11	20	100.9	0.0	92.6	92.8	85.0
Kidney	C64	743	101	90	200	235	117	63.0	69.9	66.2	45.2	22.5
Renal pelvis	C65	67	3	5	19	28	12	101.6	82.7	51.6	57.7	72.2
Ureter	C66	68	2	5	31	23	7	101.0	103.0	57.0	44.0	45.7
Urinary bladder	C67	1 750	84	92	350	656	568	83.3	80.0	74.1	69.8	44.9
Other urinary organs	C68	26	1	6	4	6	9	102.0	34.9	55.2	61.6	61.9
Eye	C69	40	16	8	8	4	4	56.9	90.3	107.4	61.7	79.9
Brain & nervous system	C70-72	1 906	551	256	453	463	183	56.2	59.2	43.9	26.2	16.2
Thyroid	C73	868	421	154	129	122	42	98.1	97.9	85.8	71.7	39.0
Adrenal gland	C74	123	64	13	22	18	6	88.2	95.0	73.4	31.6	82.7
Other endocrine	C75	330	176	48	57	38	11	86.5	85.7	74.1	69.6	51.8
Hodgkin lymphoma	C81	99	46	7	24	19	3	85.3	88.1	55.1	24.6	53.4

Table 4b (Continued).

Site	ICD-10	Cases included	Number of cases by age group					Relative survival by age group % 5-year survival				
			< 45	45-54	55-64	65-74	> 75	< 45	45-54	55-64	65-74	> 75
Non-Hodgkin lymphoma	C82-85+C96	1 271	303	143	295	350	180	50.1	53.9	38.6	31.5	23.2
Multiple myeloma	C90	230	13	30	63	89	35	39.0	38.0	25.9	16.3	8.6
Lymphoid leukaemia	C91	338	173	29	54	60	22	28.5	28.4	32.6	38.2	20.9
Myeloid leukaemia	C92-94	605	248	74	121	118	44	35.4	36.3	20.9	13.5	14.9
Leukaemia unspecified	C95	377	122	34	65	93	63	17.4	12.1	13.4	8.0	7.7

Table 5. Comparison of 5-year absolute and relative survival of cases diagnosed between 1988–1991 and 1992–1995, Shanghai, China

Site	ICD-10	% 5-year absolute survival		% 5-year relative survival	
		1988–1991	1992–1995	1988–1991	1992–1995
Lip	C00	73.1	59.5	86.0	73.9
Tongue	C01-02	41.8	54.8	47.5	61.5
Oral cavity	C03-06	45.0	53.4	52.1	63.4
Salivary gland	C07-08	56.3	65.9	64.1	73.4
Oropharynx	C09-10	46.8	52.6	55.3	60.4
Nasopharynx	C11	50.0	51.9	53.3	56.0
Hypopharynx	C12-13	18.5	24.3	22.3	29.7
Oesophagus	C15	9.0	13.1	11.2	16.0
Stomach	C16	20.1	24.8	23.9	29.3
Small intestine	C17	27.7	24.0	31.4	27.6
Colon	C18	37.7	43.0	43.5	50.6
Rectum	C19-20	37.1	40.8	42.8	47.7
Liver	C22	3.9	7.5	4.4	8.6
Gall bladder	C23-24	8.0	12.7	9.5	15.2
Pancreas	C25	5.2	6.5	6.1	7.8
Larynx	C32	43.7	49.9	52.1	60.6
Lung	C33-34	9.9	12.4	11.9	15.0
Bone	C40-41	17.0	27.3	19.4	30.1
Melanoma of skin	C43	39.1	44.1	45.3	51.5
Other skin	C44	59.4	69.5	72.7	85.8
Connective tissue	C47+C49	56.3	56.7	61.0	62.4
Breast	C50	67.5	73.1	72.0	78.7
Vulva	C51	41.6	45.1	47.1	53.0
Cervix	C53	45.0	52.4	51.9	60.1
Corpus uteri	C54	72.3	79.7	76.8	85.7
Ovary	C56	41.5	42.7	44.2	45.6
Penis	C60	55.8	67.3	67.9	83.3
Prostate	C61	29.6	36.9	40.1	50.8
Testis	C62	62.4	74.3	65.8	77.5
Kidney	C64	42.2	46.5	47.7	53.3
Urinary bladder	C67	49.2	51.1	60.9	64.3
Brain & nervous system	C70-72	32.3	39.8	34.8	42.8
Thyroid	C73	75.8	85.6	79.7	89.8
Hodgkin lymphoma	C81	45.6	62.3	48.8	66.0
Non-Hodgkin lymphoma	C82-85+C96	29.8	35.1	33.4	39.2
Multiple myeloma	C90	20.7	19.5	23.3	22.3
Lymphoid leukaemia	C91	17.9	27.8	19.2	30.2
Myeloid leukaemia	C92-94	16.0	25.4	17.1	27.1

Chapter 8

Cancer survival in Tianjin, China, 1991–1999

Xishan H, Chen K, Min H, Shufen D and Jifang W

Abstract

The Tianjin cancer registry was established in 1978, and registration of cases is done by the active method. The registry contributed data on 51 cancer sites or types registered during 1991–1999 for this survival study. Follow-up has been a mixture of both active and passive methods, with median follow-up ranging from 5–77 months. The proportion with histologically verified diagnosis for various cancers ranged from 21–95% and 97–100% of total registered cases were included for survival analysis. The top-ranking cancers by 5-year age-standardized relative survival (%) were renal pelvis (101%), lip (99%), corpus uteri (91%), penis and non-melanoma skin (90%) and thyroid (89%). The corresponding survival for common cancers were lung (31%), stomach (41%), liver (25%) and breast (82%). The 5-year relative survival by age group reveals an inverse relationship for a few cancers and fluctuated for most cancers. Period survival closely predicted the survival experience of cancer cases diagnosed in that period, with the 5-year relative survival in 1991–1995 by period approach being more or less similar to survival by cohort approach in 1996–1999 for most cancers.

Tianjin cancer registry

The Tianjin cancer registry was established in 1978 at the Tianjin Cancer Institute and Hospital, Tianjin, and is partly funded by the Tianjin Health Bureau. The registry has been contributing data to the quinquennial IARC publication *Cancer Incidence in Five Continents* since Vol V [1]. Cancer is a notifiable disease, but registration of cases is done by active methods. The principal source of information is the report form filled by all physicians and medical clerks in the registry area for each new case diagnosed as malignant tumour. An active re-checking is done by the registry to review all patient records at every medical unit within the registry area to ensure completeness. The registry covers an area of 12 000 km^2 and caters to an entirely urban population of about 4 million with a sex ratio of 1010 females to 1000 males in 2000. The average annual age-standardized incidence rate is 200 per 100 000 among males and 152 per 100 000 among females with a lifetime cumulative risk of one in 5 of developing cancer in the period 1993–1997. The most common cancers among males are lung, stomach, liver and oesophagus. The rank order among females is lung, breast, stomach and liver [1].

The registry contributed data on survival from 51 cancer sites or types registered during 1991–1999 for the first time in this volume of the IARC publication on *Cancer survival in Africa, Asia, the Caribbean and Central America*. In the present volume, data on survival from 1981–1990 are also utilized to elicit the trend in cancer survival.

Data quality indices (Table 1)

The proportion of cases having a histologically verified cancer diagnosis in the series is 55%, varying from 21% (liver cancer) to 95% (myeloid leukaemia). The proportion of cases registered based on a death certificate only (DCO) and cases excluded from the study without any follow-up information or due to other reasons is negligible. For cancers of the brain and central nervous system and other endocrine glands, the exclusions comprise benign or uncertain malignant cases. Thus, in the rest of cancers, 97–100% of the total cases registered are included in the estimation of the survival probability.

Outcome of follow-up (Table 2)

Follow-up has been a mixture of both active and passive methods. These included obtaining cancer mortality information from the death certificates registered in local police station. The mortality data are periodically matched with the incident cancer database. The vital status of the unmatched incident cases is then collected by postal/telephone and house visit enquiries.

The closing date of follow-up was 31st December 2000. The median follow-up ranged from 5 months for cancer of the liver to 77 months for cancer of the placenta. The completeness of follow-up at 5 years from the incidence date is 100%, as there are no losses to follow-up.

Survival statistics

All ages and both sexes together (Table 3)

The top ranking cancers on 5-year relative survival are other endocrine gland (101%), lip (98%), penis (97%), renal pelvis (96%) and placenta (94%). The lowest survival rate is encountered with unspecified leukaemia and uterus (22%) preceded by liver (25%), bone (28%) and pancreas (30%). Salivary gland (89%) and tonsil (87%) among other head and neck cancers and anus (82%) among gastrointestinal cancers, have higher survival than others. Hodgkin lymphoma had a better survival (81%) than non-Hodgkin lymphoma (48%). The survival figures for haematopoietic malignancies are multiple myeloma (46%), lymphoid leukaemia (66%) and myeloid leukaemia (68%).

Figure 1a. Top ten cancers (ranked by survival), Tianjin, China, 1991–1999

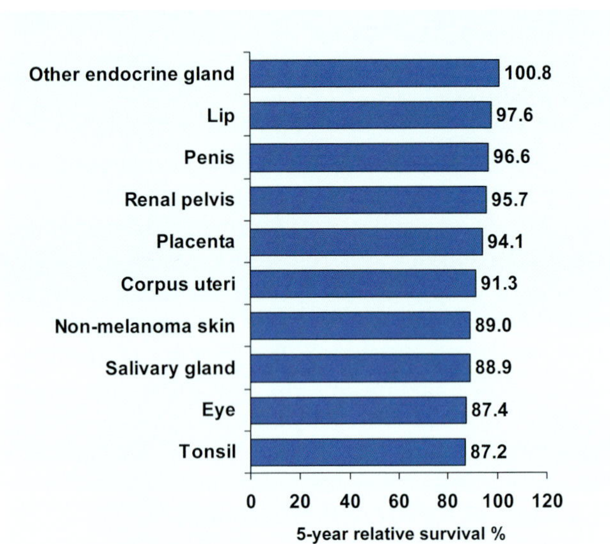

The 5-year age-standardized relative survival (ASRS) probability for all ages together is observed to be greater than or similar to the corresponding unadjusted one for a majority of cancers. Also, the 5-year ASRS (0–74 years of age) is generally higher than or similar to the corresponding ASRS (all ages) for a majority of cancers.

Sex

Male (Table 4a)

The top ranking cancers on 5-year relative survival are renal pelvis (107%), other endocrine gland (100%), lip (99%), penis (97%) and breast (91%). Survival from prostate and testicular cancers are 72% and 69%, respectively. A notably higher survival for cancers of the larynx, kidney, renal pelvis, ureter and bladder is seen among males than females.

Female (Table 4b)

Figure 1b. Top five cancers (ranked by survival), Male, Tianjin, China, 1991–1999

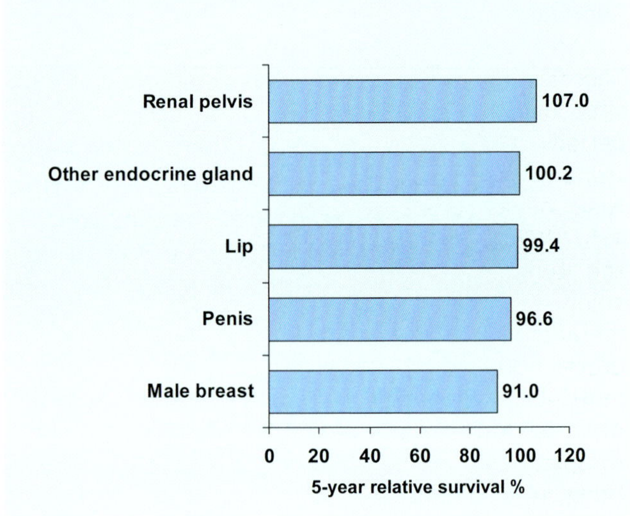

The highest 5-year relative survival is observed in cancer of the hypopharynx followed by other endocrine gland, anus, placenta, lip and non-melanoma skin cancers. Survival from cancers of the breast, cervix, corpus uteri and ovary are 85%, 62%, 91% and 64%, respectively. Survival is distinctly higher among females than males in cancers of tongue, hypopharynx, anus, mesothelioma and multiple myeloma.

Figure 1c. Top five cancers (ranked by survival), Female, Tianjin, China, 1991–1999

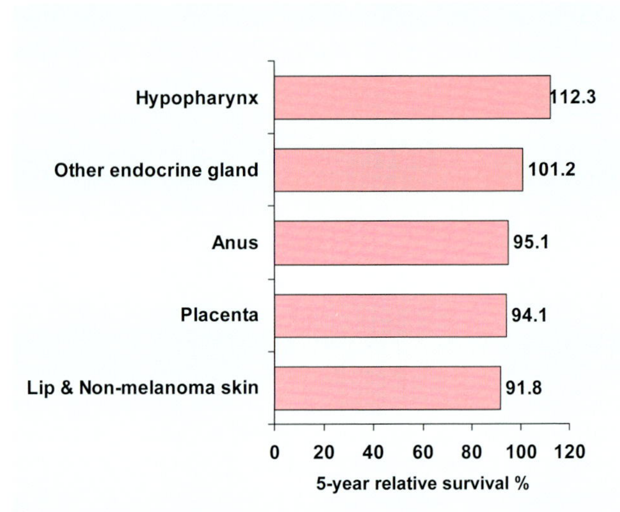

Age group (Table 4c)

The 5-year relative survival by age group reveals an inverse relationship: a decreasing survival with increasing age at diagnosis for many cancers like nasopharynx, lung, bone, breast, uterus (unspecified), thyroid, adrenal gland and non-Hodgkin lymphoma. In the rest, it is observed to fluctuate.

Survival trend (Table 5)

The data on survival trend is available for all cancer sites or types spanning 19 years in the two time periods 1981–1990 and 1991–1999. An increasing trend in the 5-year relative survival estimates to the tune of an absolute difference of 10% between 1981–1990 and 1991–1999 is observed in cancers of the tongue, salivary gland, tonsil, hypopharynx, colon, rectum, anus, gallbladder, nose/sinuses, non-melanoma skin, mesothelioma, penis, prostate, ureter, urinary bladder, eye, Hodgkin lymphoma, multiple myeloma and myeloid leukaemia. A decreasing survival is noted for cancers of the uterus (unspecified), testis, vulva, lip, oral cavity and non-Hodgkin lymphoma.

Trend of survival estimated by period and cohort approaches (Table 6)

The availability of data on registration and follow-up together for both a long and more recent period of calendar time led to the possibility of estimating up-to-date survival and trend by period approach. Survival is also estimated by cohort approach for comparison.

The 5-year relative survival estimates for the calendar period 1991–1995 by period approach seem to be approximately similar to the survival estimates obtained by cohort approach for the period 1996–1999 for most cancers. Thus, period survival closely predicts the survival experience of most cancer cases diagnosed in that period. However, this seems to vary for the earlier calendar periods, indicating some limitation in the ascertainment of follow-up in those periods, especially mortality.

References

1. Parkin DM, Whelan SL, Ferlay J and Storm H. *Cancer Incidence in Five Continents, Vol I to VIII: IARC Cancerbase No. 7*. IARCPress, Lyon, 2005.

Table 2. Number and proportion of cases by vital status and median follow-up (in months) by site: Tianjin, China, 1991–1999 cases followed-up until 2000

Site	ICD-10	Cases included	Dead		Alive		Complete FU		Median FU (in months)
			No.	%	No.	%	No.	%	
Lip	C00	53	9	17.0	44	83.0	53	100.0	49.6
Tongue	C01-02	187	80	42.8	107	57.2	187	100.0	34.4
Oral cavity	C03-06	253	111	43.9	142	56.1	253	100.0	32.4
Salivary gland	C07-08	141	28	19.9	113	80.1	141	100.0	50.6
Tonsil	C09	25	6	24.0	19	76.0	25	100.0	45.6
Nasopharynx	C11	421	198	47.0	223	53.0	421	100.0	34.4
Hypopharynx	C12-13	47	17	36.2	30	63.8	47	100.0	31.4
Oesophagus	C15	3 208	2 316	72.2	892	27.8	3 208	100.0	10.1
Stomach	C16	7 516	4 829	64.2	2 687	35.8	7 516	100.0	13.1
Small intestine	C17	181	83	45.9	98	54.1	181	100.0	25.3
Colon	C18	2 655	1 205	45.4	1 450	54.6	2 655	100.0	26.2
Rectum	C19-20	2 501	1 195	47.8	1 306	52.2	2 501	100.0	26.3
Anus	C21	46	15	32.6	31	67.4	46	100.0	28.9
Liver	C22	6 525	5 057	77.5	1 468	22.5	6 525	100.0	5.0
Gall bladder	C23-24	1 042	620	59.5	422	40.5	1 042	100.0	12.1
Pancreas	C25	1 990	1 468	73.8	522	26.2	1 990	100.0	6.9
Nose/Sinuses	C30-31	167	68	40.7	99	59.3	167	100.0	30.4
Larynx	C32	1 039	454	43.7	585	56.3	1 039	100.0	31.4
Lung	C33-34	21 403	15 546	72.6	5 857	27.4	21 403	100.0	9.0
Other thoracic organs	C37-38	244	129	52.9	115	47.1	244	100.0	18.7
Bone	C40-41	686	505	73.6	181	26.4	686	100.0	9.6
Melanoma of skin	C43	119	53	44.5	66	55.5	119	100.0	30.4
Other skin	C44	350	92	26.3	258	73.7	350	100.0	49.6
Mesothelioma	C45	84	42	50.0	42	50.0	84	100.0	20.3
Connective tissue	C47+C49	425	115	27.1	310	72.9	425	100.0	44.6
Breast	C50	5 863	1 106	18.9	4 757	81.1	5 863	100.0	48.6
Vulva	C51	57	20	35.1	37	64.9	57	100.0	33.4
Cervix	C53	567	258	45.5	309	54.5	567	100.0	37.4
Corpus uteri	C54	722	98	13.6	624	86.4	722	100.0	50.6
Uterus unspecified	C55	287	225	78.4	62	21.6	287	100.0	13.1
Ovary	C56	1 124	428	38.1	696	61.9	1 124	100.0	29.3
Other female genital org.	C57	52	19	36.5	33	63.5	52	100.0	44.1
Placenta	C58	62	4	6.5	58	93.5	62	100.0	77.1
Penis	C60	65	16	24.6	49	75.4	65	100.0	46.6
Prostate	C61	423	191	45.2	232	54.8	423	100.0	29.3
Testis	C62	73	23	31.5	50	68.5	73	100.0	38.4
Kidney	C64	1 094	491	44.9	603	55.1	1 094	100.0	26.3
Renal pelvis	C65	146	28	19.2	118	80.8	146	100.0	47.6
Ureter	C66	63	19	30.2	44	69.8	63	100.0	27.3
Urinary bladder	C67	2 020	794	39.3	1 226	60.7	2 020	100.0	33.9
Eye	C69	35	7	20.0	28	80.0	35	100.0	56.7
Brain & nervous system	C70-72	1 944	1 149	59.1	795	40.9	1 944	100.0	14.1
Thyroid	C73	618	124	20.1	494	79.9	618	100.0	45.6
Adrenal gland	C74	53	16	30.2	37	69.8	53	100.0	52.6
Other endocrine	C75	121	4	3.3	117	96.7	121	100.0	74.0
Hodgkin lymphoma	C81	123	25	20.3	98	79.7	123	100.0	55.7
Non-Hodgkin lymphoma	C82-85+C96	1 481	817	55.2	664	44.8	1 481	100.0	17.2

Table 2 (Continued).

Site	ICD-10	Cases included	Dead		Alive		Complete FU		Median FU (in months)
			No.	%	No.	%	No.	%	
Multiple myeloma	C90	217	119	54.8	98	45.2	217	100.0	17.2
Lymphoid leukaemia	C91	309	116	37.5	193	62.5	309	100.0	45.6
Myeloid leukaemia	C92-94	567	207	36.5	360	63.5	567	100.0	40.5
Leukaemia unspecified	C95	611	487	79.7	124	20.3	611	100.0	7.0

FU: follow-up

Table 3. Comparison of 1-, 3- and 5-year absolute and relative survival and 5-year age-standardized relative survival by site: Tianjin, China, 1991–1999 cases followed-up until 2000

Site	ICD-10	Cases included	% Absolute survival			% Relative survival			% ASRS at 5-years	
			1-year	3-year	5-year	1-year	3-year	5-year	all ages	0-74 years
Lip	C00	53	92.5	86.4	80.3	96.0	97.2	97.6	99.3	99.3
Tongue	C01-02	187	71.1	59.2	59.2	72.9	63.9	67.8	68.3	68.2
Oral cavity	C03-06	253	71.5	59.8	55.6	73.7	65.4	64.6	68.4	69.2
Salivary gland	C07-08	141	88.7	79.7	78.7	90.7	85.4	88.9	87.2	88.3
Tonsil	C09	25	88.0	79.0	72.7	90.4	87.1	87.2	75.6	68.3
Nasopharynx	C11	421	75.3	60.9	50.5	76.7	64.3	55.3	54.1	57.6
Hypopharynx	C12-13	47	74.5	65.4	65.4	77.2	72.9	78.6	80.9	82.3
Oesophagus	C15	3 208	46.2	28.7	26.9	48.3	32.6	33.4	36.7	40.3
Stomach	C16	7 516	52.3	36.8	34.4	54.3	40.9	41.3	41.1	44.2
Small intestine	C17	181	71.3	55.7	50.4	72.9	59.7	57.4	53.9	57.8
Colon	C18	2 655	69.5	55.6	52.5	71.6	60.9	61.4	61.3	61.9
Rectum	C19-20	2 501	73.2	55.4	48.1	75.4	60.5	56.0	53.0	58.1
Anus	C21	46	80.4	66.2	66.2	84.0	75.1	81.9	81.0	77.8
Liver	C22	6 525	32.5	22.6	21.3	33.5	24.8	25.1	25.4	25.8
Gall bladder	C23-24	1 042	49.9	40.3	39.1	51.8	45.0	47.3	47.5	50.3
Pancreas	C25	1 990	36.4	26.0	25.2	37.6	28.6	29.8	30.3	31.0
Nose/Sinuses	C30-31	167	77.2	62.9	58.5	78.9	67.4	66.6	72.6	61.6
Larynx	C32	1 039	76.1	58.5	54.0	78.8	64.9	64.6	65.1	69.7
Lung	C33-34	21 403	43.6	27.6	25.7	45.1	30.7	30.9	31.3	32.3
Other thoracic organs	C37-38	244	59.4	48.5	46.2	60.9	51.9	51.8	50.5	52.1
Bone	C40-41	686	45.3	27.6	25.0	46.5	29.5	27.8	25.7	29.8
Melanoma of skin	C43	119	77.3	59.8	56.0	79.6	65.0	63.9	57.9	62.8
Other skin	C44	350	82.6	76.3	72.8	85.7	85.5	89.0	89.7	86.7
Mesothelioma	C45	84	58.3	49.8	49.8	60.1	54.4	58.5	60.6	58.1
Connective tissue	C47+C49	425	83.3	73.3	71.9	85.0	77.9	79.8	81.0	78.7
Breast	C50	5 863	91.8	84.3	79.8	92.9	87.2	84.8	82.3	85.6
Vulva	C51	57	84.2	66.7	61.2	86.5	72.6	71.3	71.6	74.3
Cervix	C53	567	71.8	58.5	53.8	73.8	63.7	62.4	68.5	70.5
Corpus uteri	C54	722	92.2	87.3	85.5	93.3	90.6	91.3	91.0	91.3
Uterus unspecified	C55	287	55.7	27.0	18.9	57.4	29.5	22.0	25.0	29.1
Ovary	C56	1 124	77.2	62.7	59.7	78.2	65.1	63.6	62.1	64.4
Other female genital org.	C57	52	80.8	66.1	60.9	81.9	68.6	64.3	49.9	67.5
Placenta	C58	62	96.8	93.3	93.3	97.0	93.8	94.1	60.1	60.0
Penis	C60	65	81.5	75.1	75.1	85.7	87.1	96.6	89.6	79.0
Prostate	C61	423	74.5	59.2	52.5	79.1	71.2	72.0	71.4	68.4
Testis	C62	73	78.1	68.8	66.8	78.8	70.0	68.6	74.9	76.4
Kidney	C64	1 094	69.6	57.8	52.6	71.7	62.9	60.6	59.0	65.7
Renal pelvis	C65	146	89.7	81.0	78.8	92.7	90.4	95.7	101.2	93.9
Ureter	C66	63	82.5	72.0	63.1	84.8	78.4	74.4	65.3	77.9
Urinary bladder	C67	2 020	76.6	63.9	59.6	80.2	73.0	74.6	73.4	81.1
Eye	C69	35	88.6	79.1	79.1	90.5	83.8	87.4	84.5	100.3
Brain & nervous system	C70-72	1 944	54.8	42.5	39.9	55.8	44.6	43.3	48.1	49.5
Thyroid	C73	618	85.3	80.8	79.4	86.7	84.3	85.4	88.6	89.1
Adrenal gland	C74	53	77.4	69.7	69.7	78.2	71.8	73.5	69.2	69.2
Other endocrine	C75	121	96.7	96.7	96.7	97.4	98.9	100.8	76.4	105.2
Hodgkin lymphoma	C81	123	91.1	83.7	77.8	92.0	86.0	81.1	81.0	81.9
Non-Hodgkin lymphoma	C82-85+C96	1 481	60.1	46.5	42.8	61.6	49.8	48.0	51.1	53.2

Table 3 (Continued).

Site	ICD-10	Cases included	% Absolute survival			% Relative survival			% ASRS at 5-years	
			1-year	3-year	5-year	1-year	3-year	5-year	all ages	0-74 years
Multiple myeloma	C90	217	60.4	44.6	40.6	61.8	47.8	45.7	46.2	46.1
Lymphoid leukaemia	C91	309	76.7	64.2	61.6	77.7	66.7	66.0	68.8	64.9
Myeloid leukaemia	C92-94	567	75.5	66.5	63.1	76.5	69.2	67.6	68.2	68.0
Leukaemia unspecified	C95	611	42.2	22.7	19.4	43.2	24.3	21.8	21.9	22.0

ASRS: age-standardized relative survival

Table 4a. Site-wise number of cases, 5-year absolute and relative survival by sex: Tianjin, China, 1991–1999 cases followed-up until 2000

Site	ICD-10	Cases included	Male			Female		
			% 5-year survival			% 5-year survival		
			No.	Abs	Rel	No.	Abs	Rel
Lip	C00	53	41	79.9	99.4	12	83.3	91.8
Tongue	C01-02	187	97	54.0	62.4	90	64.9	73.5
Oral cavity	C03-06	253	139	54.6	65.9	114	56.9	63.2
Salivary gland	C07-08	141	75	79.3	90.9	66	77.5	86.2
Tonsil	C09	25	12	63.9	84.6	13	83.1	89.5
Nasopharynx	C11	421	299	47.9	53.3	122	56.1	59.8
Hypopharynx	C12-13	47	41	60.4	73.7	6	100.0	112.3
Oesophagus	C15	3 208	2 198	27.5	35.0	1 010	25.5	30.0
Stomach	C16	7 516	5 286	34.7	42.9	2 230	33.6	37.8
Small intestine	C17	181	96	49.8	58.0	85	51.1	56.8
Colon	C18	2 655	1 399	53.9	64.7	1 256	51.0	57.8
Rectum	C19-20	2 501	1 304	49.6	59.3	1 197	46.6	52.5
Anus	C21	46	21	51.3	65.6	25	78.9	95.1
Liver	C22	6 525	4 606	22.7	27.0	1 919	18.0	20.8
Gall bladder	C23-24	1 042	525	38.3	48.3	517	40.0	46.3
Pancreas	C25	1 990	1 121	26.8	32.6	869	23.1	26.3
Nose/Sinuses	C30-31	167	108	57.5	66.8	59	60.7	66.4
Larynx	C32	1 039	682	55.6	68.4	357	51.1	57.6
Lung	C33-34	21 403	12 575	27.5	33.8	8 828	23.2	26.7
Other thoracic organs	C37-38	244	149	45.7	52.0	95	47.2	51.8
Bone	C40-41	686	360	25.3	28.8	326	24.6	26.7
Melanoma of skin	C43	119	68	57.4	67.6	51	54.0	59.1
Other skin	C44	350	200	68.7	86.9	150	78.2	91.8
Mesothelioma	C45	84	51	45.0	54.6	33	57.4	64.5
Connective tissue	C47+C49	425	252	70.0	79.7	173	74.6	80.0
Breast	C50	5 863	44	77.6	91.0	5 819	79.8	84.7
Vulva	C51	57				57	61.2	71.3
Cervix	C53	567				567	53.8	62.4
Corpus uteri	C54	722				722	85.5	91.3
Uterus unspecified	C55	287				287	18.9	22.0
Ovary	C56	1 124				1 124	59.7	63.6
Other female genital org.	C57	52				52	60.9	64.3
Placenta	C58	62				62	93.3	94.1
Penis	C60	65	65	75.1	96.6			
Prostate	C61	423	423	52.5	72.0			
Testis	C62	73	73	66.8	68.6			
Kidney	C64	1 094	732	54.4	63.9	362	49.2	54.2
Renal pelvis	C65	146	93	85.2	107.0	53	67.5	76.4
Ureter	C66	63	36	71.7	84.6	27	43.1	51.0
Urinary bladder	C67	2 020	1 552	61.4	78.0	468	53.5	64.0
Eye	C69	35	19	77.2	89.6	16	81.0	84.7
Brain & nervous system	C70-72	1 944	1 005	40.0	43.5	939	39.8	43.1
Thyroid	C73	618	172	72.7	81.3	446	82.0	86.9
Adrenal gland	C74	53	30	66.4	70.5	23	73.9	77.1
Other endocrine	C75	121	58	94.8	100.2	63	98.4	101.2
Hodgkin lymphoma	C81	123	78	77.1	80.9	45	79.2	81.6

Table 4a (Continued).

Site	ICD-10	Cases included	Male % 5-year survival			Female % 5-year survival		
			No.	Abs	Rel	No.	Abs	Rel
Non-Hodgkin lymphoma	C82-85+C96	1 481	835	44.2	50.4	646	41.0	44.9
Multiple myeloma	C90	217	143	31.9	36.2	74	57.6	63.9
Lymphoid leukaemia	C91	309	185	63.9	69.4	124	58.1	60.9
Myeloid leukaemia	C92-94	567	339	62.6	68.3	228	63.7	66.6
Leukaemia unspecified	C95	611	350	19.3	22.2	261	19.6	21.3

Abs: absolute survival; Rel: relative survival

Table 4b. Site-wise number of cases and relative survival by age group: Tianjin, China, 1991–1999 cases followed-up until 2000

Site	ICD-10	Cases included	Number of cases by age group					Relative survival by age group % 5-year survival				
			< 45	45-54	55-64	65-74	> 75	< 45	45-54	55-64	65-74	> 75
Lip	C00	53	2	6	12	24	9	100.8	104.3	98.9	89.0	113.3
Tongue	C01-02	187	20	30	52	61	24	71.0	67.9	71.1	62.4	73.6
Oral cavity	C03-06	253	34	28	59	90	42	76.8	80.3	67.8	53.0	65.4
Salivary gland	C07-08	141	39	19	32	30	21	95.6	82.7	82.3	97.2	79.2
Tonsil	C09	25	1	4	10	8	2	0.0	102.6	97.5	45.6	206.8
Nasopharynx	C11	421	96	89	117	93	26	61.1	60.2	58.7	43.8	42.1
Hypopharynx	C12-13	47	3	4	11	23	6	101.3	77.2	79.8	77.3	75.3
Oesophagus	C15	3 208	60	180	642	1 324	1 002	42.9	47.6	42.1	31.7	27.0
Stomach	C16	7 516	596	725	1 705	2 835	1 655	46.9	47.2	42.4	42.1	35.0
Small intestine	C17	181	22	33	47	65	14	59.4	51.8	52.2	67.4	46.8
Colon	C18	2 655	282	298	628	939	508	62.7	65.6	60.1	61.6	62.9
Rectum	C19-20	2 501	287	305	627	830	452	55.4	57.3	58.8	59.6	45.3
Anus	C21	46	4	6	3	20	13	75.6	86.4		82.8	85.4
Liver	C22	6 525	574	861	1 754	2 198	1 138	26.6	27.2	24.7	25.0	24.8
Gall bladder	C23-24	1 042	41	73	222	436	270	51.4	53.5	49.1	49.0	42.3
Pancreas	C25	1 990	131	196	517	759	387	38.7	30.6	30.6	28.1	30.7
Nose/Sinuses	C30-31	167	42	21	44	43	17	75.9	47.4	55.7	64.8	106.0
Larynx	C32	1 039	40	77	318	402	202	72.0	74.0	68.1	67.5	48.5
Lung	C33-34	21 403	764	1 640	5 680	9 162	4 157	36.9	36.1	30.7	30.5	29.8
Other thoracic organs	C37-38	244	62	29	59	60	34	60.0	52.3	50.6	47.0	49.2
Bone	C40-41	686	173	66	137	190	120	49.2	37.7	22.1	15.8	14.2
Melanoma of skin	C43	119	25	12	31	31	20	58.7	43.1	73.8	84.1	39.2
Other skin	C44	350	42	39	69	116	84	88.6	92.8	81.7	86.6	101.5
Mesothelioma	C45	84	16	8	17	27	16	62.9	77.4	44.8	53.2	69.6
Connective tissue	C47+C49	425	155	58	82	78	52	80.4	72.8	70.9	89.2	92.6
Breast	C50	5 863	1 731	1 594	1 295	901	342	88.3	85.1	84.2	84.1	68.1
Vulva	C51	57	4	7	19	12	15	76.0	65.8	71.3	84.2	61.8
Cervix	C53	567	41	42	111	235	138	79.1	72.5	62.1	62.4	54.4
Corpus uteri	C54	722	116	186	243	150	27	91.7	92.8	90.6	90.8	89.6
Uterus unspecified	C55	287	23	34	59	90	81	49.3	32.0	26.4	15.8	13.9
Ovary	C56	1 124	316	256	245	229	78	77.4	62.7	55.9	56.4	51.2
Other female genital org.	C57	52	12	11	11	16	2	82.7	89.4	74.9	31.1	0.0
Placenta	C58	62	54	6	2	0	0	96.6	102.1	0.0		
Penis	C60	65	10	5	8	21	21	81.1	62.3	68.4	103.5	133.2
Prostate	C61	423	8	4	57	183	171	38.1	39.5	61.7	77.6	74.5
Testis	C62	73	52	5	10	4	2	82.7	61.9	29.2		0.0
Kidney	C64	1 094	115	169	292	342	176	71.0	73.1	61.4	61.1	38.2
Renal pelvis	C65	146	6	15	37	65	23	101.3	89.6	96.9	87.2	126.2
Ureter	C66	63	4	5	22	25	7	101.0		65.1	97.0	40.2
Urinary bladder	C67	2 020	113	149	386	773	599	90.8	81.3	84.6	75.2	62.6
Eye	C69	35	16	2	3	10	4	80.2	102.2	106.5	110.4	38.9
Brain & nervous system	C70-72	1 944	596	272	408	480	188	58.4	48.8	39.8	28.2	32.0
Thyroid	C73	618	212	119	113	112	62	98.0	93.6	83.5	67.5	59.9
Adrenal gland	C74	53	25	9	7	12	0	80.9	80.5	61.8	60.3	
Other endocrine	C75	121	67	25	17	11	1	99.5	98.8	108.3	111.7	0.0
Hodgkin lymphoma	C81	123	68	18	18	13	6	82.9	67.2	90.2	100.7	
Non-Hodgkin lymphoma	C82-85+C96	1 481	322	202	344	401	212	57.3	55.8	50.1	43.0	31.8

Table 4b (Continued).

Site	ICD-10	Cases included	Number of cases by age group					Relative survival by age group % 5-year survival				
			< 45	45-54	55-64	65-74	> 75	< 45	45-54	55-64	65-74	> 75
Multiple myeloma	C90	217	31	32	61	73	20	37.4	48.9	49.3	46.1	52.5
Lymphoid leukaemia	C91	309	168	33	44	46	18	62.8	62.8	66.5	74.0	91.1
Myeloid leukaemia	C92-94	567	267	88	90	93	29	70.8	65.2	60.8	68.4	72.8
Leukaemia unspecified	C95	611	233	62	101	126	89	22.4	20.4	24.6	19.4	21.9

Table 5. Comparison of 5-year absolute and relative survival of cases diagnosed between 1981–1990 and 1991–1999, Tianjin, China

Site	ICD-10	% 5-year absolute survival		% 5-year relative survival	
		1981–1990	1991–1999	1981–1990	1991–1999
Lip	C00	84.8	80.3	103.3	97.6
Tongue	C01-02	46.7	59.2	53.9	67.8
Oral cavity	C03-06	61.1	55.6	68.9	64.6
Salivary gland	C07-08	67.5	78.7	72.3	88.9
Tonsil	C09	37.5	72.7	40.4	87.2
Nasopharynx	C11	50.8	50.5	55.1	55.3
Hypopharynx	C12-13	49.3	65.4	56.4	78.6
Oesophagus	C15	23.1	26.9	27.9	33.4
Stomach	C16	28.5	34.4	33.4	41.3
Small intestine	C17	50.0	50.4	55.2	57.4
Colon	C18	43.8	52.5	49.4	61.4
Rectum	C19-20	40.4	48.1	45.8	56.0
Anus	C21	42.9	66.2	49.2	81.9
Liver	C22	15.1	21.3	17.4	25.1
Gall bladder	C23-24	31.7	39.1	36.6	47.3
Pancreas	C25	20.3	25.2	23.4	29.8
Nose/Sinuses	C30-31	47.6	58.5	52.2	66.6
Larynx	C32	53.1	54.0	60.9	64.6
Lung	C33-34	24.5	25.7	28.2	30.9
Other thoracic organs	C37-38	42.9	46.2	46.7	51.8
Bone	C40-41	24.8	25.0	27.6	27.8
Melanoma of skin	C43	54.1	56.0	62.5	63.9
Other skin	C44	57.6	72.8	69.1	89.0
Mesothelioma	C45	29.6	49.8	32.9	58.5
Connective tissue	C47+C49	67.6	71.9	73.8	79.8
Breast	C50	75.4	79.8	80.1	84.8
Vulva	C51	67.7	61.2	77.6	71.3
Cervix	C53	55.3	53.8	62.0	62.4
Corpus uteri	C54	77.5	85.5	82.8	91.3
Uterus unspecified	C55	36.6	18.9	41.8	22.0
Ovary	C56	52.4	59.7	55.7	63.6
Other female genital org.	C57	56.8	60.9	60.2	64.3
Placenta	C58	85.0	93.3	86.0	94.1
Penis	C60	61.1	75.1	76.7	96.6
Prostate	C61	41.0	52.5	56.0	72.0
Testis	C62	73.1	66.8	75.9	68.6
Kidney	C64	48.6	52.6	55.5	60.6
Renal pelvis	C65	80.0	78.8	90.5	95.7
Ureter	C66	54.5	63.1	59.3	74.4
Urinary bladder	C67	53.8	59.6	63.9	74.6
Eye	C69	65.1	79.1	71.0	87.4
Brain & nervous system	C70-72	38.8	39.9	40.9	43.3
Thyroid	C73	78.2	79.4	82.1	85.4
Adrenal gland	C74	60.0	69.7	64.5	73.5
Other endocrine	C75	89.2	96.7	92.1	100.8
Hodgkin lymphoma	C81	59.8	77.8	61.4	81.1
Non-Hodgkin lymphoma	C82-85+C96	44.5	42.8	49.2	48.0

Table 5 (Continued).

Site	ICD-10	% 5-year absolute survival		% 5-year relative survival	
		1981–1990	1991–1999	1981–1990	1991–1999
Multiple myeloma	C90	19.2	40.6	22.2	45.7
Lymphoid leukaemia	C91	58.2	61.6	61.6	66.0
Myeloid leukaemia	C92-94	44.5	63.1	46.9	67.6
Leukaemia unspecified	C95	13.1	19.4	14.4	21.8

Table 6. Up-to-date 5-year relative survival estimates using cohort and period approaches by site and calendar period: Tianjin, China, 1981–1999 cases followed-up until 2000

Site	ICD-10	Period approach			Cohort approach		
		1986–90	1991–95	1986–99	1986–90	1991–95	1996–99
Tongue	C01-02	52.1	74.6	69.7	46.9	59.3	78.2
Oral cavity	C03-06	72.6	62.2	68.4	58.3	76.2	61.6
Salivary gland	C07-08	82.0	82.2	89.4	60.0	80.8	87.9
Nasopharynx	C11	57.5	57.3	59.2	44.6	64.1	54.0
Oesophagus	C15	29.9	35.2	34.9	18.7	37.1	33.0
Stomach	C16	34.9	42.4	42.1	23.4	42.5	39.7
Small intestine	C17	59.9	68.3	59.5	39.0	67.2	66.1
Colon	C18	47.8	58.5	63.9	38.1	57.3	54.8
Rectum	C19-20	46.8	53.8	58.8	31.4	57.0	47.8
Liver	C22	16.8	25.2	26.4	10.2	23.7	23.7
Gall bladder	C23-24	37.4	42.2	52.6	27.0	42.3	38.7
Pancreas	C25	21.6	28.8	31.7	15.0	29.5	27.0
Larynx	C32	59.6	63.8	67.1	53.3	67.1	60.5
Lung	C33	28.6	33.6	31.0	17.9	35.5	30.9
Other thoracic organs	C37-38	50.4	48.5	52.5	36.2	54.9	48.9
Bone	C40-41	23.9	28.9	30.8	23.5	31.2	30.4
Melanoma of skin	C43	62.1	75.2	58.3	51.9	68.8	67.5
Other skin	C44	64.9	87.4	91.9	65.6	73.2	90.9
Breast	C50	79.9	85.2	85.4	72.7	84.9	83.3
Cervix	C53	63.4	64.4	67.1	57.2	69.3	63.1
Corpus uteri	C54	85.5	93.3	91.8	73.1	91.0	91.3
Ovary	C56	30.6	62.8	66.6	40.7	56.8	60.3
Prostate	C61	46.5	66.5	78.5	44.6	63.5	63.9
Testis	C62	86.9	67.5	73.6	64.8	85.4	60.3
Kidney	C64	41.1	60.0	61.1	64.5	54.8	61.5
Urinary bladder	C67	62.4	74.7	74.9	56.4	69.7	73.9
Brain & nervous system	C70-72	34.5	46.2	42.2	37.8	43.5	43.9
Thyroid	C73	80.9	85.6	84.3	79.5	84.0	86.0
Non-Hodgkin lymphoma	C82-85+C96	48.7	49.9	49.8	42.1	54.3	45.6
Multiple myeloma	C90	22.0	26.0	51.1	17.3	25.5	29.3
Lymphoid leukaemia	C91	70.1	77.6	59.1	39.1	77.4	72.7
Myeloid leukaemia	C92-94	53.3	77.2	60.9	25.3	63.4	74.1
Leukaemia unspecified	C95	16.3	18.4	22.2	11.3	17.6	22.3

Chapter 9

Cancer survival in Costa Rica, 1995–2000

Ortiz-Barboza A, Gomez L, Cubero C, Bonilla G and Mena H

Abstract

The Costa Rica national tumour registry was founded in 1976 and nationwide data collection commenced in 1980. Cancer registration is predominantly done by passive methods. The registry contributed data on survival for invasive cancers of breast and cervix and *in situ* cancer of the cervix registered during 1995–2000. Follow-up has been carried out predominantly by passive methods, with median follow-up ranging from 31–47 months. The proportion of cases with histological confirmation of cancer diagnosis was 92% for invasive cancers and almost 100% for in-situ cancer of the cervix; death certificates only (DCOs) comprised 3%, and 78-86% of total cases registered were included for survival analysis. The one-, three- and five-year relative survival were 93%, 77% and 68%, respectively for breast cancer; the corresponding figures for invasive cervix cancer were 83%, 61% and 54%, respectively. The five-year relative survival for in-situ cervix cancer was 99%. A decreasing survival with increasing age group at diagnosis was noted for in-situ cancer of the cervix, while it fluctuated for invasive breast and cervix cancers. A decreasing survival with increasing clinical extent of disease was noted for invasive breast and cervix cancers.

National tumour registry

The population-based cancer registry in Costa Rica, known as the Costa Rica national tumour registry, was founded in 1976 to collect data on cancer incidence and prevalence in the entire country. It is based at the statistics department of the Ministry of Health, which funds the registry, and started nationwide data collection in 1980. It has contributed data to the quinquennial IARC publication *Cancer Incidence in Five Continents* since volume V [1]. An executive decree makes it compulsory to report cancer cases diagnosed in the country. Cancer registration is predominantly done by passive methods. The principal sources of data are notification sheets in addition to the pathology, clinical laboratory and the hospital discharge reports. The registry covers an area of 51 100 km^2 and caters to a population of about 3.8 million in 2000 with a sex ratio of 1003 females to 1000 males. The average annual age-standardized incidence rate is 204 per 100 000 among males and 191 per 100 000 among females in 1995–1996. The top-ranking cancers among males are stomach, non-melanoma skin, prostate and lung. Among females, the order is non-melanoma skin, breast, stomach and cervix.

The registry contributed data on survival for invasive cancers of breast and cervix and *in situ* cancer of the cervix registered during 1995–2000 for the first time in this volume of the IARC publication on *Cancer Survival in Africa, Asia, the Caribbean and Central America*.

Data quality indices (Table 1)

The proportion of cases with histological confirmation of cancer diagnosis in this series is 92% for invasive cancers and almost 100% for *in situ* cancer of the cervix. The proportion of invasive cancer cases registered based on a death certificate only (DCO) is 3%. The exclusion rate of cases without any follow-up information is 12% for invasive cancers and 22% for *in situ* cervix cancer. Thus, 78–86% of the total cases registered are included in the estimation of the survival probability.

Outcome of follow-up (Table 2)

Follow-up has been carried out predominantly by passive methods. Death certificates mentioning cancer are obtained from the National Institute of Statistics and Census. These are matched with the cancer registry database by record linkage techniques using personal identification numbers. The vital status of each unmatched incident cases is then ascertained by matching with the Civil Registry database and reviewing clinical histories.

The closing date of follow-up was 31st December 2003. The median follow-up varied between 31 and 45 months for invasive cervix and breast cancers, respectively; it was 47 months for *in situ* cervix cancer. Complete follow-up at five years from the incidence date ranged between 74–83%. The losses to follow-up have generally occurred evenly in the different time intervals from incidence date; from <1 year to more than 5 years.

Survival statistics

All ages and both sexes together (Table 3)

The one-, three- and five-year relative survival estimates are 93%, 77% and 68%, respectively in invasive breast cancer; the corresponding figures for invasive cervix cancer are 83%, 61% and 54%, respectively. The five-year relative survival for *in situ* cervix cancer is 99%.

The 5-year age-standardized relative survival (ASRS) probability for all ages together is less than the corresponding unadjusted one for invasive breast and cervix cancers. Both the estimates were similar in *in situ* cervix cancer. The 5-year ASRS (0–74 years of age) is higher than the corresponding ASRS (all ages) for invasive cancers but lower for *in situ* cervix cancer.

Sex

Male (Table 4a)

The 5-year relative survival of breast cancer patients is higher among males than females.

Female (Table 4a)

The 5-year relative survival from invasive breast cancer (68%) is higher than for cervix cancer (54%). *In situ* cervix cancer has the highest survival (99%).

Age group (Table 4b)

The 5-year relative survival by age group is seen to fluctuate, with no definite pattern or trend emerging for invasive cancers of breast and cervix. However, a decreasing survival with increasing age group at diagnosis is forthcoming for *in situ* cancer of the cervix.

Extent of disease (Table 5; Figure 1)

The majority of invasive breast (34%) and cervix cancer (40%) cases are classified as having regional spread of disease at the time of diagnosis.

Localized cancers comprised 31% of breast and 22% of cervix cancer cases. The extent of disease was unknown in 14% of breast and 33% of cervix cancers. The 5-year absolute survival by extent of disease followed the expected pattern: highest for localized cases, followed by regional and distant metastasis cases among known categories of extent of disease.

Figure 1a. Absolute survival (%) by extent of disease, Costa Rica, 1995–2000, cancer of the breast

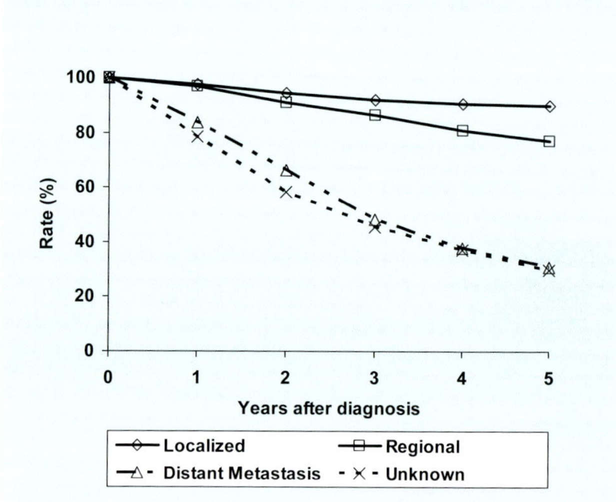

Figure 1b. Absolute survival (%) by extent of disease, Costa Rica, 1995–2000, cancer of the cervix

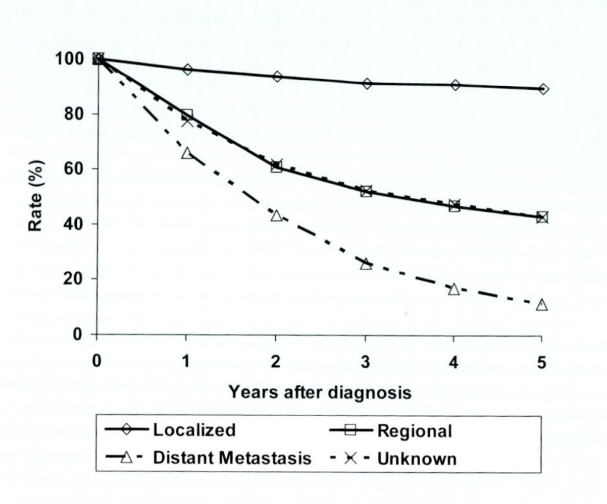

References

1. Parkin DM, Whelan SL, Ferlay J and Storm H. *Cancer Incidence in Five Continents, Vol I to VIII: IARC Cancerbase No. 7.* IARCPress, Lyon, 2005.

Table 1. Data quality indices - Proportion of histologically verified and death certificate only cases, number and proportion of included and excluded cases by site: Costa Rica, 1995–2000 cases followed-up until 2003

Site	ICD-10	Total registered	% HV	% DCO	Excluded cases DCO	Excluded cases Follow-up	Excluded cases Others	Excluded cases Total	Excluded cases %	Included cases No.	Included cases %
Breast	C50	2 854	92.4	2.5	72	316	4	392	13.7	2 462	86.3
Cervix	C53	1 807	91.4	3.3	60	259	3	322	17.8	1 485	82.2
In-situ cervix	D06	3 009	99.7	0.0	0	658	1	659	21.9	2 350	78.1

HV: histologically verified; DCO: death certificate only

Table 2. Number and proportion of cases with complete/incomplete follow-up (in years) and median follow-up (in months) by site: Costa Rica, 1995–2000 cases followed-up until 2003

Site	ICD-10	Cases included	Complete FU (Alive/dead at end of FU) No.	Complete FU (Alive/dead at end of FU) %	Incomplete FU: lost to FU No.	Incomplete FU: lost to FU %	% lost to FU: years from diagnosis < 1	1-3	3-5	> 5	% with complete FU at 5 years	Median FU (in months)
Breast	C50	2 462	1 866	75.8	596	24.2	7.1	4.5	5.8	6.8	82.6	45.3
Cervix	C53	1 485	1 001	67.4	484	32.6	9.9	8.6	7.8	6.3	73.7	30.9
In-situ cervix	D06	2 350	792	33.7	1 558	66.3	12.4	20.9	19.4	13.6	47.3	46.9

FU: follow-up

Table 3. Comparison of 1-, 3- and 5-year absolute and relative survival and 5-year age-standardized relative survival by site: Costa Rica, 1995–2000 cases followed-up until 2003

Site	ICD-10	Cases included	% Absolute survival 1-year	3-year	5-year	% Relative survival 1-year	3-year	5-year	% ASRS at 5-years all ages	0-74 years
Breast	C50	2 462	91.7	73.8	63.4	92.9	76.6	67.7	66.0	69.6
Cervix	C53	1 485	81.9	59.6	51.5	82.7	61.2	53.8	50.0	53.5
In-situ cervix	D06	2 350	99.6	99.0	97.3	99.9	99.9	98.8	98.5	96.0

ASRS: age-standardized relative survival

Table 4a. Site-wise number of cases, 5-year absolute and relative survival by sex: Costa Rica, 1995–2000 cases followed-up until 2003

Site	ICD-10	Cases included	Male % 5-year survival			Female % 5-year survival		
			No.	Abs	Rel	No.	Abs	Rel
Breast	C50	2 462	15	72.8	90.8	2 447	63.3	67.5
Cervix	C53	1 485				1 485	51.5	53.8
In-situ cervix	D06	2 350				2 350	97.3	98.8

Abs: absolute survival; Rel: relative survival

Table 4b. Site-wise number of cases and relative survival by age group: Costa Rica, 1995–2000 cases followed-up until 2003

Site	ICD-10	Cases included	Number of cases by age group					Relative survival by age group % 5-year survival				
			< 45	45-54	55-64	65-74	> 75	< 45	45-54	55-64	65-74	> 75
Breast	C50	2 462	597	671	478	451	265	62.6	70.3	72.9	74.6	49.8
Cervix	C53	1 485	652	311	224	174	124	65.9	54.4	44.2	42.4	24.5
In-situ cervix	D06	2 350	1 820	287	140	82	21	74.4	80.6	71.4	59.4	57.2

Table 5. Proportion of cases and 5-year absolute survival by extent of disease and site: Costa Rica, 1995–2000

Site	ICD-10	Cases included	% of cases by extent of disease				% 5-year absolute survival			
			Localized	Regional	Dist. met.	Unknown	Localized	Regional	Dist. met.	Unknown
Breast	C50	2 462	31.2	34.0	20.3	14.5	89.9	77.1	31.0	29.9
Cervix	C53	1 485	22.4	40.5	4.0	33.1	89.5	43.1	11.3	43.2

Dis. met.: distant metastasis

Chapter 10

Cancer survival in Cuba, 1994–1995

Garrote LF, Alvarez YG, Babie PT, Yi MG, Alvarez MG and Cicili ML

Abstract

The population-based cancer registry in Cuba is a national cancer registry established in 1964; cancer registration is entirely done by passive methods. Data on survival from 13 cancer sites or types registered during 1994–1995 are reported. Follow-up has been carried out predominantly by passive methods, with median follow-up ranging from 13–54 months. The proportion with histologically verified diagnosis for various cancers ranged between 34–100%; death certificates only (DCOs) comprised 8–50%; 50–89% of total registered cases were included for the survival analysis. The 5-year age-standardized relative survival for selected cancers were breast (69%), colon (41%), cervix (56%), urinary bladder (64%), rectum (48%) and non-Hodgkin lymphoma (49%). The 5-year relative survival by age group showed no distinct pattern or trend, and was fluctuating. A decreasing survival with increasing clinical extent of disease was noted for all cancers studied. The data on survival trend revealed that the 5-year relative survival of most cancers diagnosed in 1994–1995 was greater than that in 1988–1989.

National cancer registry

The population-based cancer registry in Cuba is a national cancer registry started within the framework of the national health system in 1964 to describe the annual cancer burden in the country. Its central office is based at the National Institute of Oncology and Radiobiology, Havana. It has contributed data to the quinquennial IARC publication *Cancer Incidence in Five Continents* in volumes III, IV and VI [1]. A health ministry resolution of 1986 makes it mandatory for physicians to report cancer cases diagnosed in the country. Cancer registration is entirely done by passive methods. The principal source of data is the cancer report form in the Hospital Statistics Department in addition to the pathology, clinical laboratory and the hospital discharge reports. The registry caters to a population of about 11.2 million in 2002 with a sex ratio of 997 females to 1000 males. The average annual age-standardized incidence rate is 203.6 per 100 000 among males and 179.6 per 100 000 among females in 2002. The top ranking cancers among males are lung, non-melanoma skin, prostate and larynx. Among females, the order is breast, non-melanoma skin, cervix and lung.

The registry contributed data on survival for 16 cancer site or type in the first volume of the IARC publication on *Cancer Survival in Developing Countries* [2]. Data on survival from 13 cancer sites or types registered during 1994–1995 are reported in this volume.

Data quality indices (Table 1)

The proportion of cases with histological confirmation of cancer diagnosis in this series is 64%, varying between 100% for lymphomas and 34% for cancer of the colon. The proportion of cases registered based on a death certificate only (DCO) is 32% , ranging from 8% in cancer of the anus to 50% in colon cancer. Cases excluded due to lack of follow-up information were negligible. The exclusion of cases from the survival analysis is the greatest in colon cancer (50%) and the least for cancer of the anus (11%). Thus, 50–89% of the total cases registered are included in the estimation of survival probability.

Outcome of follow-up (Table 2)

Follow-up has been carried out predominantly by passive methods. A copy of the national death certificate file is obtained every year from the national statistical department of the Ministry of Health and is matched with the cancer registry database using record linkage techniques. The vital status of the unmatched incident cases are then ascertained by matching with the national identity registry, repeated scrutiny of hospital records and some minimal postal enquiries.

The closing date of follow-up was 31st December 1999. The median follow-up varied from 13 months in tongue cancer to 54 months for breast cancer. Complete follow-up at five years from the incidence date ranged between 94–99%. The losses to follow-up generally occurred in the first year of follow-up.

Survival statistics

All ages and both sexes together (Table 3)

The 5-year relative survival was the highest in cancer of the larynx (53%) among head and neck cancers. The corresponding survival estimates for cancers of the colon, rectum and anus were 41%, 49% and 58%, respectively. Hodgkin lymphoma had a better survival (52%) than non-Hodgkin lymphoma (47%).

Figure 1a. Top five cancers (ranked by survival), Cuba, 1994-1995

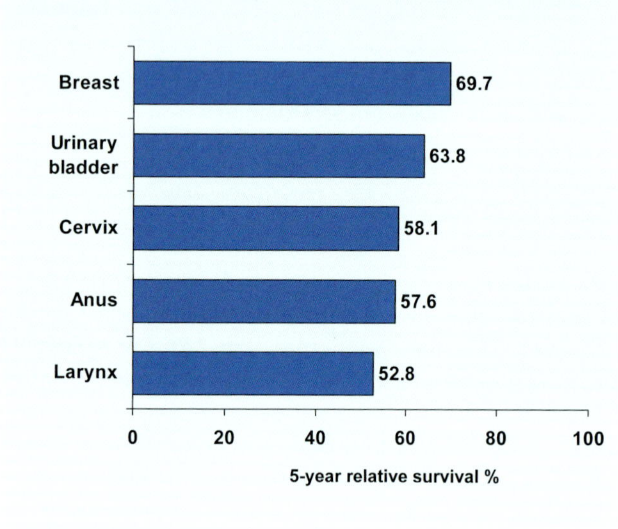

The 5-year age-standardized relative survival (ASRS) probability for all ages together is either greater than or similar to the corresponding unadjusted one for a majority of cancers. The 5-year ASRS (0–74 years of age) is observed to be either higher than or similar to the corresponding ASRS (all ages) for all cancers.

Sex

Male (Table 4a)

The 5-year relative survival was the highest for cancer of the urinary bladder (63%) followed in order by larynx (53%), anus (51%), Hodgkin and non-Hodgkin lymphomas and rectum (46%).

Figure 1b. Top five cancers (ranked by survival), Male, Cuba, 1994–1995

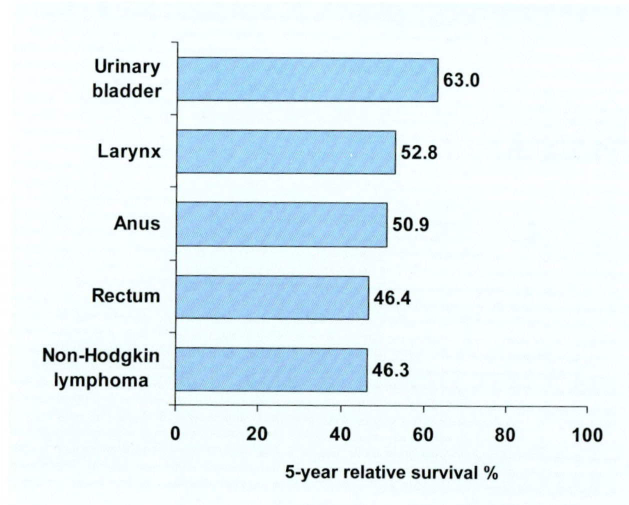

Female (Table 4a)

The top-ranking cancers in terms of 5-year relative survival were breast (70%), urinary bladder and tonsil (67%) and anus (60%). Survival from cervix cancer was 58%. Survival was markedly higher among females than males for cancers of the tongue, oral cavity, oropharynx including tonsil, anus and Hodgkin lymphoma.

Figure 1c. Top five cancers (ranked by survival), Female, Cuba, 1994–1995

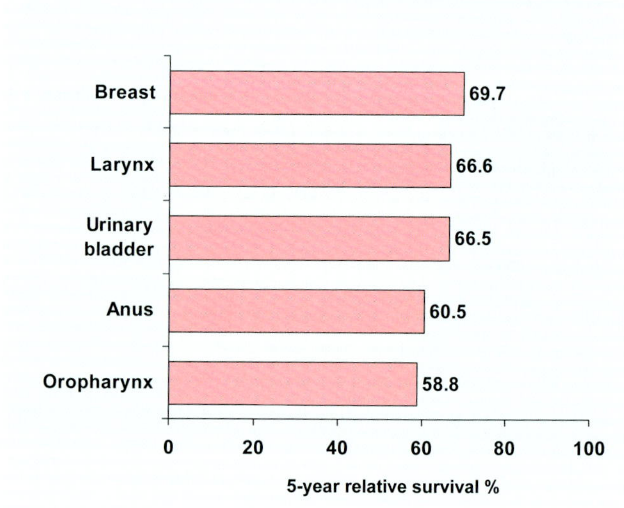

Age group (Table 4b)

The 5-year relative survival by age group was seen to fluctuate, with no definite pattern or trend emerging.

Extent of disease (Table 5; Figure 2)

Among cancers except tongue cancer, a majority of cases have been diagnosed with a localized disease at diagnosis, from 51% for cancer of the larynx to 28% in cancer of the colon. Regional disease among tongue cancers constituted 40%. The extent of disease was unknown in 18–42%. The 5-year absolute survival by extent of disease followed the expected pattern: highest for localized cases followed by regional and distant metastasis cases among known categories of extent of disease.

Figure 2. Absolute survival (%) from selected cancers by extent of disease, Cuba, 1994–1995

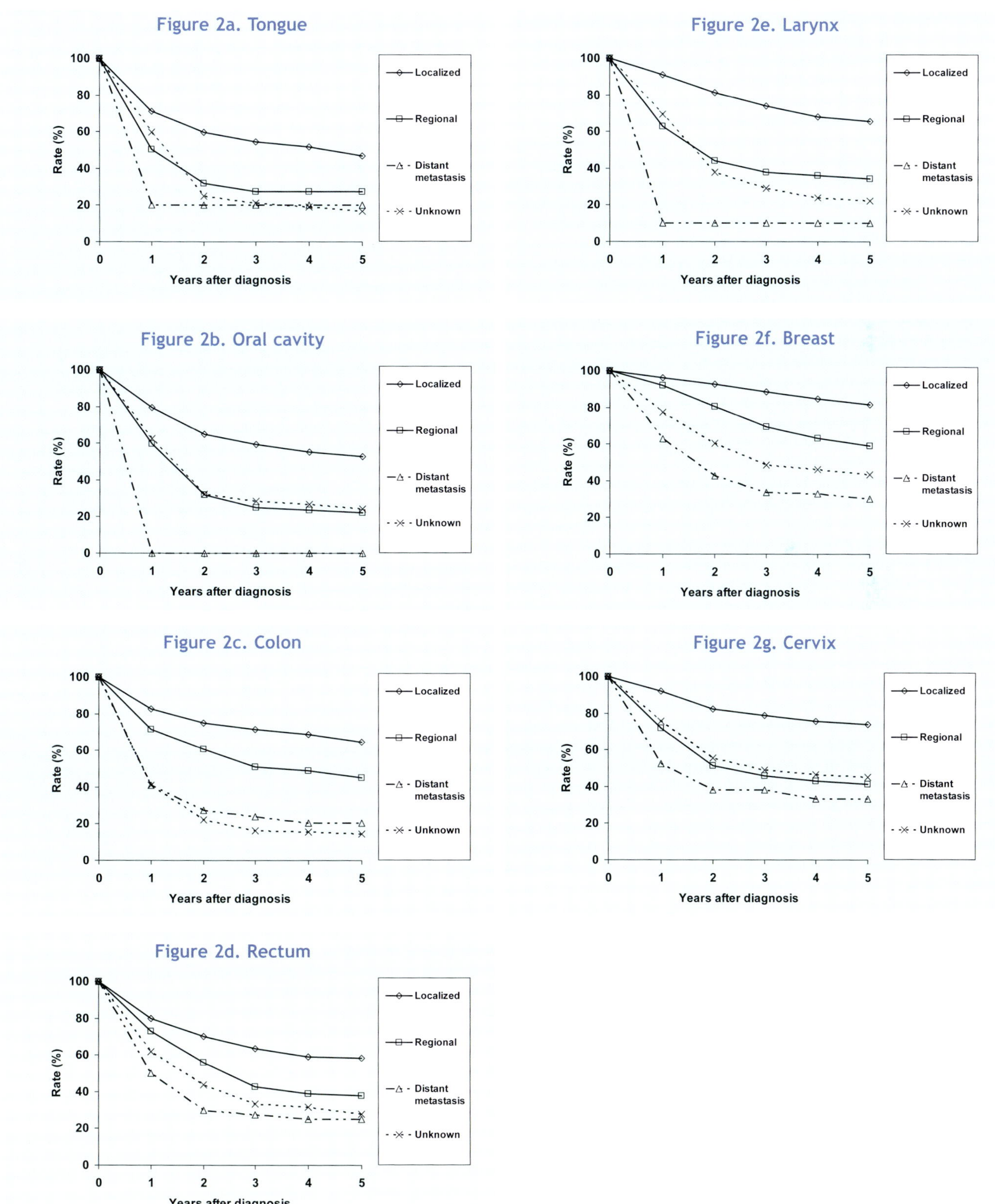

Survival trend (Table 6)

The data on trends in cancer survival are available for 9 cancers registered in two time periods between 1988–1989 [2] and 1994–1995. The 5-year relative survival of most cancers diagnosed between 1994–1995 is greater than those registered in 1988–1989. The absolute difference exceeded 10% in cancers of tongue, oropharynx (including tonsil) and non-Hodgkin lymphoma. Hodgkin lymphoma and cancer of the oral cavity experienced a decrease in survival in 1994–1995 compared to 1988–1989.

References

1. Parkin DM, Whelan SL, Ferlay J and Storm H. *Cancer Incidence in Five Continents, Vol I to VIII: IARC Cancerbase No. 7*. IARCPress, Lyon, 2005.

2. Garrote LF, Boschmonar MG, Alvarez YG, Cicilli ML, Garcia AM and Rodriguez RC. Cancer survival in Cuba. In: *Cancer Survival in Developing Countries* (eds) R Sankaranarayanan, RJ Black and DM Parkin. IARC Scientific Publications No. 145. IARCPress, Lyon, 1998, pp 51–59.

Table 1. Data quality indices - Proportion of histologically verified and death certificate only cases, number and proportion of included and excluded cases by site: Cuba, 1994–1995 cases followed-up until 1999

Site	ICD-10	Total registered	%		Excluded cases					Included cases	
			HV	DCO	DCO	Follow-up	Others	Total	%	No.	%
Tongue	C01-02	314	69.1	25.5	80	0	3	83	26.4	231	73.6
Oral cavity	C03-06	355	69.0	25.9	92	0	3	95	26.8	260	73.2
Tonsil	C09	82	62.2	32.9	27	0	1	28	34.1	54	65.9
Oropharynx	C10	60	80.0	20.0	12	0	0	12	20.0	48	80.0
Colon	C18	2 491	33.6	49.7	1238	0	5	1243	49.9	1 248	50.1
Rectum	C19-20	790	62.0	29.1	230	0	4	234	29.6	556	70.4
Anus	C21	106	84.0	8.5	9	1	2	12	11.3	94	88.7
Larynx	C32	1 165	61.6	30.7	358	0	7	365	31.3	800	68.7
Breast	C50	2 929	69.4	25.6	749	2	9	760	25.9	2 169	74.1
Cervix	C53	1 450	81.8	15.4	224	0	5	229	15.8	1 221	84.2
Urinary bladder	C67	1 182	60.2	29.5	349	0	14	363	30.7	819	69.3
Hodgkin lymphoma	C81	320	100.0	40.3	129	0	5	134	41.9	186	58.1
Non-Hodgkin lymphoma	C82-85+C96	771	100.0	39.7	306	0	1	307	39.8	464	60.2

HV: histologically verified; DCO: death certificate only

Table 2. Number and proportion of cases with complete/incomplete follow-up (in years) and median follow-up (in months) by site: Cuba, 1994–1995 cases followed-up until 1999

Site	ICD-10	Cases included	Complete FU Alive/dead at end of FU		Incomplete FU: lost to FU		% lost to FU: years from diagnosis				% with complete FU at 5 years	Median FU (in months)
			No.	%	No.	%	< 1	1-3	3-5	> 5		
Tongue	C01-02	231	220	95.2	11	4.8	3.0	0.9	0.9	0.0	95.2	13.2
Oral cavity	C03-06	260	243	93.4	17	6.6	3.1	1.9	1.2	0.4	93.8	19.2
Tonsil	C09	54	53	98.1	1	1.9	0.0	0.0	1.9	0.0	98.1	20.5
Oropharynx	C10	48	47	97.9	1	2.1	2.1	0.0	0.0	0.0	97.9	13.8
Colon	C18	1 248	1 238	99.2	10	0.8	0.2	0.2	0.3	0.1	99.3	14.4
Rectum	C19-20	556	545	98.0	11	2.0	1.1	0.4	0.5	0.0	98.0	28.9
Anus	C21	94	93	98.9	1	1.1	1.1	0.0	0.0	0.0	98.9	50.7
Larynx	C32	800	771	96.3	29	3.7	1.5	0.9	1.0	0.3	96.6	40.6
Breast	C50	2 169	2 104	97.0	65	3.0	0.9	0.3	1.4	0.4	97.4	54.5
Cervix	C53	1 221	1 152	94.4	69	5.6	2.2	1.2	1.7	0.5	94.9	50.4
Urinary bladder	C67	819	798	97.4	21	2.6	1.2	0.0	1.0	0.4	97.8	50.1
Hodgkin lymphoma	C81	186	181	97.4	5	2.6	1.6	0.5	0.5	0.0	97.4	49.2
Non-Hodgkin lymphoma	C82-85+C96	464	453	97.7	11	2.3	0.6	0.6	1.1	0.0	97.7	25.1

FU: follow-up

Table 3. Comparison of 1-, 3- and 5-year absolute and relative survival and 5-year age-standardized relative survival by site: Cuba, 1994–1995 cases followed-up until 1999

Site	ICD-10	Cases included	% Absolute survival			% Relative survival			% ASRS at 5-years	
			1-year	3-year	5-year	1-year	3-year	5-year	all ages	0-74 years
Tongue	C01-02	231	59.1	35.2	31.4	60.8	38.2	36.3	37.9	38.9
Oral cavity	C03-06	260	68.8	40.6	35.8	70.7	44.2	41.6	43.3	43.7
Tonsil	C09	54	61.1	46.3	42.0	62.4	49.1	46.4	46.1	51.2
Oropharynx	C10	48	60.0	40.7	38.1	61.4	43.8	43.3	52.6	55.8
Colon	C18	1 248	58.7	39.5	35.3	60.6	43.3	41.2	40.5	46.4
Rectum	C19-20	556	70.9	47.0	42.1	72.8	50.9	48.5	47.6	50.7
Anus	C21	94	77.5	59.2	50.7	79.5	63.7	57.6	59.8	61.7
Larynx	C32	800	78.1	53.8	46.9	79.9	57.7	52.8	54.1	58.1
Breast	C50	2 169	89.7	72.3	64.6	91.0	75.6	69.7	69.4	70.4
Cervix	C53	1 221	80.7	60.2	55.7	81.3	61.6	58.1	55.8	56.3
Urinary bladder	C67	819	74.8	59.0	53.3	77.5	65.5	63.8	64.1	68.8
Hodgkin lymphoma	C81	186	72.9	56.4	50.0	73.6	57.8	51.9	55.5	57.5
Non-Hodgkin lymphoma	C82-85+C96	464	66.3	47.5	43.5	67.4	49.9	47.3	49.4	50.3

ASRS: age-standardized relative survival

Table 4a. Site-wise number of cases, 5-year absolute and relative survival by sex: Cuba, 1994–1995 cases followed-up until 1999

Site	ICD-10	Cases included	Male % 5-year survival			Female % 5-year survival		
			No.	Abs	Rel	No.	Abs	Rel
Tongue	C01-02	231	178	26.8	31.6	53	47.3	52.3
Oral cavity	C03-06	260	173	31.2	36.1	87	45.2	52.8
Tonsil	C09	54	46	39.1	43.0	8	60.0	66.6
Oropharynx	C10	48	36	32.8	38.4	12	55.4	58.8
Colon	C18	1 248	518	32.9	38.4	730	37.1	43.2
Rectum	C19-20	556	274	39.8	46.4	282	44.4	50.4
Anus	C21	94	28	42.2	50.9	66	54.4	60.5
Larynx	C32	800	683	46.8	52.8	117	47.7	53.1
Breast	C50	2 169				2 169	64.6	69.7
Cervix	C53	1 221				1 221	55.7	58.1
Urinary bladder	C67	819	631	52.5	63.0	188	56.2	66.5
Hodgkin lymphoma	C81	186	94	44.2	46.2	92	56.2	57.9
Non-Hodgkin lymphoma	C82-85+C96	464	247	42.2	46.3	217	45.1	48.5

Abs: absolute survival; Rel: relative survival

Table 4b. Site-wise number of cases and relative survival by age group: Cuba, 1994–1995 cases followed-up until 1999

Site	ICD-10	Cases included	Number of cases by age group					Relative survival by age group % 5-year survival				
			< 45	45-54	55-64	65-74	> 75	< 45	45-54	55-64	65-74	> 75
Tongue	C01-02	231	18	30	59	60	64	50.5	37.5	34.9	37.2	32.8
Oral cavity	C03-06	260	12	35	67	72	74	51.0	41.2	47.3	36.6	39.8
Tonsil	C09	54	8	11	8	18	9	76.0	37.7	40.3	64.9	0.0
Oropharynx	C10	48	1	9	15	14	9	100.8	68.7	21.4	55.2	33.6
Colon	C18	1 248	74	124	247	345	458	51.8	40.8	43.3	49.7	31.7
Rectum	C19-20	556	40	79	113	167	157	52.0	52.9	52.6	47.5	42.9
Anus	C21	94	5	17	22	20	30	60.6	46.0	46.6	84.0	58.8
Larynx	C32	800	50	130	238	244	138	80.7	63.5	49.5	51.3	38.9
Breast	C50	2 169	424	515	502	435	293	71.7	67.0	70.7	72.6	65.4
Cervix	C53	1 221	531	284	184	155	67	65.3	55.3	46.7	54.5	53.0
Urinary bladder	C67	819	31	82	157	241	308	74.4	80.6	71.4	59.4	57.2
Hodgkin lymphoma	C81	186	108	15	22	25	16	63.6	61.4	43.9	18.4	20.3
Non-Hodgkin lymphoma	C82-85+C96	464	122	80	87	97	78	56.7	54.9	41.8	37.5	43.4

Rel: relative survival

Table 5. Proportion of cases and 5-year absolute survival by extent of disease and site: Cuba, 1994–1995

Site	ICD-10	Cases included	% of cases by extent of disease				% 5-year absolute survival			
			Localized	Regional	Dist. met.	Unknown	Localized	Regional	Dist. met.	Unknown
Tongue	C01-02	231	35.5	39.8	2.2	22.5	46.7	27.3	20.0	16.8
Oral cavity	C03-06	260	44.2	34.6	0.4	20.8	52.6	22.2	0.0	24.4
Colon	C18	1 248	28.0	20.3	9.6	42.1	64.7	45.0	20.5	14.6
Rectum	C19-20	556	38.8	25.4	7.2	28.6	58.5	38.0	25.0	27.7
Larynx	C32	800	51.3	23.0	1.3	24.5	65.5	34.5	10.0	22.2
Breast	C50	2 169	43.5	33.3	4.9	18.3	81.6	58.9	30.2	43.3
Cervix	C53	1 221	41.3	34.3	1.7	22.7	73.9	41.5	33.3	45.0

Dis. met.: distant metastasis

Table 6. Comparison of 5-year absolute and relative survival of cases diagnosed between 1988–1989 and 1994–1995, Cuba

Site	ICD-10	% 5-year absolute survival		% 5-year relative survival	
		1988–1989	1994–1995	1988–1989	1994–1995
Tongue	C01-02	19.0	31.4	25.5	36.3
Oral cavity	C03-06	38.5	35.8	49.1	41.6
Oropharynx	C10	27.0	38.1	33.7	43.3
Colon	C18	29.2	35.3	38.1	41.2
Rectum	C19-20	31.7	42.1	41.7	48.5
Breast	C50	54.0	64.6	60.8	69.7
Cervix	C53	52.3	55.7	55.9	58.1
Hodgkin lymphoma	C81	51.0	50.0	54.9	51.9
Non-Hodgkin lymphoma	C82-85+C96	31.8	43.5	37.0	47.3

FU: follow-up

Chapter 11

Cancer survival in the Gambia, 1993–1997

Bah E, Sam O, Whittle H, Ramanakumar A and Sankaranarayanan R

Abstract

The national cancer registry of the Gambia was established in 1986 as part of the Gambia Hepatitis Intervention Study in collaboration with IARC, France; Medical Research Council (MRC) Laboratories of the UK; and the Government of the Gambia at MRC, Banjul. Registration of incident cancer cases is done by active and passive methods. For this study, the registry contributed data on survival for six cancer sites or types registered during 1993–1997. Follow-up has been carried out predominantly by active methods with median follow-up ranging between 1–6 months. The proportion of histologically verified diagnosis for various cancers ranged between 1–45%, and 54–82% of total registered cases were included for survival analysis. Complete follow-up at five years from the incidence date ranged between 81–98% for different cancers. The 5-year age-standardized relative survival for selected cancers were cervix (23%), non-Hodgkin lymphoma (22%), breast (10%), stomach (4%) and liver (3%). The 5-year relative survival by age group showed fluctuations with no definite pattern or trend emerging, and with no survivors in many age intervals.

National cancer registry

The national cancer registry of the Gambia was established in 1986 as part of the Gambia Hepatitis Intervention Study in collaboration with International Agency for Research on Cancer (IARC), the Medical Research Council (MRC) Laboratories of UK and the Government of the Gambia at MRC, Banjul. It contributed data to the quinquennial IARC publication *Cancer Incidence in Five Continents* in volumes VI and VIII [1]. Cancer notification is voluntary, and registration of cases is done by passive and active methods. The principal sources of data are the medical records/registers in the hospitals in public and private sectors, pathology laboratories and other medical institutions. The registry covers the entire country of 11 300 km^2 and caters to a population of about 1 million in 1997–1998 with a sex ratio of 1038 females to 1000 males. The average annual age-standardized incidence rate is 84 per 100 000 among males and 85 per 100 000 among females in 1997–1998. The top ranking cancers among males are liver, lung and prostate. Among females, the order is cervix, liver and breast.

The registry contributed data on survival from 6 cancer sites or types for the first time in this volume of the IARC publication on *Cancer Survival in Africa, Asia, the Caribbean and Central America*. A random sample of 150 cases of liver cancer and 275 cases of cervix cancer among the total incident cases was selected for this study. For the rest of the cancers, all incident cases have been included.

Data quality indices (Table 1)

The proportion of cases with histological confirmation of cancer diagnosis in this series is 25%, varying between 1% for cancer of the liver and 45% for non-Hodgkin lymphoma. The proportion of cases registered based on a death certificate only (DCO) is negligible except for lung cancer. The exclusion of cases without any follow-up information is 25%, ranging from 1% in liver cancer to 34% in non-Hodgkin lymphoma. Thus, 54–82% of the total cases in different cancers are included in the estimation of the survival probability.

Outcome of follow-up (Table 2)

Follow-up has been carried out predominantly by active methods. Cancer mortality information obtained from accessible death certificates in registration office is matched with the registry database. The vital status of the unmatched incident cases is then ascertained by repeated scrutiny of hospital records and house visits.

The closing date of follow-up was 31st December 1999. The median follow-up varied from one month in stomach, liver and lung cancers to 6 months for cervix cancer. Complete follow-up at five years from the incidence date ranged between 81% in cancer of the lung and 98% for liver cancer. The bulk of the losses to follow-up generally occurred in the first year of follow-up.

Survival statistics

All ages and both sexes together (Table 3)

The 5-year relative survival was the highest in cancer of the lung (32%) followed by non-Hodgkin lymphoma (25%) and cervix (24%). The lowest survival rate was encountered with liver cancer (3%) and preceded by stomach cancer (5%) in the series.

The 5-year age-standardized relative survival (ASRS) probability for all ages together is either less than or similar to the corresponding unadjusted one for all the cancers except lung. The 5-year ASRS (0–74 years of age) is observed to be greater than or similar to the corresponding ASRS (all ages) for most cancers.

Sex

Male (Table 4a)

The highest 5-year relative survival was observed in lung cancer (29%). None of the breast cancer cases survived for 5 years from incidence date. The 5-year relative survival was notably higher among males than females in cancer of the stomach.

Female (Table 4a)

The 5-year relative survival estimates for breast and cervix cancers were 11% and 24% respectively. None of the stomach cancer cases survived until 5 years from incidence date. Survival from non-Hodgkin lymphoma was noticeably higher among females than males.

Age group (Table 4b)

The 5-year relative survival by age group was seen to fluctuate, with no definite pattern or trend emerging and no survivors in many age intervals.

References

1. Parkin DM, Whelan SL, Ferlay J and Storm H. *Cancer Incidence in Five Continents, Vol I to VIII: IARC Cancerbase No. 7*. IARCPress, Lyon, 2005.

Table 1. Data quality indices - Proportion of histologically verified and death certificate only cases, number and proportion of included and excluded cases by site: The Gambia, 1993–1997 cases followed-up until 1999

Site	ICD-10	Total registered	%		Excluded cases					Included cases	
			HV	DCO	DCO	Follow-up	Others	Total	%	No.	%
Stomach	C16	52	19.2	0.0	0	3	10	13	25.0	39	75.0
Liver	C22*	150	1.3	0.0	0	1	26	27	18.0	123	82.0
Lung	C33-34	48	12.5	6.3	3	4	10	17	35.4	31	64.6
Breast	C50	93	39.8	1.1	1	11	20	32	34.4	61	65.6
Cervix	C53*	275	17.5	0.4	1	29	43	73	26.5	202	73.5
Non-Hodgkin lymphoma	C82-85+C96	91	45.1	0.0	0	31	11	42	46.2	49	53.8

*HV: histologically verified; DCO: death certificate only; * random sample of total cases*

Table 2. Number and proportion of cases with complete/incomplete follow-up (in years) and median follow-up (in months) by site: The Gambia, 1993–1997 cases followed-up until 1999

Site	ICD-10	Cases included	Complete FU Alive/dead at end of FU		Incomplete FU: lost to FU		% lost to FU: years from diagnosis				% with complete FU at 5 years	Median FU (in months)
			No.	%	No.	%	< 1	1-3	3-5	> 5		
Stomach	C16	39	34	87.2	5	12.8	12.8	0.0	0.0	0.0	87.2	1.3
Liver	C22*	123	121	98.4	2	1.6	1.6	0.0	0.0	0.0	98.4	1.0
Lung	C33-34	31	25	80.6	6	19.4	19.4	0.0	0.0	0.0	80.6	0.8
Breast	C50	61	56	91.8	5	8.2	8.2	1.5	0.0	0.0	91.8	4.6
Cervix	C53*	202	193	95.5	9	4.5	4.5	0.0	0.0	0.0	95.5	5.6
Non-Hodgkin lymphoma	C82-85+C96	49	44	89.8	5	10.2	10.2	0.0	0.0	0.0	89.8	2.2

*FU: follow-up; * from a random sample of total cases*

Table 3. Comparison of 1-, 3- and 5-year absolute and relative survival and 5-year age-standardized relative survival by site: The Gambia, 1993–1997 cases followed-up until 1999

Site	ICD-10	Cases included	% Absolute survival			% Relative survival			% ASRS at 5-years	
			1-year	3-year	5-year	1-year	3-year	5-year	all ages	0-74 years
Stomach	C16	39	17.8	17.8	4.5	18.3	18.8	4.8	4.0	2.8
Liver	C22*	123	8.2	3.3	3.3	8.4	3.4	3.4	2.6	3.2
Lung	C33-34	31	25.0	25.0	25.0	25.8	28.9	32.1	49.8	19.7
Breast	C50	61	29.9	9.3	9.3	30.3	9.9	10.3	9.5	12.5
Cervix	C53*	202	44.3	22.4	22.4	44.8	23.0	23.6	22.9	21.8
Non-Hodgkin lymphoma	C82-85+C96	49	39.8	24.4	24.4	40.3	25.2	25.4	22.5	25.5

*ASRS: age-standardized relative survival; * random sample of total incident cases*

Table 4a. Site-wise number of cases, 5-year absolute and relative survival by sex: The Gambia, 1993–1997 cases followed-up until 1999

Site	ICD-10	Cases included	Male % 5-year survival			Female % 5-year survival		
			No.	Abs	Rel	No.	Abs	Rel
Stomach	C16	39	17	20.0	21.2	22	0.0	0.0
Liver	C22*	123	91	2.1	2.2	32		
Lung	C33-34	31	27	16.0	28.8	4	100.0	106.2
Breast	C50	61	2	0.0	0.0	59	9.7	10.8
Cervix	C53*	202				202	22.4	23.6
Non-Hodgkin lymphoma	C82-85+C96	49	30	17.9	18.6	19	37.8	39.2

*Abs: absolute survival; Rel: relative survival; * random sample of total cases*

Table 4b. Site-wise number of cases and relative survival by age group: The Gambia, 1993–1997 cases followed-up until 1999

Site	ICD-10	Cases included	Number of cases by age group					Relative survival by age group % 5-year survival				
			< 45	45-54	55-64	65-74	> 75	< 45	45-54	55-64	65-74	> 75
Stomach	C16	39	10	3	11	11	4	13.6	0.0	0.0		
Liver	C22*	123	50	27	26	15	5	3.7			0.0	0.0
Lung	C33-34	31	5	8	7	8	3		56.5	0.0		126.2
Breast	C50	61	26	18	9	5	3	16.3		0.0	35.5	0.0
Cervix	C53*	202	109	45	26	18	4	26.4	20.2	22.5	13.2	
Non-Hodgkin lymphoma	C82-85+C96	49	32	7	4	4	2	27.7	29.9		0.0	0.0

** random sample of total cases*

Chapter 12

Cancer survival in Barshi, India, 1993–2000

Jayant K, Nene BM, Dinshaw KA, Badwe RA, Panse NS, and Thorat RV

Abstract

The rural cancer registry of Barshi, Paranda and Bhum, was the first of its kind in India and was established in 1987. Registration of cases is carried out entirely by active methods. Data on survival from 15 cancer sites or types registered during 1993–2000 are reported in this study. Follow-up has been carried out predominantly by active methods, with median follow-up time ranging between 2–49 months for different cancers. The proportion of histologically verified diagnosis for various cancers ranged between 73–98%; death certificates only (DCOs) comprised 0–2%; 98–100% of total registered cases were included for survival analysis. Complete follow-up at five years ranged between 96–100% for different cancers. The 5-year age-standardized relative survival rates for selected cancers were non-melanoma skin (86%), penis (63%), breast (61%), cervix (32%), mouth (23%), hypopharynx (11%) and oesophagus (4%). The 5-year relative survival by age group did not display any particular pattern. Five-year relative survival trend between 1988–1992 and 1993–2000 showed a marked decrease for cancers of the tongue, hypopharynx, stomach, rectum, larynx, lung and penis; but a notable increase for breast and non-Hodgkin lymphoma.

Rural cancer registry: Barshi, Paranda and Bhum

The rural cancer registry of Barshi, Paranda and Bhum, is the first of its kind in India. It was established in 1987 at the Nargis Dutt Memorial Cancer Hospital, Barshi, in Maharashtra state. Data from the registry were published in the IARC publication *Cancer Incidence in Five Continents in volume VII* [1]. Cancer registration is entirely done by active methods. It is different from the registration practices of urban registries in that it relies heavily on interaction with the village community, health camps and other interventions apart from data collection from different medical institutions catering to the population [1,2]. The registry covers an area of 3713 km^2 and caters to a predominantly rural population of about 0.5 million in 2001 with a sex ratio of 926 females to 1000 males. The average annual age-standardized incidence rate is 44 per 100 000 among males and 52 per 100 000 among females with a lifetime cumulative risk of one in 16 of developing cancer for both sexes in the period 1999–2001 [3]. The top ranking cancers among males are hypopharynx followed by penis and oesophagus. Among females, the order is cervix, breast and oral cavity.

The registry contributed data on survival from cancer of the cervix registered in 1988–1992 for the first volume of the IARC publication on *Cancer Survival in Developing Countries* [4]. Data on survival from 15 cancer sites or types registered during 1993–2000 are reported in this second volume.

Data quality indices (Table 1)

The proportion of cases with histological confirmation of cancer diagnosis in this series is 87%, varying between 98% for myeloid leukaemia and cancer of the penis and 73% for cancer of the stomach. The proportion of cases registered as death certificates only (DCOs) is <1%, ranging between 0% for most cancers and 2% in liver/lung cancers. There are no cases without any follow-up. The exclusion of cases from the survival analysis ranged between none for most cancers and 2% for cancers of oesophagus, liver and lung. Thus, 98–100% of the total cases registered are included in the estimation of the survival probability.

Outcome of follow-up (Table 2)

Follow-up has been carried out predominantly by active methods. These included abstraction of cancer mortality information from hospitals and village death records. The abstracted data are first matched with the incident cancer database. The follow-up information for the unmatched incident cases is then obtained through postal enquiries and house visits.

The closing date of follow-up was 31st December 2003. The median follow-up (in months) ranged between 1.6 for liver cancer to 49.2 for cancer of non-melanoma skin. Complete follow-up at five years from the incidence date ranged between 96-100%. The losses to follow-up are very minimal and have occurred at varying intervals of time ranging from <1 year to >5 years.

Survival statistics

All ages and both sexes together (Table 3)

Non-melanoma skin cancer had the highest 5-year relative survival (83%), while none survived that period with liver cancer. The highest survival among head and neck cancers was observed in oral cavity (24%) followed by hypopharynx (11%) and tongue (10%). For the gastrointestinal tract cancers, the order is rectum (13%), stomach (6%) and oesophagus (5%). The survival figure for non-Hodgkin lymphoma is 25% and myeloid leukaemia is 15%.

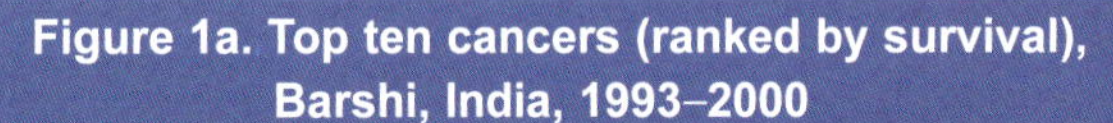

Figure 1a. Top ten cancers (ranked by survival), Barshi, India, 1993–2000

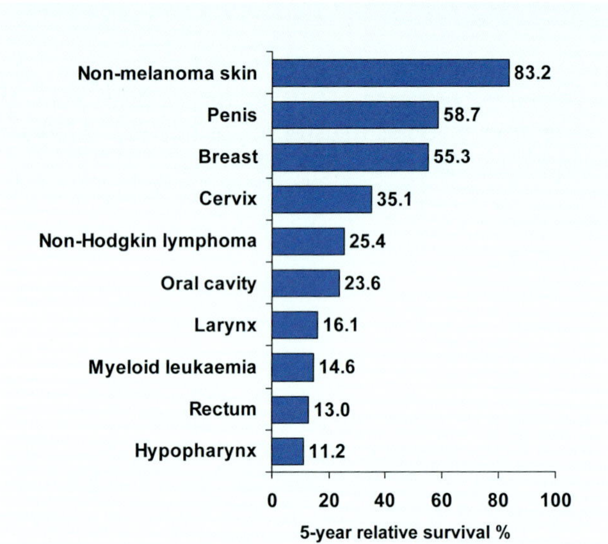

The 5-year age-standardized relative survival (ASRS) probability for all ages together is lesser than the corresponding unadjusted for a majority of cancers. The 5-year ASRS (0–74 years of age) is observed to be higher than the corresponding ASRS (all ages) with a few exceptions.

Sex

Male (Table 4a)

The 5-year relative survival was the highest for non-melanoma skin cancer (81%) followed by penis (59%). Survival from cancers of the hypopharynx and larynx was noticeably higher among males than females.

Figure 1b. Top five cancers (ranked by survival), Male, Barshi, India, 1993–2000

Non-melanoma skin 80.7
Penis 58.7
Breast 50.4
Oral cavity 22.0
Non-Hodgkin lymphoma 20.8
0 20 40 60 80 100
5-year relative survival %

Female (Table 4a)

The top-ranking cancers in terms of 5-year relative survival were non-melanoma skin (89%), breast (55%), cervix (35%) and non-Hodgkin lymphoma (33%). Survival was markedly higher among females than males for cancers of the tongue, oesophagus and stomach, and non-Hodgkin lymphoma.

Figure 1c. Top five cancers (ranked by survival), Female, Barshi, India, 1993–2000

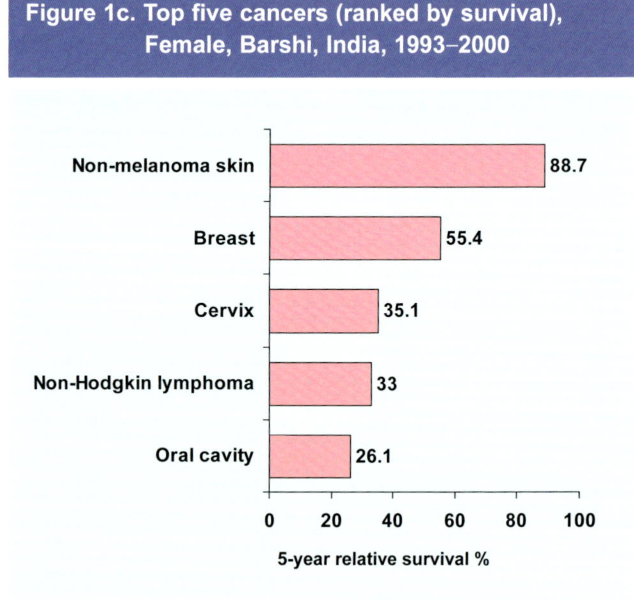

Age group (Table 4b)

The 5-year relative survival by age group does not display any particular pattern. This may be due to scanty number of cases in many age groups for most cancers.

Survival trend (Table 5)

The data on trends in survival are available for 15 cancer sites covering 13 years in two time periods between 1988–1992 [4] and 1993–2000. The completeness of follow-up at 5 years from incidence date was between 98–100% in both periods. The absolute difference in 5-year relative survival between 1988–1992 and 1993–2000 showed a marked decrease for cancers of tongue, hypopharynx, stomach, rectum, larynx, lung and penis. A notable increase in 5-year relative survival was seen in female breast cancer and non-Hodgkin lymphoma. In the rest, there has been little change.

Acknowledgements

The authors are thankful to the registry staff, Dr. A.M. Budukh, Dr.F.Y. Khan, Mr. S.R. Mathapati, Mr. N.V. Kesare, Mr. N.P. Gaikwad, Mr. D.R. Pise, Mr. T.S. Dudhankar and Mr. B.D. Honmane, for their diligent work.

References

1. Parkin DM, Whelan SL, Ferlay J and Storm H. *Cancer Incidence in Five Continents, Vol I to VIII: IARC Cancerbase No. 7*. IARCPress, Lyon, 2005.

2. Jayant K, Rao RS, Nene BM, Dale PS. *Population-based Rural Cancer Registry. Annual Report 1987–1988*, Tata Memorial Centre, Bombay, 1989.

3. *National Cancer Registry Programme. Consolidated report of population-based cancer registries: 1999–2001*. Indian Council of Medical Research, New Delhi, 2004.

4. Jayant K, Nene BM, Dinshaw KA, Budukh AM. Survival from cervical cancer in Barshi registry, rural India. In: *Cancer Survival in Developing Countries* (eds) R Sankaranarayanan, RJ Black and DM Parkin. IARC Scientific Publications No. 145. IARCPress, Lyon, 1998, pp 69–77.

Table 1. Data quality indices - Proportion of histologically verified and death certificate only cases, number and proportion of included and excluded cases by site: Barshi, India, 1993–2000 cases followed-up until 2003

Site	ICD-10	Total registered	%		Excluded cases					Included cases	
			HV	DCO	DCO	Follow-up	Others	Total	%	No.	%
Tongue	C01-02	47	87.2	0.0	0	0	0	0	0.0	47	100.0
Oral cavity	C03-06	55	94.5	0.0	0	0	0	0	0.0	55	100.0
Hypopharynx	C12-13	80	92.5	0.0	0	0	0	0	0.0	80	100.0
Oesophagus	C15	99	82.8	1.0	1	0	1	2	2.0	97	98.0
Stomach	C16	45	73.3	0.0	0	0	0	0	0.0	45	100.0
Rectum	C19-20	49	91.8	0.0	0	0	0	0	0.0	49	100.0
Liver	C22	48	83.3	2.1	1	0	0	1	2.1	47	97.9
Larynx	C32	33	87.9	0.0	0	0	0	0	0.0	33	100.0
Lung	C33-34	48	81.3	2.1	1	0	0	1	2.1	47	97.9
Other skin	C44	39	97.4	0.0	0	0	0	0	0.0	39	100.0
Breast	C50	124	91.1	0.0	0	0	0	0	0.0	124	100.0
Cervix	C53	407	94.8	0.0	0	0	1	1	0.2	406	99.8
Penis	C60	43	97.7	0.0	0	0	0	0	0.0	43	100.0
Non-Hodgkin lymphoma	C82-85+C96	36	91.7	0.0	0	0	0	0	0.0	36	100.0
Myeloid leukaemia	C92-94	40	97.5	0.0	0	0	0	0	0.0	40	100.0

HV: histologically verified; DCO: death certificate only

Table 2. Number and proportion of cases with complete/incomplete follow-up (in years) and median follow-up (in months) by site: Barshi, India, 1993–2000 cases followed-up until 2003

Site	ICD-10	Cases included	Complete FU Alive/dead at end of FU		Incomplete FU: lost to FU		% lost to FU: years from diagnosis				% with complete FU at 5 years	Median FU (in months)
			No.	%	No.	%	< 1	1-3	3-5	> 5		
Tongue	C01-02	47	47	100.0	0	0.0	0.0	0.0	0.0	0.0	100.0	9.5
Oral cavity	C03-06	55	53	96.4	2	3.6	0.0	1.8	1.8	0.0	96.4	10.1
Hypopharynx	C12-13	80	79	98.8	1	1.3	0.0	0.0	1.3	0.0	98.8	7.5
Oesophagus	C15	97	96	99.0	1	1.0	0.0	0.0	0.0	1.0	100.0	3.9
Stomach	C16	45	43	95.6	2	4.4	2.2	0.0	2.2	0.0	95.6	2.8
Rectum	C19-20	49	48	98.0	1	2.0	2.0	0.0	0.0	0.0	98.0	9.4
Liver	C22	47	47	100.0	0	0.0	0.0	0.0	0.0	0.0	100.0	1.6
Larynx	C32	33	32	97.0	1	3.0	3.0	0.0	0.0	0.0	97.0	12.1
Lung	C33-34	47	45	95.7	2	4.3	2.1	2.1	0.0	0.0	95.7	3.4
Other skin	C44	39	39	100.0	0	0.0	0.0	0.0	0.0	0.0	100.0	49.2
Breast	C50	124	119	96.0	5	4.0	0.0	0.0	3.2	0.8	96.8	41.4
Cervix	C53	406	403	99.3	3	0.7	0.2	0.0	0.2	0.2	99.5	24.4
Penis	C60	43	42	97.7	1	2.3	0.0	0.0	2.3	0.0	97.7	38.3
Non-Hodgkin lymphoma	C82-85+C96	36	36	100.0	0	0.0	0.0	0.0	0.0	0.0	100.0	9.8
Myeloid leukaemia	C92-94	40	40	100.0	0	0.0	0.0	0.0	0.0	0.0	100.0	4.0

FU: follow-up

Table 3. Comparison of 1-, 3- and 5-year absolute and relative survival and 5-year age-standardized relative survival by site: Barshi, India, 1993–2000 cases followed-up until 2003

Site	ICD-10	Cases included	% Absolute survival			% Relative survival			% ASRS at 5-years	
			1-year	3-year	5-year	1-year	3-year	5-year	all ages	0-74 years
Tongue	C01-02	47	46.8	8.5	8.5	48.5	9.5	9.9	10.4	11.8
Oral cavity	C03-06	55	45.5	30.6	21.7	46.7	32.4	23.6	22.9	26.1
Hypopharynx	C12-13	80	32.5	11.3	8.4	34.1	13.1	11.2	11.0	10.0
Oesophagus	C15	97	19.6	4.1	4.1	20.4	4.7	5.2	4.2	5.3
Stomach	C16	45	16.9	4.8	4.8	17.4	5.5	6.5	6.5	6.0
Rectum	C19-20	49	46.4	16.9	11.2	47.8	18.4	13.0	9.2	14.7
Liver	C22	47	2.1	0.0	0.0	2.2	0.0	0.0	0.0	0.0
Larynx	C32	33	53.8	19.0	12.7	56.6	22.3	16.1	12.7	15.7
Lung	C33-34	47	18.3	4.6	4.6	19.0	5.2	5.2	3.8	5.3
Other skin	C44	39	87.2	71.8	65.0	91.2	83.3	83.2	86.2	75.3
Breast	C50	124	81.5	55.6	49.2	83.3	59.6	55.3	61.4	52.7
Cervix	C53	406	70.7	38.3	32.2	72.0	40.4	35.1	32.1	35.7
Penis	C60	43	81.4	51.2	44.7	85.6	59.9	58.7	63.1	64.1
Non-Hodgkin lymphoma	C82-85+C96	36	41.7	27.8	22.2	42.5	30.0	25.4	24.1	25.9
Myeloid leukaemia	C92-94	40	37.5	27.5	13.6	37.9	28.5	14.6	19.5	19.5

ASRS: age-standardized relative survival

Table 4a. Site-wise number of cases, 5-year absolute and relative survival by sex: Barshi, India, 1993–2000 cases followed-up until 2003

Site	ICD-10	Cases included	Male	% 5-year survival		Female	% 5-year survival	
			No.	Abs	Rel	No.	Abs	Rel
Tongue	C01-02	47	33	3.0	3.7	14	21.4	23.4
Oral cavity	C03-06	55	35	20.1	22.0	20	24.2	26.1
Hypopharynx	C12-13	80	71	9.7	13.0	9	0.0	0.0
Oesophagus	C15	97	57	0.0	0.0	40	10.0	12.8
Stomach	C16	45	28	0.0	0.0	17	11.8	16.0
Rectum	C19-20	49	32	9.5	11.3	17	14.1	15.7
Liver	C22	47	44	0.0	0.0	3	0.0	0.0
Larynx	C32	33	28	15.1	19.0	5	0.0	0.0
Lung	C33-34	47	31	3.6	3.9	16		
Other skin	C44	39	23	60.9	80.7	16	72.3	88.7
Breast	C50	124	3	33.3	50.4	121	49.6	55.4
Cervix	C53	406				406	32.2	35.1
Penis	C60	43	43	44.7	58.7			
Non-Hodgkin lymphoma	C82-85+C96	36	26	17.9	20.8	10	30.0	33.0
Myeloid leukaemia	C92-94	40	28	12.9	14.0	12	16.7	17.2

Abs: absolute survival; Rel: relative survival

Table 4b. Site-wise number of cases and relative survival by age group: Barshi, India, 1993–2000 cases followed-up until 2003

Site	ICD-10	Cases included	Number of cases by age group					Relative survival by age group % 5-year survival				
			< 45	45-54	55-64	65-74	> 75	< 45	45-54	55-64	65-74	> 75
Tongue	C01-02	47	7	6	18	15	1	14.5	17.5	13.1	0.0	0.0
Oral cavity	C03-06	55	17	13	11	10	4	28.2	22.0	51.0	0.0	0.0
Hypopharynx	C12-13	80	9	8	22	31	10	11.4	13.2	5.3	13.8	19.4
Oesophagus	C15	97	7	16	32	32	10	0.0	6.6		8.7	0.0
Stomach	C16	45	8	7	14	13	3	0.0	0.0		11.6	
Rectum	C19-20	49	14	10	10	11	4	0.0	42.8	0.0	21.8	0.0
Liver	C22	47	2	10	18	11	6	0.0	0.0	0.0	0.0	0.0
Larynx	C32	33	7	5	6	9	6	29.4	29.9	0.0	16.4	0.0
Lung	C33-34	47	8	10	10	12	7	15.3	0.0	0.0		0.0
Other skin	C44	39	5	5	13	11	5	40.8	84.6	78.7	91.7	116.7
Breast	C50	124	26	42	29	22	5	42.4	61.3	40.3	75.1	116.7
Cervix	C53	406	109	106	115	67	9	37.9	37.0	40.4	19.7	0.0
Penis	C60	43	8	3	10	16	6	51.2	106.3	46.0	62.8	64.3
Non-Hodgkin lymphoma	C82-85+C96	36	14	7	8	7	0	29.1		42.0	13.4	
Myeloid leukaemia	C92-94	40	23	10	3	4	0	12.3	7.1	79.8	0.0	

Table 5. Comparison of 5-year absolute and relative survival of cases diagnosed between 1988–1992 and 1993–2000, Barshi, India

Site	ICD-10	% 5-year absolute survival		% 5-year relative survival	
		1988–1992	1993–2000	1988–1992	1993–2000
Tongue	C01-02	13.6	8.5	26.4	9.9
Oral cavity	C03-06	18.7	21.7	28.1	23.6
Hypopharynx	C12-13	19.9	8.4	40.1	11.2
Oesophagus	C15	6.3	4.1	11.3	5.2
Stomach	C16	13.3	4.8	16.9	6.5
Rectum	C19-20	17.3	11.2	24.0	13.0
Liver	C22	5.0	0.0	6.4	0.0
Larynx	C32	19.6	12.7	36.1	16.1
Lung	C33-34	14.3	4.6	20.1	5.2
Other skin	C44	52.4	65.0	88.3	83.2
Breast	C50	32.4	49.2	45.1	55.3
Cervix	C53	28.4	32.2	37.3	35.1
Penis	C60	46.7	44.7	73.8	58.7
Non-Hodgkin lymphoma	C82-85+C96	8.9	22.2	11.2	25.4
Myeloid leukaemia	C92-94	6.7	13.6	7.5	14.6

Chapter 13

Cancer survival in Bhopal, India, 1991–1995

Dikshit R, Kanhere S and Surange S

Abstract

The Bhopal population-based cancer registry was established in 1986 under the national cancer registry programme to investigate the after-effect of a gas leak in 1984. Cancer registration is done entirely by active methods. The registry is contributing data on survival for 16 cancer sites or types registered during 1991–1995. Follow-up of cases was done by active methods with median follow-up time ranging between 8–44 months for different cancers. The proportion with histologically verified diagnosis for various cancers ranged between 61–100%; death certificates only (DCOs) comprised 0–2%; 50–92% of total registered cases were included for survival analysis. The 5-year age-standardized relative survival rates for common cancers were mouth (34%), cervix (31%), breast (25%), tongue (12%), oesophagus (3%) and lung (1%). The 5-year relative survival by age group showed that survival was the highest in the youngest age group (45 years and below) for a majority of cancers. A decreasing survival with increasing clinical extent of disease was noted for most cancers studied.

Bhopal cancer registry

The Bhopal population-based cancer registry is the only one of its kind in the central part of India. It was established in 1986 as a special purpose registry at the Gandhi medical college, Bhopal, under the national cancer registry programme, to investigate the after-effect of the gas leak in 1984. Data from the registry have been regularly published by the Indian Council of Medical Research [1]. The method of cancer registration is entirely done by active methods. The registry staff visits the various medical institutions in and around Bhopal city for data collection by direct interview of cases and/or from medical records [2]. The registry covers an area of 285 km^2 and caters to an entirely urban population of about 1.4 million in 2001 with a sex ratio of 893 females to 1000 males. The average annual age-standardized incidence rate is 114 per 100 000 among males and 104 per 100 000 among females with a lifetime cumulative risk of one in 10 of developing cancer for both sexes in the period 1999–2001. The leading site of cancer among males is the lung followed by oral cavity and oesophagus. The ranking among females is breast followed by cervix and oral cavity [1].

The registry is contributing data on survival from cancer for the first time in this volume of the IARC monograph on *Cancer Survival in Africa, Asia, the Caribbean and Central America*. Data on survival from 16 cancer sites or types registered during 1991–1995 are reported.

Data quality indices (Table 1)

The proportion of cases with histological confirmation of cancer diagnosis in this series is 84%, from 100% for non-Hodgkin lymphoma and lymphoid leukaemia to 61% for lung cancer. Cases without any follow-up comprised 19%, with a low of 6% (colon cancer) and a high of 48% (non-Hodgkin lymphoma). The exclusion of cases from the survival analysis ranged between 8% and 50%. Thus, 50–92% of the total cases registered are included in the estimation of the survival probability.

Outcome of follow-up (Table 2)

Follow-up has been carried out predominantly by active methods. These included abstraction of cancer mortality information from the hospitals and the vital statistics division records. The abstracted data are first matched with the incident cancer database. The follow-up information for the unmatched incident cases is then obtained through house visits.

The closing date of follow-up was 31st December 2000. The median follow-up (in months) ranged between 8.3 for cancer of the oesophagus and 44.1 for cancer of the cervix. No partial information is available on follow-up within five years from the incidence date. Cases with no follow-up have been excluded; hence, all the reported cases have a complete follow-up at five years from the incidence date.

Survival statistics

All ages and both sexes together (Table 3)

The 5-year relative survival is the highest in cervix cancer (35%) and the lowest in lung cancer (1%). The survival figures for head and neck cancers are oral cavity (34%), tongue (11%) and hypopharynx (2%). The rank order among the gastrointestinal tract cancers is rectum (9%), colon (7%), oesophagus (4%) and stomach (3%). The survival from non-Hodgkin lymphoma is 11%, lymphoid leukaemia is 10% and myeloid leukaemia is 17%.

Figure 1a. Top ten cancers (ranked by survival), Bhopal, India, 1991–1995

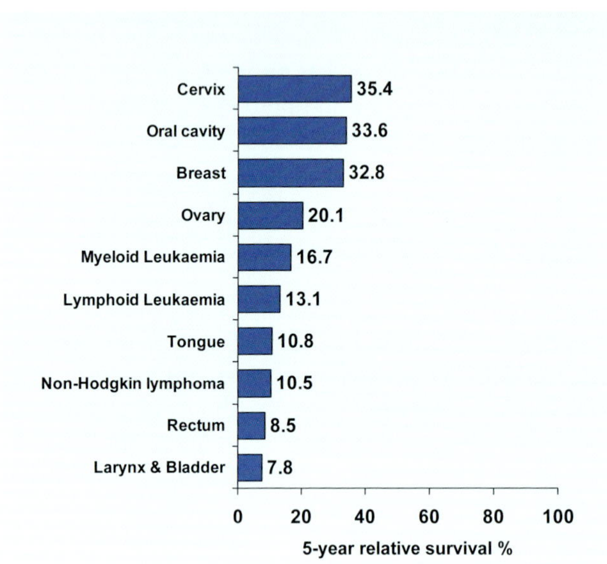

The 5-year age-standardized relative survival (ASRS) probability for all ages together was observed to be less than the corresponding unadjusted one barring a few exceptions. The 5-year ASRS (0–74 years of age) was observed to be higher than the corresponding ASRS (all ages) for all cancers.

Sex
Male (Table 4a)

The 5-year relative survival was the highest for male breast cases (75%; 3 cases) followed by oral cavity (35%) and lymphoid leukaemia (16%). Survival from cancer of the urinary bladder and lymphoid leukaemia was noticeably higher among males than females.

Figure 1b. Top five cancers (ranked by survival), Male, Bhopal, India, 1991–1995

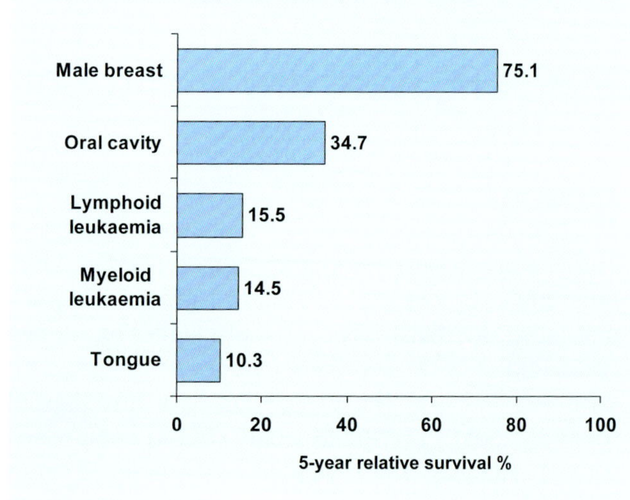

Female (Table 4a)

Non-Hodgkin lymphoma (61%; 5 cases) tops the ranking by 5-year relative survival; the others in order are cervix (35%), breast (32%) and oral cavity (31%). Survival was distinctly higher among females than males with non-Hodgkin lymphoma.

Figure 1c. Top five cancers (ranked by survival), Female, Bhopal, India, 1991–1995

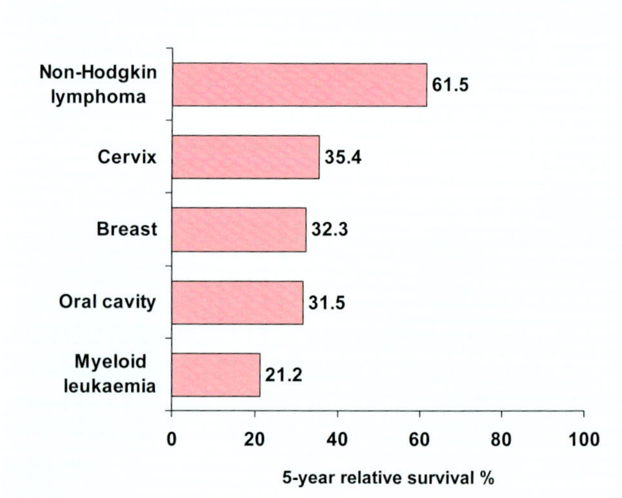

Age group (Table 4b)

The 5-year relative survival analysis by age group indicates that no case aged 75 years and above at diagnosis has survived 5 years after diagnosis. The number of cases was also the least in this age group. Survival was the highest in the younger age group of 45 years and below for a majority of cancers.

Extent of disease (Table 5; Figure 2)

A majority of cases with tongue and oral cavity cancers were diagnosed with a regional spread of disease (56%). For cancers of the colon and rectum, most cases presented with a localized disease (38% and 41%). For breast cancer, both localized (43%) and regional (44%) disease constituted equal proportions. Two thirds of ovarian cancers were diagnosed at a localized stage and 70% of cervix cancers had a regional spread. The extent of disease was unknown in 1–17%. The 5-year absolute survival by extent of disease revealed that none of the cases with distant metastasis at diagnosis survived 5 years for any cancer. Breast cancer cases with unknown extent of disease and ovarian cancer cases with regional spread had a higher or same 5-year survival probability as that of a localized disease.

Acknowledgements

The authors are grateful to all the staff of Bhopal Cancer Registry for their excellent work.

References

1. *National Cancer Registry Programme. Consolidated report of population-based cancer registries: 1999–2001.* Indian Council of Medical Research, New Delhi, 2004.

2. *Bhopal Cancer Registry. Incidence of cancer morbidity and mortality in Bhopal Urban Agglomerate: 1995–1999.* Gandhi Medical College, Bhopal, 2003.

Figure 2. Absolute survival (%) from selected cancers by extent of disease, Bhopal, India

Figure 2a. Tongue

Figure 2e. Breast

Figure 2b. Oral cavity

Figure 2f. Cervix

Figure 2c. Colon

Figure. 2g. Ovary

Figure 2d. Rectum

Table 1. Data quality indices - Proportion of histologically verified and death certificate only cases, number and proportion of included and excluded cases by site: Bhopal, India, 1991–1995 cases followed-up until 2000

Site	ICD-10	Total registered	%		Excluded cases					Included cases	
			HV	DCO	DCO	Follow-up	Others	Total	%	No.	%
Tongue	C01-02	151	90.1	0.7	1	20	3	24	15.9	127	84.1
Oral cavity	C03-06	204	89.2	0.0	0	32	0	32	15.7	172	84.3
Hypopharynx	C12-13	131	92.4	0.0	0	13	0	13	9.9	118	90.1
Oesophagus	C15	189	83.1	1.6	3	22	1	26	13.8	163	86.2
Stomach	C16	87	65.5	0.0	0	11	1	12	13.8	75	86.2
Colon	C18	52	90.4	1.9	1	3	0	4	7.7	48	92.3
Rectum	C19-20	52	80.8	1.9	1	11	1	13	25.0	39	75.0
Larynx	C32	70	87.1	1.4	1	9	0	10	14.3	60	85.7
Lung	C33-34	253	60.5	1.6	4	31	2	37	14.6	216	85.4
Breast	C50	348	87.9	0.6	2	84	1	87	25.0	261	75.0
Cervix	C53	380	83.4	0.3	1	46	1	48	12.6	332	87.4
Ovary	C56	104	82.7	0.0	0	34	1	35	33.7	69	66.3
Urinary bladder	C67	52	84.6	0.0	0	6	0	6	11.5	46	88.5
Non-Hodgkin lymphoma	C82-85+C96	60	100.0	0.0	0	29	1	30	50.0	30	50.0
Lymphoid leukaemia	C91	45	100.0	0.0	0	13	0	13	28.9	32	71.1
Myeloid leukaemia	C92-94	85	96.5	2.4	2	8	0	10	11.8	75	88.2

HV: histologically verified; DCO: death certificate only

Table 2. Number and proportion of cases by vital status and median follow-up (in months) by site: Bhopal, India, 1991–1995 cases followed-up until 2000

Site	ICD-10	Cases included	Dead		Alive		Complete FU		Median FU (in months)
			No.	%	No.	%	No.	%	
Tongue	C01-02	127	124	97.6	3	2.4	127	100.0	12.7
Oral cavity	C03-06	172	145	84.3	27	15.7	172	100.0	34.0
Hypopharynx	C12-13	118	117	99.2	1	0.8	118	100.0	11.8
Oesophagus	C15	163	161	98.8	2	1.2	163	100.0	8.3
Stomach	C16	75	75	100.0	0	0.0	75	100.0	8.7
Colon	C18	48	47	97.9	1	2.1	48	100.0	13.1
Rectum	C19-20	39	36	92.3	3	7.7	39	100.0	12.6
Larynx	C32	60	59	98.3	1	1.7	60	100.0	18.8
Lung	C33-34	216	215	99.5	1	0.5	216	100.0	8.5
Breast	C50	261	216	82.8	45	17.2	261	100.0	42.5
Cervix	C53	332	288	86.7	44	13.3	332	100.0	44.1
Ovary	C56	69	64	92.8	5	7.2	69	100.0	26.0
Urinary bladder	C67	46	46	100.0	0	0.0	46	100.0	13.1
Non-Hodgkin lymphoma	C82-85+C96	30	28	93.3	2	6.7	30	100.0	8.4
Lymphoid leukaemia	C91	32	30	93.8	2	6.3	32	100.0	9.9
Myeloid leukaemia	C92-94	75	71	94.7	4	5.3	75	100.0	19.0

FU: follow-up

Table 3. Comparison of 1-, 3- and 5-year absolute and relative survival and 5-year age-standardized relative survival by site: Bhopal, India, 1991–1995 cases followed-up until 2000

Site	ICD-10	Cases included	% Absolute survival			% Relative survival			% ASRS at 5-years	
			1-year	3-year	5-year	1-year	3-year	5-year	all ages	0-74 years
Tongue	C01-02	127	52.8	20.5	9.4	54.8	22.6	10.8	11.7	13.1
Oral cavity	C03-06	172	80.2	45.9	29.1	83.0	50.4	33.6	33.9	37.5
Hypopharynx	C12-13	118	50.8	16.9	1.7	52.7	18.6	2.0	1.7	2.0
Oesophagus	C15	163	36.2	12.9	3.1	37.6	14.1	3.5	2.7	3.6
Stomach	C16	75	38.7	5.3	2.7	39.8	5.8	2.9	2.8	3.8
Colon	C18	48	52.1	25.0	6.3	53.9	27.1	7.0	3.2	5.2
Rectum	C19-20	39	56.4	25.6	7.7	58.0	27.2	8.5	4.0	6.5
Larynx	C32	60	61.7	23.3	6.7	63.6	25.4	7.8	12.5	15.7
Lung	C33-34	216	33.3	6.9	0.9	34.7	7.7	1.1	0.8	1.0
Breast	C50	261	83.1	62.1	30.7	84.5	64.8	32.8	25.3	30.6
Cervix	C53	332	88.9	66.0	33.1	90.3	68.8	35.4	30.8	34.5
Ovary	C56	69	63.8	47.8	18.8	64.8	49.7	20.1	15.8	18.9
Urinary bladder	C67	46	54.3	17.4	6.5	57.1	19.6	7.8	6.0	9.7
Non-Hodgkin lymphoma	C82-85+C96	30	33.3	16.7	10.0	33.9	17.3	10.5	8.8	9.9
Lymphoid leukaemia	C91	32	46.9	31.3	12.5	47.5	32.1	13.1	10.4	12.6
Myeloid leukaemia	C92-94	75	61.3	33.3	16.0	62.0	34.3	16.7	12.3	14.2

ASRS: age-standardized relative survival

Table 4a. Site-wise number of cases, 5-year absolute and relative survival by sex: Bhopal, India, 1991–1995 cases followed-up until 2000

Site	ICD-10	Cases included	Male % 5-year survival			Female % 5-year survival		
			No.	Abs	Rel	No.	Abs	Rel
Tongue	C01-02	127	112	8.9	10.3	15	13.3	14.4
Oral cavity	C03-06	172	110	30.0	34.7	62	27.4	31.5
Hypopharynx	C12-13	118	103	1.9	2.3	15	0.0	0.0
Oesophagus	C15	163	99	4.0	4.6	64	1.6	1.7
Stomach	C16	75	47	4.3	4.7	28	0.0	0.0
Colon	C18	48	31	6.5	7.4	17	5.9	6.2
Rectum	C19-20	39	21	4.8	5.4	18	11.1	11.7
Larynx	C32	60	51	5.9	6.9	9	11.1	12.6
Lung	C33-34	216	183	1.1	1.3	33	0.0	0.0
Breast	C50	261	3	66.7	75.1	258	30.2	32.3
Cervix	C53	332				332	33.1	35.4
Ovary	C56	69				69	18.8	20.1
Urinary bladder	C67	46	36	8.3	10.1	10	0.0	0.0
Non-Hodgkin lymphoma	C82-85+C96	30	25	0.0	0.0	5	60.0	61.5
Lymphoid leukaemia	C91	32	27	14.8	15.5	5	0.0	0.0
Myeloid leukaemia	C92-94	75	50	14.0	14.5	25	20.0	21.2

Abs: absolute survival; Rel: relative survival

Table 4b. Site-wise number of cases and relative survival by age group: Bhopal, India, 1991–1995 cases followed-up until 2000

Site	ICD-10	Cases included	Number of cases by age group					Relative survival by age group % 5-year survival				
			< 45	45-54	55-64	65-74	> 75	< 45	45-54	55-64	65-74	> 75
Tongue	C01-02	127	16	29	43	27	12	44.9	7.4	8.2	0.0	0.0
Oral cavity	C03-06	172	20	57	43	39	13	61.5	35.5	40.5	14.1	0.0
Hypopharynx	C12-13	118	16	31	38	22	11	0.0	3.5	3.1	0.0	0.0
Oesophagus	C15	163	18	43	46	38	18	11.4	7.4	0.0	0.0	0.0
Stomach	C16	75	10	29	15	16	5	20.3	0.0	0.0	0.0	0.0
Colon	C18	48	8	14	14	8	4	12.7	15.1	0.0	0.0	0.0
Rectum	C19-20	39	7	10	15	6	1	14.6	10.5	7.8	0.0	0.0
Larynx	C32	60	5	15	30	6	4	20.6	0.0	3.9	44.2	0.0
Lung	C33-34	216	20	44	74	58	20	0.0	4.9	0.0	0.0	0.0
Breast	C50	261	80	90	61	22	8	44.5	29.0	35.1	5.9	0.0
Cervix	C53	332	114	109	70	30	9	51.7	33.5	20.8	17.9	0.0
Ovary	C56	69	29	18	13	7	2	28.0	17.3	8.7	22.9	0.0
Urinary bladder	C67	46	1	11	16	9	9	0.0	9.6	7.2	15.4	0.0
Non-Hodgkin lymphoma	C82-85+C96	30	12	9	6	3	0	16.9	11.7	0.0	0.0	
Lymphoid leukaemia	C91	32	25	2	3	1	1	12.2	0.0	39.2	0.0	0.0
Myeloid leukaemia	C92-94	75	54	10	8	1	2	18.8	10.7	14.1	0.0	0.0

Table 5. Proportion of cases and 5-year absolute survival by extent of disease and site: Bhopal, India, 1991–1995

Site	ICD-10	Cases included	% of cases by extent of disease				% 5-year absolute survival			
			Localized	Regional	Dist. met.	Unknown	Localized	Regional	Dist. met.	Unknown
Tongue	C01-02	127	39.4	55.9	0.0	4.7	16.0	5.6		0.0
Oral cavity	C03-06	172	40.7	55.8	0.6	2.9	45.7	17.7	0.0	20.0
Colon	C18	48	37.5	27.1	18.8	16.7	11.1	7.7	0.0	0.0
Rectum	C19-20	39	41.0	33.3	15.4	10.3	12.5	7.7	0.0	0.0
Breast	C50	261	42.9	44.1	5.7	7.3	41.1	22.6	0.0	42.1
Cervix	C53	332	28.3	70.5	0.3	0.9	60.6	22.7	0.0	0.0
Ovary	C56	69	66.7	8.7	13.0	11.6	21.7	33.3	0.0	12.5

Dis. met.: distant metastasis

Chapter 14

Cancer survival in Chennai (Madras), India, 1990–1999

Swaminathan R, Rama R, Nalini S and Shanta V

Abstract

The Madras metropolitan tumour registry was established in 1981, and registration of incident cancer cases is entirely done by active method. Data on survival for 20 cancer sites or types registered during 1990–1999 are reported. Follow-up has been carried out predominantly by active methods with a median follow-up time ranging between 2–28 months for different cancers. The proportion of histologically verified diagnosis for various cancers ranged between 45–100%; death certificates only (DCOs) comprised 0–5%; 68–95% of total registered cases were included for survival analysis. Complete follow-up at five years ranged between 83–96%. The 5-year age-standardized relative survival rates for common cancers were cervix (60%), breast (47%), stomach (8%), oesophagus (9%), lung (6%) and mouth (36%). The 5-year relative survival by age group portrayed either an inverse relationship or fluctuated. A majority of cases were diagnosed with regional spread of disease, and survival decreased with increasing extent of disease. The absolute difference in 5-year relative survival of most cancers diagnosed in 1984–1989 and 1990–1999 ranged between 2–3%, with lesser survival in the latest period in most instances.

Madras metropolitan tumour registry

The population-based cancer registry in Chennai (Madras), known as the Madras metropolitan tumour registry (MMTR), is one of the oldest in India. It was established in 1981 at the Cancer Institute (WIA), a Regional Cancer Centre, where a hospital cancer registry has been established since 1955. MMTR has been contributing data to the quinquennial IARC publication *Cancer Incidence in Five Continents* since volume V [1]. The method of cancer registration is entirely done by active methods [2]. Over 200 sources of registration comprising hospitals in the government and private sectors, nursing homes, pathology laboratories, imaging centres and hospices are visited for data collection. The registry caters to an entirely urban population of about 4.3 million in 2005 with a sex ratio of 940 females to 1000 males. The average annual age-standardized incidence rate is 112 per 100 000 among males and 121 per 100 000 among females, with a lifetime cumulative risk of one in 8 of developing cancer for both sexes in the period 1999–2001 [3]. The top-ranking cancers among males are stomach followed by lung and oesophagus. Among females, the order is cervix, breast and ovary.

The registry contributed data on survival from the top ten cancers in the region and cancers associated with tobacco in the first volume of the IARC publication on *Cancer Survival in Developing Countries* [4]. Data on survival from 20 cancer sites or types registered during 1990–1999 are reported in this second volume.

Data quality indices (Table 1)

The proportion of cases with histological confirmation of cancer diagnosis in this series is 79%, varying between 99.6% for lymphoid leukaemia and 45% for cancer of the pancreas. The proportion of cases registered as death certificates only (DCOs) was 2%, ranging between 0% in lip cancer and 23% in leukaemia unspecified. The exclusion of cases from the survival analysis was the greatest among unspecified leukaemia (32%) and the least for cancer of the tonsil (5%). Thus, 68–95% of the total cases registered are included in the estimation of the survival probability.

Outcome of follow-up (Table 2)

Follow-up has been carried out predominantly by active methods. These included abstraction of mortality information, irrespective of the stated cause of death in the death certificate, from the hospitals and the vital statistics division of Chennai corporation records. The abstracted data are first matched with the incident cancer database. The follow-up information for the unmatched incident cases is then obtained through one or more of the following ways: repeated scrutiny of records in the respective sources of registration, postal/telephone enquiries and house visits.

The closing date of follow-up was 31st December 2001. The median follow-up (in months) ranged between 1.5 for unspecified leukaemia to 27.5 for cancer of the cervix. Complete follow-up at five years from the incidence date ranged from 96.3% (cancer of the pancreas) to 79.2% (ovarian cancer). The losses to follow-up generally occurred in the first year of follow-up for a majority of cancers. However, a substantial proportion of cases have been known to be alive for varying periods of time between 1–5 years and more than 5 years. This minimizes the bias in the estimation of survival probability in the respective years.

Survival statistics

All ages and both sexes together (Table 3)

The 5-year relative survival is the highest for lip cancer (47%) and the lowest for cancer of the hypopharynx (15%) among the cancers of the head and neck. Cancers of the stomach, pancreas and oesophagus had the survival figures of 10%, 9% and 8%, respectively. Hodgkin lymphoma had a better survival rate (41%) than non-Hodgkin lymphoma (24%). The survival figures for leukaemias are lymphoid (25%), myeloid (16%) and unspecified (12%).

Figure 1a. Top ten cancers (ranked by survival), Chennai, India, 1990–1999

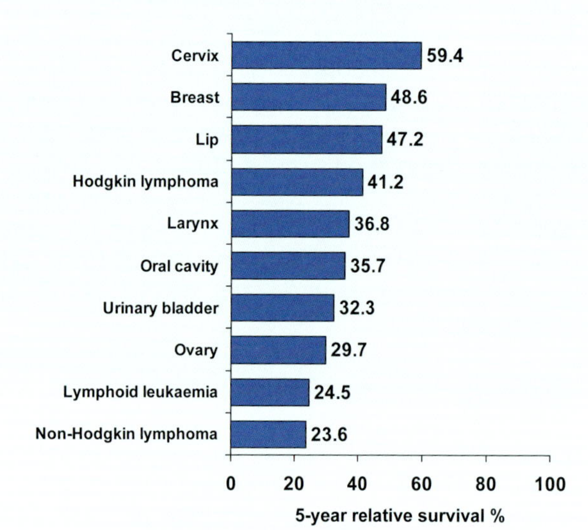

The 5-year age-standardized relative survival (ASRS) probability for all ages together is less than or similar to the corresponding unadjusted for a majority of cancers. The 5-year ASRS (0–74 years of age) is observed to be higher than the corresponding ASRS (all ages) with a few exceptions.

Sex

Male (Table 4a)

The 5-year relative survival was the highest for lip cancer (52%) followed in order by Hodgkin lymphoma (38%), larynx and oral cavity (37%). Survival from lip cancer was noticeably higher among males than females (41%).

Figure 1b. Top five cancers (ranked by survival), Male, Chennai, India, 1990–1999

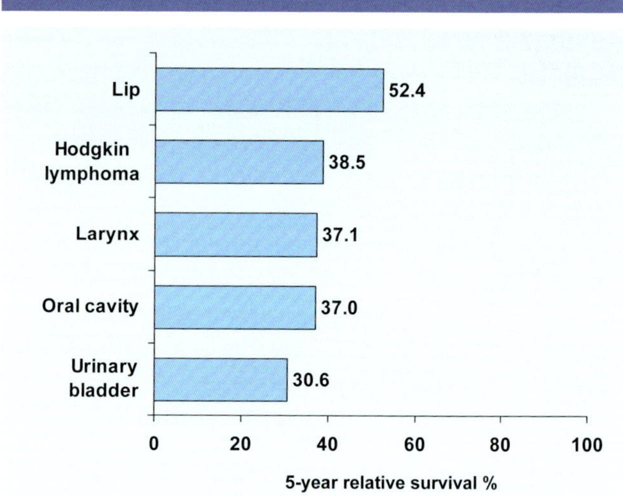

Female (Table 4a)

The top ranking cancers on 5-year relative survival are cervix (59%), breast (49%), Hodgkin lymphoma (47%) and lip (41%). The survival is markedly higher among females (32%) than males (14%) for cancer of the tonsil.

Figure 1c. Top five cancers (ranked by survival), Female, Chennai, India, 1990–1999

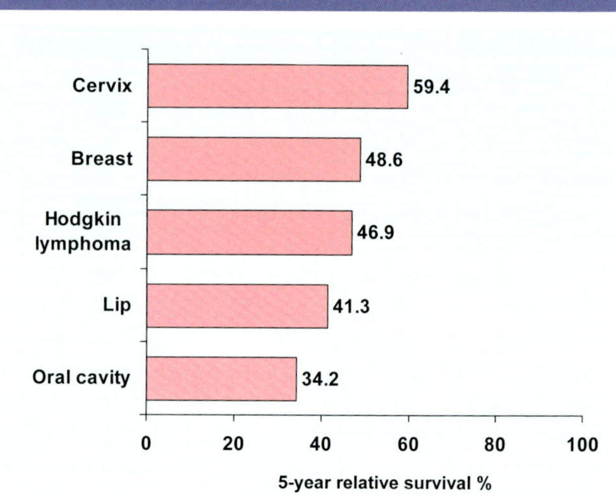

Age group (Table 4b)

The 5-year relative survival by age group portrays an inverse relationship: a decreasing survival with increasing age at diagnosis for cancers of the hypopharynx, stomach, larynx, lung and ovary. In the majority, it is seen to fluctuate, especially with an increase in the age group of 75+ years compared to that of 65–74 years.

Extent of disease (Table 5; Figure 2)

A majority of cases have been diagnosed with a regional spread of disease among all the selected cancers: from 62% (cancer of the ovary) to 89% (oral cavity). Correspondingly, a meagre 1% (ovary) to 7% (larynx) had a localized disease at diagnosis. The highest proportion of cases with distant metastasis at diagnosis is observed for breast cancer (13%). The extent of disease was unknown in 4–18%. The 5-year absolute survival by extent of disease followed the expected pattern: highest for localized cases followed by regional and distant metastasis cases among known categories of extent of disease.

Figure 2. Absolute survival (%) from selected cancers by extent of disease, Chennai, India

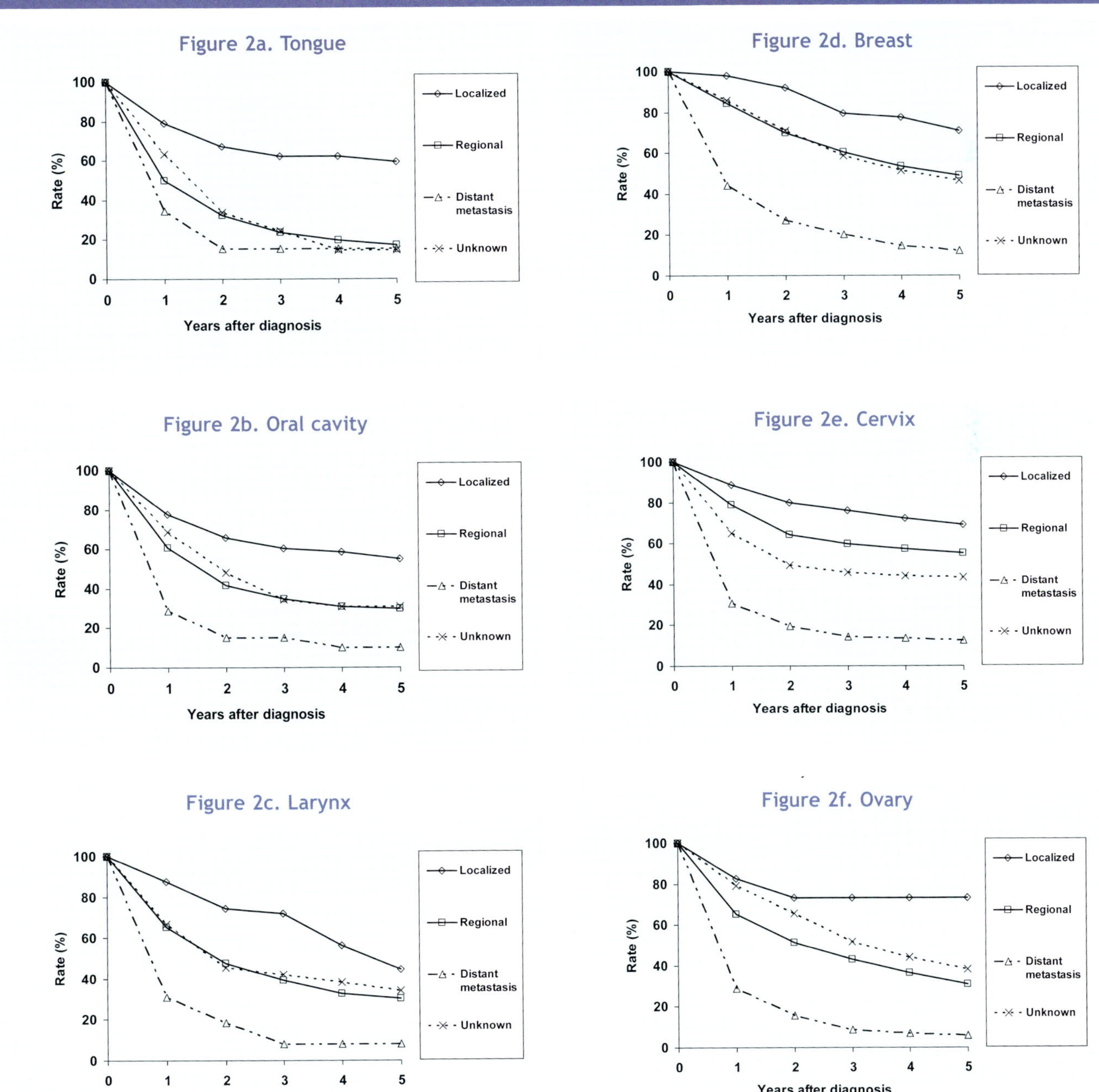

Survival trend (Table 6)

The data on trend in survival are available for 17 cancers spanning 16 years in two time periods between 1984–1989 [4] and 1990–1999. The completeness of follow-up at 5 years from incidence date was higher in 1990–1999 than 1984–1989 for a majority of cancers. In the rest, there was not much change. The absolute difference in 5-year relative survival of most cancers diagnosed between 1984–1989 and 1990–1999 ranged 2–3%, with a lesser survival in the latest period in most instances. This may be attributable to the increase in the completeness of follow-up for cases diagnosed in 1990–1999 due to the matching of incident cases with all deaths occurring in the city of Chennai, irrespective of the cause of death, since 1992. A notable increase in survival in 1990–1999 compared to 1984–1989 was observed only for cancer of the urinary bladder.

Acknowledgements

The authors express their sincere thanks to the staff of MMTR and the institutions providing data to MMTR, without which this study would not have become a reality.

References

1. Parkin DM, Whelan SL, Ferlay J and Storm H. *Cancer Incidence in Five Continents, Vol I to VIII: IARC Cancerbase No. 7.* IARCPress, Lyon, 2005.

2. Shanta V, Gajalakshmi CK, Swaminathan R, Ravichandran K, Vasanthi L. Cancer registration in Madras Metropolitan Tumour Registry, India. *Eur J Cancer*. 1994; 30: 974–978.

3. Shanta V, Swaminathan R. *Cancer incidence and mortality in Chennai, India: 1999–2001.* National Cancer Registry Programme, Cancer Institute (WIA), Chennai, 2004.

4. Shanta V, Gajalakshmi CK, Swaminathan R. Cancer survival in Chennai (Madras), India. In: *Cancer Survival in Developing Countries* (eds) R Sankaranarayanan, RJ Black and DM Parkin. IARC Scientific Publications No. 145. IARCPress, Lyon, 1998, pp 89–100.

Table 1. Data quality indices - Proportion of histologically verified and death certificate only cases, number and proportion of included and excluded cases by site: Chennai, India, 1990–1999 cases followed-up to 2001

Site	ICD-10	Total registered	%		Excluded cases					Included cases	
			HV	DCO	DCO	Follow-up	Others	Total	%	No.	%
Lip	C00	92	76.1	0.0	0	6	0	6	6.5	86	93.5
Tongue	C01-02	1 073	78.4	1.1	12	73	0	85	7.9	988	92.1
Oral cavity	C03-06	1 776	75.7	0.5	9	105	0	114	6.4	1 662	93.6
Tonsil	C09	262	80.5	0.0	0	12	0	12	4.6	250	95.4
Oropharynx	C10	172	77.9	2.3	4	10	0	14	8.1	158	91.9
Hypopharynx	C12-13	1 087	85.1	0.2	2	68	0	70	6.4	1 017	93.6
Oesophagus	C15	2 243	76.2	2.4	53	174	0	227	10.1	2 016	89.9
Stomach	C16	3 078	65.5	5.0	154	243	0	397	12.9	2 681	87.1
Pancreas	C25	376	44.7	4.0	15	33	0	48	12.8	328	87.2
Larynx	C32	792	84.0	1.4	11	59	0	70	8.8	722	91.2
Lung	C33-34	2 066	63.7	2.8	58	202	0	260	12.6	1 806	87.4
Breast	C50	3 595	85.4	2.0	72	456	0	528	14.7	3 067	85.3
Cervix	C53	4 776	86.3	1.0	50	288	0	338	7.1	4 438	92.9
Ovary	C56	932	70.9	2.4	22	102	0	124	13.3	808	86.7
Urinary bladder	C67	517	79.1	1.5	8	67	0	75	14.5	442	85.5
Hodgkin lymphoma	C81	330	98.8	1.2	4	28	0	32	9.7	298	90.3
Non-Hodgkin lymphoma	C82-85+C96	1 008	98.0	1.7	17	123	0	140	13.9	868	86.1
Lymphoid leukaemia	C91	481	99.6	0.4	2	46	0	48	10.0	433	90.0
Myeloid leukaemia	C92-94	504	99.0	0.8	4	35	0	39	7.7	465	92.3
Leukaemia unspecified	C95	125	76.8	23.2	29	11	0	40	32.0	85	68.0

HV: histologically verified; DCO: death certificate only

Table 2. Number and proportion of cases with complete/incomplete follow-up (in years) and median follow-up (in months) by site: Chennai, India, 1990–1999 cases followed-up to 2001

Site	ICD-10	Cases included	Complete FU Alive/dead at end of FU		Incomplete FU: lost to FU		% lost to FU: years from diagnosis				% with complete FU at 5 years	Median FU (in months)
			No.	%	No.	%	< 1	1-3	3-5	> 5		
Lip	C00	86	56	65.1	30	34.9	7.0	2.3	0.0	25.6	90.7	27.3
Tongue	C01-02	988	747	75.6	241	24.4	13.1	2.6	1.2	7.5	83.1	9.8
Oral cavity	C03-06	1 662	1 221	73.5	441	26.5	10.3	2.2	1.8	12.2	85.6	12.9
Tonsil	C09	250	230	92.0	20	8.0	4.8	0.8	0.0	2.4	94.4	10.3
Oropharynx	C10	158	151	95.6	7	4.4	0.6	0.6	0.0	3.2	98.7	11.0
Hypopharynx	C12-13	1 017	892	87.7	125	12.3	9.0	0.7	0.3	2.3	90.0	8.7
Oesophagus	C15	2 016	1 818	90.2	198	9.8	6.7	0.9	0.4	1.8	92.0	6.9
Stomach	C16	2 681	2 397	89.4	284	10.6	7.3	0.9	0.9	1.5	90.9	6.1
Pancreas	C25	328	314	95.7	14	4.3	3.1	0.3	0.3	0.6	96.3	4.3
Larynx	C32	722	598	82.8	124	17.2	6.7	0.8	0.3	9.4	92.2	17.4
Lung	C33-34	1 806	1 619	89.6	187	10.4	8.0	0.7	0.3	1.4	91.1	5.8
Breast	C50	3 067	2 351	76.7	716	23.3	12.4	2.9	2.0	6.0	82.6	26.9
Cervix	C53	4 438	2 752	62.0	1 686	38.0	11.0	3.7	2.5	20.8	82.8	27.5
Ovary	C56	808	625	77.4	183	22.6	14.7	4.6	1.4	1.9	79.2	11.4
Urinary bladder	C67	442	367	83.0	75	17.0	10.9	1.6	0.2	4.3	87.3	11.7
Hodgkin lymphoma	C81	298	245	82.2	53	17.8	6.4	1.7	1.0	8.7	90.9	21.0
Non-Hodgkin lymphoma	C82-85+C96	868	732	84.3	136	15.7	10.9	1.3	0.6	2.9	87.2	9.4
Lymphoid leukaemia	C91	433	372	85.9	61	14.1	2.8	3.2	3.5	4.6	90.5	8.5
Myeloid leukaemia	C92-94	465	400	86.0	65	14.0	8.6	1.3	0.4	3.7	89.7	4.5
Leukaemia unspecified	C95	85	74	87.1	11	12.9	10.5	0.0	0.0	2.4	89.4	1.5

FU: follow-up

Table 3. Comparison of 1-, 3- and 5-year absolute and relative survival and 5-year age-standardized relative survival by site: Chennai, India, 1990–1999 cases followed-up to 2001

Site	ICD-10	Cases included	% Absolute survival			% Relative survival			% ASRS at 5-years	
			1-year	3-year	5-year	1-year	3-year	5-year	all ages	0-74 years
Lip	C00	86	74.7	51.1	40.7	77.1	56.0	47.2	47.4	49.0
Tongue	C01-02	988	51.6	25.7	19.4	53.3	28.4	23.0	23.2	23.4
Oral cavity	C03-06	1 662	60.9	35.3	30.5	62.9	38.8	35.7	35.6	36.7
Tonsil	C09	250	43.4	19.7	13.7	45.0	22.1	16.8	17.3	15.6
Oropharynx	C10	158	47.9	23.9	15.3	49.9	26.7	18.4	19.3	20.7
Hypopharynx	C12-13	1 017	43.6	21.0	12.5	44.9	23.1	14.5	13.8	15.0
Oesophagus	C15	2 016	32.1	12.4	6.9	33.2	13.8	8.3	9.3	8.6
Stomach	C16	2 681	34.5	13.2	8.6	35.7	14.6	10.1	8.0	10.3
Pancreas	C25	328	26.6	11.6	7.9	27.5	12.7	9.1	6.9	8.7
Larynx	C32	722	65.6	40.4	30.7	68.0	44.9	36.8	36.0	38.0
Lung	C33-34	1 806	31.9	12.0	6.5	33.0	13.2	7.6	6.4	7.1
Breast	C50	3 067	79.2	54.7	43.7	81.0	58.3	48.6	47.1	47.7
Cervix	C53	4 438	77.0	58.4	54.0	78.4	61.8	59.4	60.2	59.6
Ovary	C56	808	60.3	37.3	27.4	61.4	39.5	29.7	24.9	28.5
Urinary bladder	C67	442	58.2	30.7	23.2	61.2	35.7	29.8	25.7	32.0
Hodgkin lymphoma	C81	298	61.2	46.4	39.4	61.8	47.7	41.1	36.8	37.8
Non-Hodgkin lymphoma	C82-85+C96	868	50.2	30.3	21.6	51.3	32.1	23.6	21.5	23.2
Lymphoid leukaemia	C91	433	41.9	27.8	23.8	42.3	28.4	24.5	13.6	16.4
Myeloid leukaemia	C92-94	465	36.3	21.3	14.7	36.9	22.2	15.8	16.6	14.9
Leukaemia unspecified	C95	85	26.7	17.1	10.9	27.4	17.8	11.6	9.1	11.2

ASRS: age-standardized relative survival

Table 4a. Site-wise number of cases, 5-year absolute and relative survival by sex: Chennai, India, 1990–1999 cases followed-up to 2001

Site	ICD-10	Cases included	Male % 5-year survival			Female % 5-year survival		
			No.	Abs	Rel	No.	Abs	Rel
Lip	C00	86	47	46.3	52.4	39	34.4	41.3
Tongue	C01-02	988	761	18.1	21.8	227	23.9	26.6
Oral cavity	C03-06	1 662	874	30.9	37.0	788	30.1	34.2
Tonsil	C09	250	213	11.2	14.0	37	27.2	31.6
Oropharynx	C10	158	135	15.9	19.1	23	13.0	15.4
Hypopharynx	C12-13	1 017	757	11.9	14.2	260	14.2	15.6
Oesophagus	C15	2 016	1 229	5.6	7.0	787	9.2	10.5
Stomach	C16	2 681	1 828	8.3	10.0	853	9.2	10.3
Pancreas	C25	328	231	6.8	7.7	97	10.7	12.2
Larynx	C32	722	651	30.8	37.1	71	30.0	33.6
Lung	C33-34	1 806	1 527	6.1	7.2	279	8.7	9.7
Breast	C50	3 067				3 067	43.7	48.6
Cervix	C53	4 438				4 438	54.0	59.4
Ovary	C56	808				808	27.4	29.7
Urinary bladder	C67	442	318	23.2	30.6	124	23.6	27.9
Hodgkin lymphoma	C81	298	213	36.8	38.5	85	45.5	46.9
Non-Hodgkin lymphoma	C82-85+C96	868	558	20.1	22.1	310	24.5	26.3
Lymphoid leukaemia	C91	433	282	23.1	23.9	151	25.3	25.9
Myeloid leukaemia	C92-94	465	262	14.2	15.4	203	15.3	16.2
Leukaemia unspecified	C95	85	50	10.5	11.1	35	11.2	11.9

Abs: absolute survival; Rel: relative survival

Table 4b. Site-wise number of cases and relative survival by age group: Chennai, India, 1990–1999 cases followed-up to 2001

Site	ICD-10	Cases included	Number of cases by age group					Relative survival by age group % 5-year survival				
			< 45	45-54	55-64	65-74	> 75	< 45	45-54	55-64	65-74	> 75
Lip	C00	86	9	28	27	18	4	85.3	52.9	40.8	26.4	48.2
Tongue	C01-02	988	120	269	321	216	62	37.0	25.6	19.3	14.9	28.6
Oral cavity	C03-06	1 662	216	408	577	353	108	48.4	44.6	31.6	25.4	30.5
Tonsil	C09	250	26	67	80	65	12	18.6	16.5	13.0	16.2	48.5
Oropharynx	C10	158	12	44	55	29	18	34.2	18.0	19.9	10.3	14.0
Hypopharynx	C12-13	1 017	172	259	326	200	60	21.2	17.2	13.2	8.9	4.1
Oesophagus	C15	2 016	236	530	689	430	131	11.6	7.1	6.3	10.5	12.0
Stomach	C16	2 681	445	635	848	561	192	16.9	12.5	8.3	6.7	2.3
Pancreas	C25	328	65	83	95	61	24	12.8	15.3	5.1	5.7	
Larynx	C32	722	88	172	262	149	51	64.9	36.4	31.1	33.0	28.1
Lung	C33-34	1 806	230	448	654	386	88	16.5	8.8	5.7	4.1	4.7
Breast	C50	3 067	931	860	696	418	162	58.4	47.0	44.4	37.5	48.4
Cervix	C53	4 438	1 150	1 405	1 235	515	133	63.4	59.9	55.8	58.0	69.4
Ovary	C56	808	270	206	195	116	21	49.3	24.4	18.9	11.6	
Urinary bladder	C67	442	45	77	111	143	66	41.6	30.5	24.2	35.5	15.1
Hodgkin lymphoma	C81	298	228	27	22	14	7	47.0	37.9	12.0	0.0	27.7
Non-Hodgkin lymphoma	C82-85+C96	868	418	139	163	117	31	30.6	20.7	20.6	5.0	6.7
Lymphoid leukaemia	C91	433	379	8	21	20	5	27.5	0.0	7.2	0.0	0.0
Myeloid leukaemia	C92-94	465	279	65	59	52	10	20.9	9.8	8.9	4.6	30.8
Leukaemia unspecified	C95	85	51	7	9	13	5	18.6	0.0	12.9	0.0	0.0

Table 5. Proportion of cases and 5-year absolute survival by extent of disease and site: Chennai, India, 1990–1999

Site	ICD-10	Cases included	% of cases by extent of disease				% 5-year absolute survival			
			Localized	Regional	Dist. met.	Unknown	Localized	Regional	Dist. met.	Unknown
Tongue	C01-02	988	4.4	86.8	2.6	6.2	59.2	17.3	15.4	14.7
Oral cavity	C03-06	1 662	3.5	88.7	2.7	5.0	54.9	30.0	10.0	30.9
Larynx	C32	722	6.6	85.5	3.6	4.3	44.3	30.3	9.2	34.1
Breast	C50	3 067	1.7	67.9	13.0	17.5	70.8	48.9	12.3	46.6
Cervix	C53	4 438	6.4	86.0	3.7	3.9	69.1	55.3	12.4	43.4
Ovary	C56	808	1.5	62.5	19.4	16.6	73.4	30.8	6.0	38.1

Dis. met.: distant metastasis

Table 6. Comparison of 5-year absolute and relative survival of cases diagnosed between 1984–1989 and 1990–1999, Chennai, India

Site	ICD-10	% Complete FU at 5 years		% 5-year absolute survival		% 5-year relative survival	
		1984–1989	1990–1999	1984–1989	1990–1999	1984–1989	1990–1999
Lip	C00	92.3	90.7	40.1	40.7	46.1	47.2
Tongue	C01-02	85.9	83.1	22.7	19.4	25.8	23.0
Oral cavity	C03-06	82.3	85.6	28.8	30.5	32.8	35.7
Oropharynx	C10	80.7	98.7	18.2	15.3	20.9	18.4
Hypopharynx	C12-13	82.7	90.0	15.5	12.5	17.5	14.5
Oesophagus	C15	87.9	92.0	5.6	6.9	6.5	8.3
Stomach	C16	87.7	90.9	6.9	8.6	7.8	10.1
Pancreas	C25	86.4	96.3	4.4	7.9	5.0	9.1
Larynx	C32	84.7	92.2	33.9	30.7	39.0	36.8
Lung	C33-34	86.5	91.1	6.6	6.5	7.5	7.6
Breast	C50	88.3	82.6	45.9	43.7	49.5	48.6
Cervix	C53	84.5	82.8	56.3	54.0	60.0	59.4
Urinary bladder	C67	89.1	87.3	19.1	26.3	22.8	32.3
Hodgkin lymphoma	C81	91.7	90.9	40.2	39.4	40.2	41.1
Non-Hodgkin lymphoma	C82-85+C96	79.9	87.2	19.4	21.6	21.1	23.6
Lymphoid leukaemia	C91	75.2	90.5	24.5	23.8	25.4	24.5
Myeloid leukaemia	C92-94	85.9	89.7	16.0	14.7	17.0	15.8

FU: follow-up

Chapter 15

Cancer survival in Karunagappally, India, 1991–1997

Jayalekshmi P, Gangadharan P and Sebastian P

Abstract

The rural cancer registry of Karunagappally was established in 1990 to study cancer occurrence due to high natural background radiation in the coastal area of Kerala state. Cancer registration was done by active methods. The registry contributed data on survival for 22 cancer sites or types registered during 1991–1997. Follow-up has been carried out predominantly by active methods, with median follow-up time ranging between 3–57 months for various cancers. The proportion of histologically verified diagnosis for different cancers ranged between 39–100%; death certificates only (DCOs) comprised 0–25%; 75–100% of total registered cases were included for survival analysis. The 5-year age-standardized relative survival rates for common cancers were lung (6%), breast (45%), cervix (55%), mouth (42%), oesophagus (14%) and tongue (31%). Five-year relative survival by age group showed no distinct pattern or trend for most cancers. A majority of cases are diagnosed with a regional spread of disease among cancers of the tongue (48%), oral cavity (66%), hypopharynx (54%), larynx (46%), cervix (61%) and breast (53%); survival decreases with increasing extent of disease.

Rural cancer registry

The rural cancer registry of Karunagappally was established in 1990 as a special purpose registry by the regional cancer centre of Trivandrum, with funding support from the Department of Atomic Energy, Government of India to study cancer occurrence in relation to the high natural background radiation present in the coastal area of Kerala state, which has monazite-rich sands that emit gamma radiation. The registry covers an area of 212 km^2 and caters to a mixed rural (96%) and urban (4%) population of 0.4 million with a sex ratio of 1025 females to 1000 males. It has been contributing data to the quinquennial IARC publication *Cancer Incidence in Five Continents* since volume VII [1]. The method of cancer registration is entirely done by active methods. There are no dedicated cancer hospitals or laboratories for tissue diagnosis within the registry area. Over 50 sources of registration, comprising hospitals in the government and private sectors, nursing homes, pathology laboratories, imaging centres and hospices, are visited for data collection. In addition, the enumerators undertake field visits to trace new cancer cases. The average annual age-standardized incidence rate is 112 per 100 000 among males and 81 per 100 000 among females with a lifetime cumulative risk of one in 8 for males and one in 11 for females of developing cancer in 1993–2001. The top-ranking cancers among males are lung, followed by oral cavity and oesophagus. Among females, the order is breast, cervix and oral cavity [2].

The registry has contributed data on survival from 22 cancer sites or types for this second volume of the IARC publication on *Cancer Survival in Africa, Asia, the Caribbean and Central America*.

Data quality indices (Table 1)

The proportion of cases with a histological confirmation of cancer diagnosis in this series is 71%, varying between 39–100%. The proportion of cases registered as death certificates only (DCOs) is 11%, ranging between 0–25%. The exclusion of cases from the survival analysis was the greatest in cancer of the brain and nervous system (25%); it was none for many cancers. Thus, 75–100% of the total cases registered are included in the estimation of the survival probability.

Outcome of follow-up (Table 2)

Follow-up has been carried out predominantly by active methods. These included abstraction of cancer mortality information from the vital statistics division records. The abstracted data are first matched with the incident cancer database. The follow-up information for the unmatched incident cases is then obtained through repeated scrutiny of records in the respective sources of registration, postal/telephone enquiries and house visits. Further, the monthly cancer follow-up clinics held by oncologists from the Regional Cancer Centre in the field office and the pain and palliative care clinics held bi-weekly have helped to obtain maximal follow-up information.

The closing date of follow-up was 31st December 1999. The median follow-up (in months) ranged between 3 for myeloid leukaemia to 59 for cancer of the thyroid. Complete follow-up at five years from the incidence date ranged from 91% (prostate cancer) to 100%. The losses to follow-up occurred in the first year of follow-up for a majority of cancers.

Survival statistics

All ages and both sexes together (Table 3)

The 5-year relative survival is the highest for thyroid cancer (88%) and the lowest for cancer of the liver (3%) among the cancers studied. The survival figures for other head and neck cancers are oral cavity (41%), larynx (35%), tongue (32%) and hypopharynx (15%). Survival rates from gastrointestinal cancers were rectum (33%) and oesophagus, stomach and pancreas (3%). The survival figures for Non-Hodgkin lymphoma was 30%, lymphoid leukaemia was 37% and myeloid leukaemia 8%.

Figure 1a. Top ten cancers (ranked by survival), Kurunagappally, India, 1991–1997

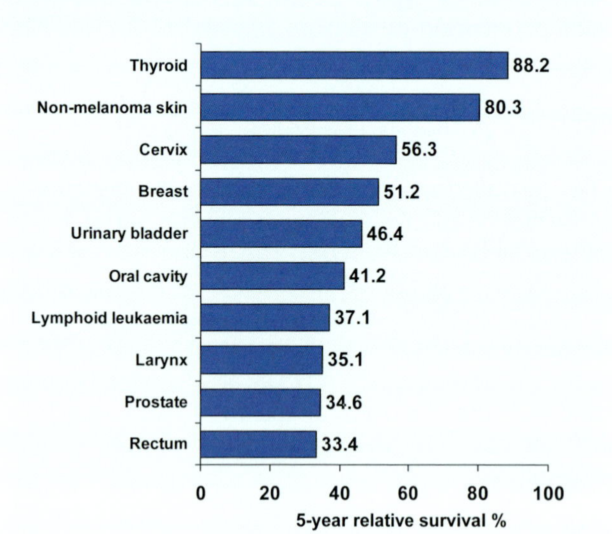

The 5-year age-standardized relative survival (ASRS) probability for all ages together is either less than or very similar to the corresponding unadjusted one for most cancers. The 5-year ASRS (0–74 years of age) is observed to be higher than the corresponding ASRS (all ages) for the majority.

Sex

Male (Table 4a)

The 5-year relative survival is the highest for non-melanoma skin cancer (83%) followed in order by thyroid (60%) and urinary bladder (49%). Survival from lymphoid and myeloid leukaemias is noticeably higher among males than females.

Figure 1b. Top five cancers (ranked by survival), Male, Kurunagappally, India, 1991–1997

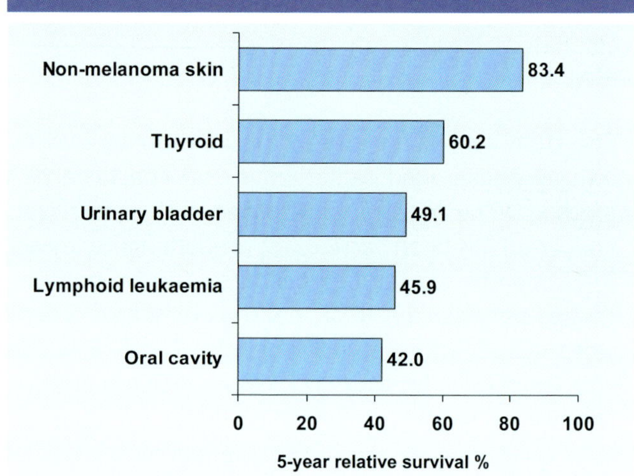

Female (Table 4a)

The top ranking cancers on 5-year relative survival probabilities are thyroid (93%), non-melanoma skin (75%), cervix (56%) and breast (51%). Survival is markedly higher among females than males for cancers of the tongue, hypopharynx and thyroid.

Figure 1c. Top five cancers (ranked by survival), Female, Kurunagappally, India, 1991–1997

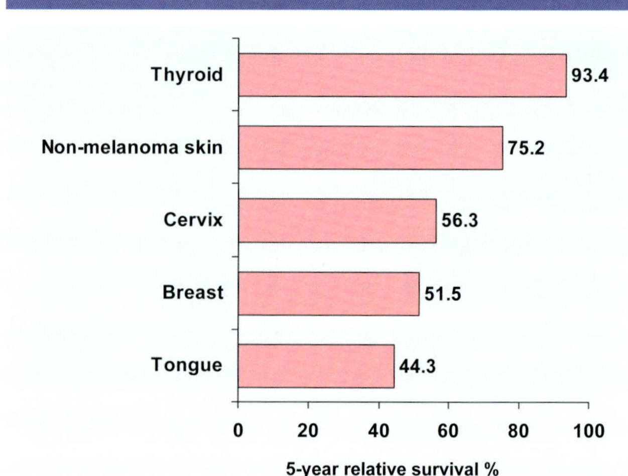

Age group (Table 4b)

The 5-year relative survival probabilities by age group do not show any distinct pattern or trend for most cancers.

Extent of disease (Table 5; Figure 2)

A majority of cases have been diagnosed with a regional spread of disease among cancers of the tongue (48%), oral cavity (66%), hypopharynx (54%), larynx (46%), cervix (61%) and breast (53%). For ovarian cancer, there are more cases in the distant metastasis category (54%) than others. The extent of disease was unknown in 7–17%. The 5-year absolute survival by extent of disease followed the expected pattern: highest for localized disease followed by regional and distant metastasis among known categories of extent of disease for most cancers.

References

1. Parkin DM, Whelan SL, Ferlay J and Storm H. *Cancer Incidence in Five Continents, Vol I to VIII: IARC Cancerbase No. 7*. IARCPress, Lyon, 2005.

2. *Rural Cancer Registry of Karunagappally. Cancer morbidity and mortality in Karunagappally: 1993–2001*. Regional Cancer Centre, Thiruvananthapuram, 2004.

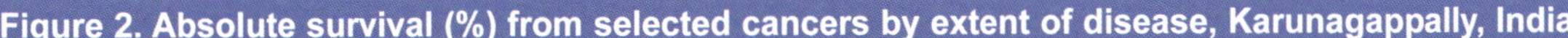

Figure 2. Absolute survival (%) from selected cancers by extent of disease, Karunagappally, India

Figure 2a. Tongue

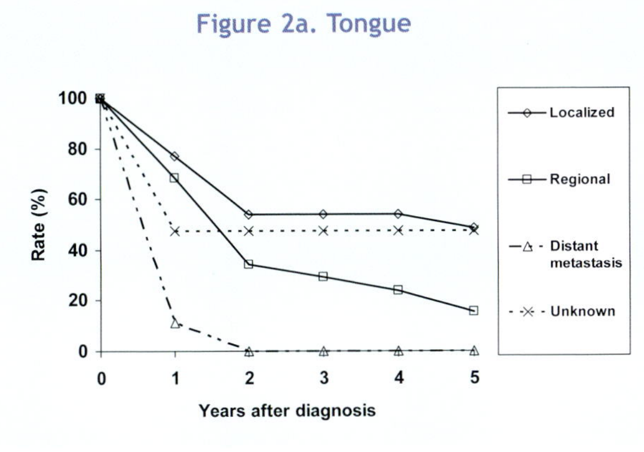

Figure 2b. Oral cavity

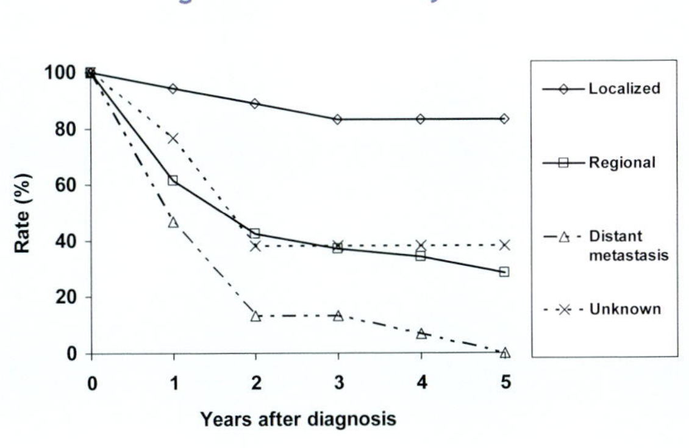

Figure 2c. Hypopharynx

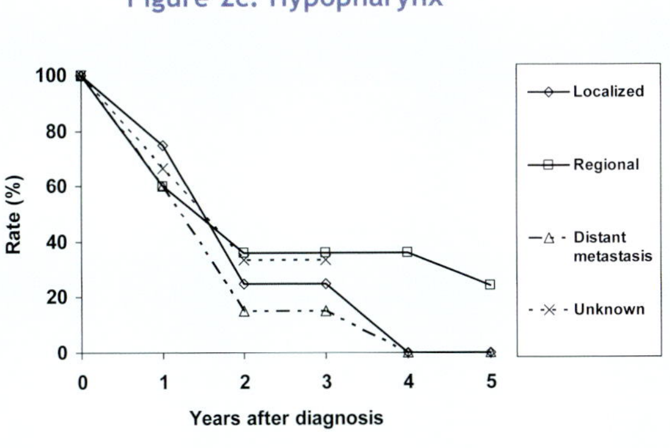

Figure 2d. Larynx

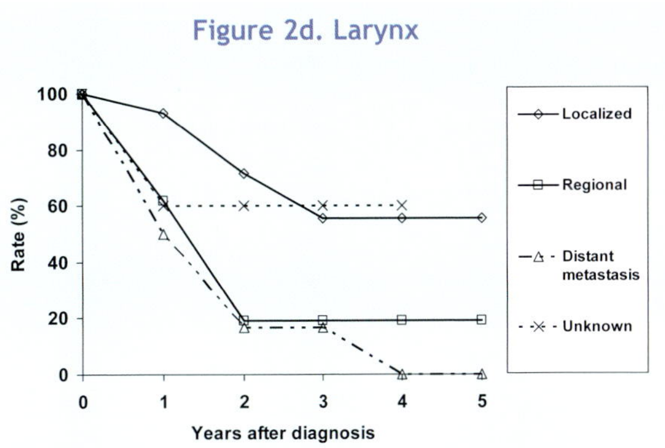

Figure 2e. Breast

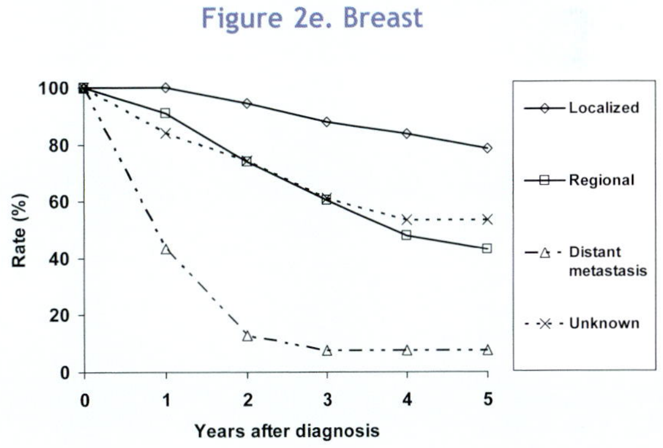

Figure 2f. Cervix

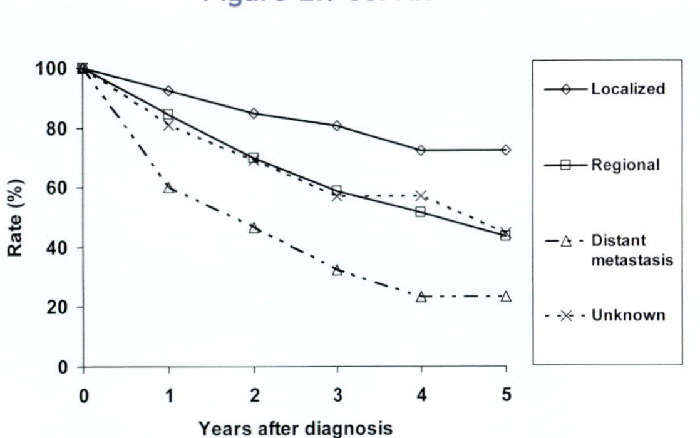

Table 1. Data quality indices - Proportion of histologically verified and death certificate only cases, number and proportion of included and excluded cases by site: Karunagappally, India, 1991–1997 cases followed-up until 1999

Site	ICD-10	Total registered	%		Excluded cases					Included cases	
			HV	DCO	DCO	Follow-up	Others	Total	%	No.	%
Tongue	C01-02	88	83.0	1.1	1	1	0	2	2.3	86	97.7
Oral cavity	C03-06	130	82.3	3.1	4	2	1	7	5.4	123	94.6
Hypopharynx	C12-13	33	93.9	0.0	0	0	0	0	0.0	33	100.0
Oesophagus	C15	111	70.3	1.8	2	2	1	5	4.5	106	95.5
Stomach	C16	86	50.0	8.1	7	2	0	9	10.5	77	89.5
Rectum	C19-20	39	76.9	2.6	1	0	0	1	2.6	38	97.4
Liver	C22	55	76.4	1.8	1	0	0	1	1.8	54	98.2
Pancreas	C25	41	39.0	0.0	0	0	0	0	0.0	41	100.0
Larynx	C32	48	87.5	2.1	1	1	0	2	4.2	46	95.8
Lung	C33-34	248	56.9	7.7	19	5	4	28	11.3	220	88.7
Other skin	C44	28	100.0	0.0	0	1	0	1	3.6	27	96.4
Breast	C50	193	93.8	1.0	2	1	0	3	1.6	190	98.4
Cervix	C53	180	85.0	3.9	7	3	0	10	5.6	170	94.4
Ovary	C56	35	88.6	0.0	0	0	0	0	0.0	35	100.0
Prostate	C61	34	67.6	0.0	0	2	0	2	5.9	32	94.1
Urinary bladder	C67	39	79.5	0.0	0	0	1	1	2.6	38	97.4
Brain & nervous system	C70-72	61	50.8	24.6	15	0	0	15	24.6	46	75.4
Thyroid	C73	75	92.0	1.3	1	0	0	1	1.3	74	98.7
Non-Hodgkin lymphoma	C82-85+C96	69	100.0	0.0	0	0	0	0	0.0	69	100.0
Multiple myeloma	C90	28	89.3	0.0	0	0	0	0	0.0	28	100.0
Lymphoid leukaemia	C91	38	100.0	0.0	0	0	0	0	0.0	38	100.0
Myeloid leukaemia	C92-94	30	100.0	0.0	0	0	0	0	0.0	30	100.0

HV: histologically verified; DCO: death certificate only

Table 2. Number and proportion of cases with complete/incomplete follow-up (in years) and median follow-up (in months) by site: Karunagappally, India, 1991–1997 cases followed-up until 1999

Site	ICD-10	Cases included	Complete FU Alive/dead at end of FU		Incomplete FU: lost to FU		% lost to FU: years from diagnosis				% with complete FU at 5 years	Median FU (in months)
			No.	%	No.	%	< 1	1-3	3-5	> 5		
Tongue	C01-02	86	84	97.7	2	2.3	1.2	0.0	1.2	0.0	97.7	15.6
Oral cavity	C03-06	123	119	96.7	4	3.3	1.6	0.8	0.8	0.0	96.7	18.7
Hypopharynx	C12-13	33	31	93.9	2	6.1	6.1	0.0	0.0	0.0	93.9	12.6
Oesophagus	C15	106	105	99.1	1	0.9	0.9	0.0	0.0	0.0	99.1	6.5
Stomach	C16	77	77	100.0	0	0.0	0.0	0.0	0.0	0.0	100.0	5.1
Rectum	C19-20	38	38	100.0	0	0.0	0.0	0.0	0.0	0.0	100.0	32.0
Liver	C22	54	53	98.1	1	1.9	1.9	0.0	0.0	0.0	98.1	3.5
Pancreas	C25	41	41	100.0	0	0.0	0.0	0.0	0.0	0.0	100.0	4.0
Larynx	C32	46	45	97.8	1	2.2	0.0	2.2	0.0	0.0	97.8	17.6
Lung	C33-34	220	217	98.6	3	1.4	1.4	0.0	0.0	0.0	98.6	5.2
Other skin	C44	27	25	92.6	2	7.4	3.7	0.0	3.7	0.0	92.6	59.0
Breast	C50	190	188	98.9	2	1.1	0.5	0.0	0.0	0.5	99.5	36.1
Cervix	C53	170	169	99.4	1	0.6	0.0	0.6	0.0	0.0	99.4	38.5
Ovary	C56	35	35	100.0	0	0.0	0.0	0.0	0.0	0.0	100.0	20.3
Prostate	C61	32	29	90.6	3	9.4	6.3	3.1	0.0	0.0	90.6	34.1
Urinary bladder	C67	38	37	97.4	1	2.6	2.6	0.0	0.0	0.0	97.4	18.6
Brain & nervous system	C70-72	46	45	97.8	1	2.2	0.0	2.2	0.0	0.0	97.8	19.9
Thyroid	C73	74	73	98.6	1	1.4	1.4	0.0	0.0	0.0	98.6	57.0
Non-Hodgkin lymphoma	C82-85+C96	69	69	100.0	0	0.0	0.0	0.0	0.0	0.0	100.0	12.1
Multiple myeloma	C90	28	27	96.4	1	3.6	3.6	0.0	0.0	0.0	96.4	17.4
Lymphoid leukaemia	C91	38	38	100.0	0	0.0	0.0	0.0	0.0	0.0	100.0	20.3
Myeloid leukaemia	C92-94	30	30	100.0	0	0.0	0.0	0.0	0.0	0.0	100.0	2.9

FU: follow-up

Table 3. Comparison of 1-, 3- and 5-year absolute and relative survival and 5-year age-standardized relative survival by site: Karunagappally, India, 1991–1997 cases followed-up until 1999

Site	ICD-10	Cases included	% Absolute survival			% Relative survival			% ASRS at 5-years	
			1-year	3-year	5-year	1-year	3-year	5-year	all ages	0-74 years
Tongue	C01-02	86	62.6	35.3	25.9	65.1	39.4	31.9	31.1	29.6
Oral cavity	C03-06	123	65.6	41.1	33.1	68.3	46.5	41.2	42.3	45.3
Hypopharynx	C12-13	33	62.5	29.6	12.6	64.3	32.0	14.6	18.4	15.5
Oesophagus	C15	106	27.0	3.9	2.9	28.3	4.4	3.5	14.1	18.5
Stomach	C16	77	22.1	5.2	2.6	23.1	5.9	3.3	3.0	4.1
Rectum	C19-20	38	76.3	49.4	26.5	79.2	55.7	33.4	43.6	32.6
Liver	C22	54	34.6	9.2	2.3	35.7	10.3	2.8	4.3	4.5
Pancreas	C25	41	12.2	2.4	2.4	12.6	2.7	3.0	2.8	4.3
Larynx	C32	46	69.6	33.3	29.6	72.5	37.2	35.1	32.3	28.3
Lung	C33-34	220	22.2	7.0	5.3	23.1	7.8	6.4	5.6	7.8
Other skin	C44	27	84.9	69.5	65.3	88.3	78.3	80.3	88.0	83.7
Breast	C50	190	85.8	59.0	46.8	87.2	62.2	51.2	44.8	54.4
Cervix	C53	170	82.9	59.4	46.7	85.7	66.0	56.3	54.8	57.8
Ovary	C56	35	62.9	36.4	26.0	64.1	38.3	28.1	24.1	27.8
Prostate	C61	32	93.5	49.0	22.1	101.2	63.3	34.6	41.1	32.6
Urinary bladder	C67	38	65.3	37.9	34.6	69.0	45.0	46.4	44.5	48.4
Brain & nervous system	C70-72	46	65.2	36.3	19.2	65.9	37.1	19.8	15.1	16.2
Thyroid	C73	74	91.8	84.7	81.2	93.6	89.5	88.2	86.0	90.0
Non-Hodgkin lymphoma	C82-85+C96	69	52.2	34.6	25.5	54.4	38.8	30.4	36.0	39.8
Multiple myeloma	C90	28	63.6	25.4	10.2	66.3	28.3	12.3	12.4	13.4
Lymphoid leukaemia	C91	38	60.5	36.3	36.3	61.1	37.0	37.1	36.3	45.6
Myeloid leukaemia	C92-94	30	30.0	16.0	8.0	30.5	16.4	8.3	6.7	8.2

ASRS: age-standardized relative survival

Table 4a. Site-wise number of cases, 5-year absolute and relative survival by sex: Karunagappally, India, 1991–1997 cases followed-up until 1999

Site	ICD-10	Cases included	Male % 5-year survival			Female % 5-year survival		
			No.	Abs	Rel	No.	Abs	Rel
Tongue	C01-02	86	57	21.8	26.4	31	34.5	44.3
Oral cavity	C03-06	123	77	34.0	42.0	53	31.7	39.7
Hypopharynx	C12-13	33	28	7.7	9.1	5	40.0	44.1
Oesophagus	C15	106	74	1.5	2.0	37	5.7	6.3
Stomach	C16	77	65	1.6	1.9	21	6.3	8.5
Rectum	C19-20	38	23	26.5	34.7	16	26.7	31.7
Liver	C22	54	49	2.2	2.6	6		
Pancreas	C25	41	29	3.4	4.3	12	0.0	0.0
Larynx	C32	46	48	29.6	35.1	0		
Lung	C33-34	220	216	5.0	6.1	32	7.6	8.7
Other skin	C44	27	17	68.5	83.4	11	60.0	75.2
Breast	C50	190	1	0.0	0.0	192	47.1	51.5
Cervix	C53	170				180	46.7	56.3
Ovary	C56	35				35	26.0	28.1
Prostate	C61	32	34	22.1	34.6			
Urinary bladder	C67	38	37	36.7	49.1	2	0.0	0.0
Brain & nervous system	C70-72	46	35	21.9	22.6	26	16.5	17.1
Thyroid	C73	74	14	48.2	60.2	61	88.0	93.4
Non-Hodgkin lymphoma	C82-85+C96	69	53	25.6	30.6	16	22.7	26.8
Multiple myeloma	C90	28	16			12	18.8	22.4
Lymphoid leukaemia	C91	38	24	44.8	45.9	14	21.4	21.8
Myeloid leukaemia	C92-94	30	19	21.1	21.8	11	0.0	0.0

Abs: absolute survival; Rel: relative survival

Table 4b. Site-wise number of cases and relative survival by age group: Karunagappally, India, 1991–1997 cases followed-up until 1999

Site	ICD-10	Cases included	Number of cases by age group					Relative survival by age group % 5-year survival				
			< 45	45-54	55-64	65-74	> 75	< 45	45-54	55-64	65-74	> 75
Tongue	C01-02	86	6	22	26	24	8	24.5	32.4	22.5	40.3	48.6
Oral cavity	C03-06	123	13	23	39	35	13	52.9	50.1	38.5	43.3	0.0
Hypopharynx	C12-13	33	6	3	17	6	1	0.0		11.4	21.9	
Oesophagus	C15	106	1	17	39	40	9	102.4	6.3	0.0	3.8	0.0
Stomach	C16	77	5	11	29	23	9	0.0	9.7	0.0	6.2	0.0
Rectum	C19-20	38	6	6	11	13	2	24.2	31.6	26.9	42.1	
Liver	C22	54	16	13	9	13	3	0.0	0.0	13.9	0.0	0.0
Pancreas	C25	41	4	15	10	10	2	0.0	0.0	0.0	13.0	0.0
Larynx	C32	46	2	14	12	16	2	0.0	46.7	44.2	23.2	
Lung	C33-34	220	13	38	89	66	14	31.6	5.8	6.8	2.2	0.0
Other skin	C44	27	4	4	5	12	2	102.8	79.4	89.1	66.2	96.5
Breast	C50	190	78	41	42	22	7	53.0	51.2	44.7	75.8	0.0
Cervix	C53	170	19	36	55	47	13	55.1	60.4	56.3	60.8	26.8
Ovary	C56	35	13	6	10	5	1	29.8	26.1	33.6	25.1	0.0
Prostate	C61	32	0	3	6	13	10		0.0	0.0	46.9	45.3
Urinary bladder	C67	38	1	7	12	13	5		28.2	60.2	47.1	38.9
Brain & nervous system	C70-72	46	30	9	4	2	1	23.4	21.2	0.0	0.0	0.0
Thyroid	C73	74	43	7	12	8	4	99.0	88.8	75.5	79.0	0.0
Non-Hodgkin lymphoma	C82-85+C96	69	17	11	14	19	8	48.0	48.8	41.0	8.5	0.0
Multiple myeloma	C90	28	3	5	8	9	3	0.0			14.2	0.0
Lymphoid leukaemia	C91	38	33	1	3	0	1	36.6				0.0
Myeloid leukaemia	C92-94	30	17	4	5	3	1	11.9		0.0	0.0	

Table 5. Proportion of cases and 5-year absolute survival by extent of disease and site: Karunagappally, India, 1991–1997

Site	ICD-10	Cases included	% of cases by extent of disease				% 5-year absolute survival			
			Localized	Regional	Dist. met.	Unknown	Localized	Regional	Dist. met.	Unknown
Tongue	C01-02	86	30.2	47.7	10.5	11.6	48.7	15.4	0.0	47.4
Oral cavity	C03-06	123	14.6	65.9	12.2	7.3	83.0	28.5	0.0	38.2
Hypopharynx	C12-13	33	12.1	54.5	24.2	9.1	0.0	24.0	0.0	38.2
Larynx	C32	46	30.4	45.7	13.0	10.9	55.6	19.0	0.0	
Breast	C50	190	18.4	53.2	12.1	16.3	78.6	43.1	7.8	53.4
Cervix	C53	170	15.3	60.6	8.8	15.3	72.1	43.5	23.1	44.3
Ovary	C56	35	17.1	11.4	54.3	17.1	100.0	0.0	8.8	44.4

Dis. met.: distant metastasis

Chapter 16

Cancer survival in Mumbai (Bombay), India, 1992–1999

Yeole BB, Kurkure AP and Sunny L

Abstract

The Bombay cancer registry is the second oldest population-based cancer registry in Asia, and the first of its kind in India. It was established in 1963, and registration of cases is done by active methods. Data on survival from 28 cancer sites or types registered during 1992–1999 are reported. Follow-up has been carried out predominantly by active methods, with median follow-up ranging between 1–51 months for different cancers. The proportion of histologically verified diagnosis for various cancers ranged between 41–100%; death certificates only (DCOs) comprised 0–15%; 84–99% of total registered cases were included for survival analysis. Complete follow-up at five years ranged from 85–92% for different cancers. The 5-year age-standardized relative survival rates for common cancers were breast (48%), cervix (44%), lung (11%), oesophagus (14%), oral cavity (35%) and non-Hodgkin lymphoma (34%). The 5-year relative survival by age group portrayed either an inverse relationship or was fluctuating. Cases with a regional spread of disease were the highest for cancers of the tongue, oral cavity, larynx and cervix; survival decreased with the increasing extent of disease for all cancers studied.

Mumbai cancer registry

The Mumbai cancer registry, formerly known as the Bombay cancer registry, is the second-oldest population-based cancer registry in Asia and the first of its kind in India. It was established in 1963 and has been contributing data to the quinquennial IARC publication *Cancer Incidence in Five Continents* since volume II [1]. Cancer registration is still done by active methods. Over 150 sources of registration, comprising hospitals in the government and private sectors, nursing homes, pathology laboratories, imaging centres and hospices, are visited for data collection. The registry caters to an entirely urban population of about 12 million with a sex ratio of 815 females to 1000 males. The average annual age-standardized incidence rate is 116 per 100 000 among males and 122 per 100 000 among females with a lifetime cumulative risk of one in 7 of developing cancer for both sexes in the period 1999–2001 [2]. The top ranking cancers among males are lung followed by oral cavity and larynx. Among females, the order is breast, cervix and ovary.

The registry contributed data on survival for the cancers of the female breast and uterine cervix in the first volume of the IARC publication on *Cancer Survival in Developing Countries* [3]. Data on survival from 28 cancer sites or types registered during 1992–1999 are reported in this second volume.

Data quality indices (Table 1)

The proportion of cases with histologically verified cancer diagnosis in our series is 78%, varying between 99.9% for lymphoid leukaemia and 41% for the pancreas. The proportion of cases registered as death certificates only (DCOs) is 6.5% ranging between 0.1% in lymphoid leukaemia and 15.2% in pancreas. The exclusion of cases from the survival analysis is the greatest among the cancer of the pancreas (15.8%) and the least among lymphoid leukaemia (0.5%). Thus, 84–99% of the total cases registered among selected cancers are included in the estimation of the survival probability.

Outcome of follow-up (Table 2)

Follow-up has been carried out predominantly by active methods. These include abstraction of mortality information from the hospitals and municipal corporation records. The abstracted data are matched with the incident cancer database. Unmatched incident cases are then subjected to one or more of the following to obtain the vital status information: repeated scrutiny of records in the respective sources of registration, postal/telephone enquiries and house visits.

The closing date of follow-up was 31st December 1999 for cases registered in 1992–1994 and 31st December

2003 for cases registered in 1995–1999. The median follow-up (in months) ranged between <1 for unspecified leukaemia to 50.9 for lip cancer. Complete follow-up information at five years from the incidence date ranged from 92.8% (cancer of the lung) to 81.7% (cancer of the penis). The cases lost to follow-up also displayed a pattern: the proportion of lost to follow-up was generally the highest in the extremities of the classified follow-up intervals (within the first year and five or more years of follow-up) for all cancers. This minimizes the bias of estimation of 5-year survival probability, as a sizeable proportion of cases lost to follow-up after five years would have had a complete follow-up until 5 years from the incidence date.

Survival statistics

All ages and both sexes together (Table 3)

The 5-year relative survival is the highest for lip cancer (64%) and the lowest for cancer of the tonsil (17%) among the cancers of the head and neck. Cancers of the pancreas, stomach and oesophagus (15%) had the poorest survival, compared to cancer of the anus (39%) among the gastrointestinal tract cancers. Survival from cancers of the urinary system was 42% for urinary bladder and 36% for kidney. Hodgkin lymphoma had a better survival (52%) than non-Hodgkin lymphoma (34%). The best survival figures for leukaemias were lymphoid (16%), followed by myeloid (15%) and unspecified (7%).

Figure 1a. Top ten cancers (ranked by survival), Mumbai, India, 1992–1999

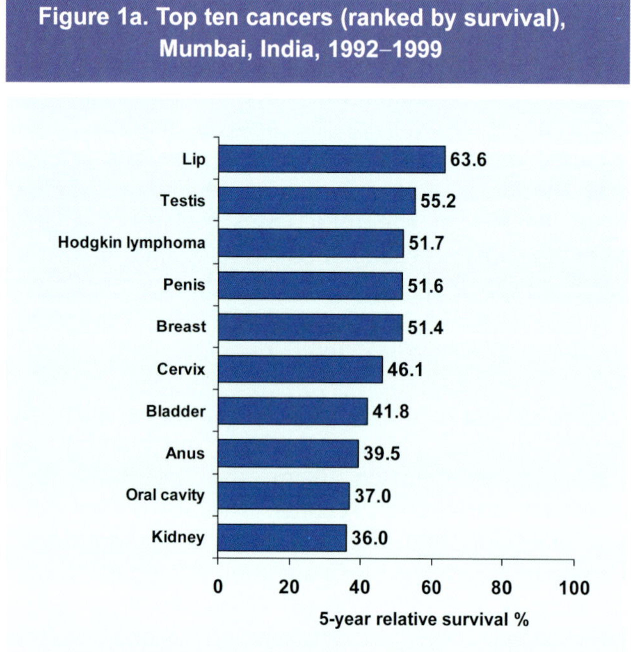

The 5-year age-standardized relative survival (ASRS) probability for all ages together is generally less than or similar to the corresponding unadjusted one with a few exceptions. Also, the 5-year ASRS (0–74 years of age) is generally higher than the corresponding ASRS (all ages) for most cancers.

Sex

Male (Table 4a)

The 5-year relative survival was the highest for lip cancer (60%) followed in order by Hodgkin lymphoma (56%), testis (55%) and penis (52%). Survival from Hodgkin lymphoma was noticeably higher among males (56%) than females (41%).

Figure 1b. Top five cancers (ranked by survival), Male, Mumbai, India, 1992–1999

Lip 59.7
Hodgkin lymphoma 56.5
Testis 55.2
Penis 51.6
Bladder 41.4
0 20 40 60 80 100
5-year relative survival %

Female (Table 4a)

The top-ranking cancers in terms of 5-year relative survival are lip (70%), breast (51%), cervix (46%) and anus (42%). The survival is markedly higher among females than males for cancers of the lip, tongue and tonsil.

Figure 1c. Top five cancers (ranked by survival), Female, Mumbai, India, 1992–1999

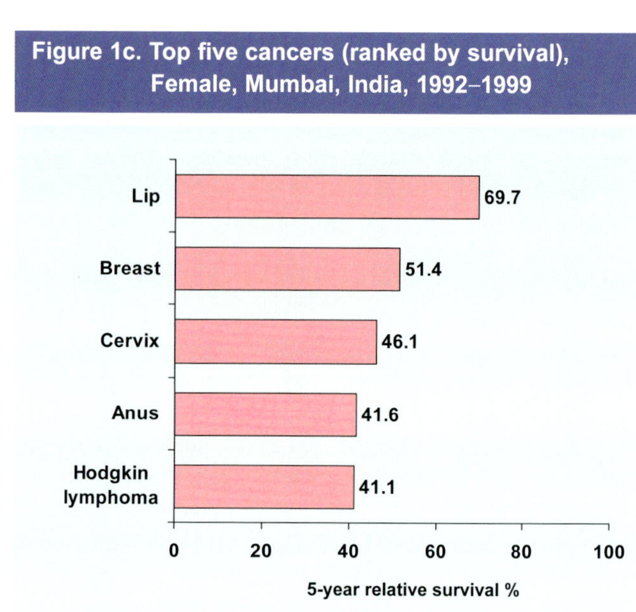

Age group (Table 4b)

The 5-year relative survival by age group portrays an inverse relationship: a decreasing survival with increasing age at diagnosis for cancers of the tongue, nasopharynx, oesophagus, stomach, colon, rectum, larynx, lung, breast, cervix, prostate, bladder and non-Hodgkin lymphoma. In the rest, it fluctuates.

Extent of disease (Table 5; Figure 2)

A majority of cases of the following cancers have been diagnosed with localized disease: lip (52%), rectum (46%) and colon (39%). In breast cancer, there was no difference in the proportion of cases with localized (40%) and regional (41%) spread of disease. Ovarian cancer is the solitary instance in which most cases were diagnosed with distant metastasis (50%). Cases with a regional spread of disease were the highest among cancers of the tongue, oral cavity, larynx and cervix. The extent of disease was unknown in 4–10%. The 5-year absolute survival by extent of disease followed the expected pattern: highest for localized cases, followed by regional and distant metastasis cases among known categories of extent of disease.

Survival trend (Table 6)

The 5-year relative survival from cancers of the female breast (51%) and cervix (46%) registered in 1992–1999 has shown a slight decline compared to an earlier series (1982–1986: breast: 55.1%; cervix: 50.7%) reported in the first volume of survival publication [3]. This might be a consequence of the increased availability of complete follow-up information in the present volume (85–87%) compared to 73–75% in the earlier series.

References

1. Parkin DM, Whelan SL, Ferlay J and Storm H. *Cancer Incidence in Five Continents, Vol I to VIII: IARC Cancerbase No. 7.* IARCPress, Lyon, 2005.

2. National Cancer Registry Programme. *Consolidated report of population-based cancer registries: 1999–2001.* Indian Council of Medical Research, New Delhi, 2004.

3. Yeole BB, Jussawalla DJ, Sabnis SD and Sunny L. Survival from breast and cervical cancer in Mumbai (Bombay), India. In: *Cancer Survival in Developing Countries* (eds) R Sankaranarayanan, RJ Black and DM Parkin. IARC Scientific Publications No. 145. IARCPress, Lyon, 1998.

Figure 2. Absolute survival (%) from selected cancers by extent of disease, Mumbai (Bombay), India

Figure 2a. Lip

Figure 2f. Larynx

Figure 2b. Tongue

Figure 2g. Breast

Figure 2c. Oral cavity

Figure 2h. Cervix

Figure 2d. Colon

Figure 2i. Ovary

Figure 2e. Rectum

Table 1. Data quality indices - Proportion of histologically verified and death certificate only cases, number and proportion of included and excluded cases by site: Mumbai, India, 1992–1994 cases followed through 1999 and 1995–1999 cases followed-up until 2003

Site	ICD-10	Total registered	%		Excluded cases					Included cases	
			HV	DCO	DCO	Follow-up	Others	Total	%	No.	%
Lip	C00	168	86.3	3.0	5	2	0	7	4.2	161	95.8
Tongue	C01-02	2 240	83.8	5.1	115	14	5	134	6.0	2 106	94.0
Oral cavity	C03-06	2 895	86.1	3.8	109	17	0	126	4.4	2 769	95.6
Tonsil	C09	548	83.4	6.0	33	2	0	35	6.4	513	93.6
Oropharynx	C10	257	83.7	5.1	13	0	1	14	5.4	243	94.6
Nasopharynx	C11	254	76.8	4.3	11	0	0	11	4.3	243	95.7
Hypopharynx	C12-13	1 969	84.1	2.7	54	12	1	67	3.4	1 902	96.6
Oesophagus	C15	3 647	61.2	13.7	498	17	4	519	14.2	3 128	85.8
Stomach	C16	2 466	65.9	9.8	241	14	6	261	10.6	2 205	89.4
Colon	C18	1 711	72.4	7.0	119	11	3	133	7.8	1 578	92.2
Rectum	C19-20	1 299	75.7	5.9	76	6	0	82	6.3	1 217	93.7
Anus	C21	237	84.0	4.2	10	0	7	17	7.2	220	92.8
Pancreas	C25	1 089	40.8	15.2	165	3	4	172	15.8	917	84.2
Larynx	C32	2 151	69.7	12.0	259	6	6	271	12.6	1 880	87.4
Lung	C33-34	3 995	62.6	13.0	518	18	8	544	13.6	3 451	86.4
Breast	C50	7 751	83.5	5.2	404	34	19	457	5.9	7 294	94.1
Cervix	C53	4 683	84.9	4.4	205	32	10	247	5.3	4 436	94.7
Ovary	C56	2 151	75.1	5.1	110	5	7	122	5.7	2 029	94.3
Penis	C60	335	81.8	1.8	6	0	2	8	2.4	327	97.6
Prostate	C61	1 622	71.6	9.1	148	8	3	159	9.8	1 463	90.2
Testis	C62	394	85.5	2.5	10	1	0	11	2.8	383	97.2
Kidney	C64	857	83.8	4.0	34	3	1	38	4.4	819	95.6
Urinary bladder	C67	1 403	77.5	6.3	88	3	5	96	6.8	1 307	93.2
Hodgkin lymphoma	C81	537	99.4	0.6	3	1	5	9	1.7	528	98.3
Non-Hodgkin lymphoma	C82-85+C96	2 362	99.6	0.2	4	18	2	24	1.0	2 338	99.0
Lymphoid leukaemia	C91	1 104	99.9	0.1	1	3	1	5	0.5	1 099	99.5
Myeloid leukaemia	C92-94	1 276	99.7	0.3	4	9	2	15	1.2	1 261	98.8
Leukaemia unspecified	C95	351	98.3	1.7	6	0	0	6	1.7	345	98.3

HV: histologically verified; DCO: death certificate only

Table 2. Number and proportion of cases with complete/incomplete follow-up (in years) and median follow-up (in months) by site: Mumbai, India, 1992–1994 cases followed through 1999 and 1995–1999 cases followed-up until 2003

Site	ICD-10	No. of cases included	Complete FU Alive/dead at end of FU		Incomplete FU: loss to FU*		% lost to FU: years from diagnosis				% with complete FU at 5 years	Median FU (in months)
			No.	%	No.	%	< 1	1-3	3-5	> 5		
Lip	C00	161	109	67.7	52	32.3	12.5	1.2	0.6	18.0	85.7	50.9
Tongue	C01-02	2106	1766	83.9	340	16.1	9.4	0.4	0.0	6.3	90.2	11.3
Oral cavity	C03-06	2769	2205	79.6	564	20.4	11.1	0.3	0.1	8.9	88.5	12.7
Tonsil	C09	513	447	87.1	66	12.9	8.6	0.8	0.0	3.5	90.6	8.3
Oropharynx	C10	243	210	86.4	33	13.6	9.9	0.0	0.0	3.7	90.1	10.1
Nasopharynx	C11	243	213	87.7	30	12.3	7.4	0.4	0.0	4.5	92.2	12.5
Hypopharynx	C12-13	1902	1621	85.2	281	14.8	9.3	0.2	0.3	5.0	90.2	8.3
Oesophagus	C15	3128	2759	88.2	369	11.8	7.5	0.4	0.2	3.7	91.9	5.0
Stomach	C16	2205	1950	88.4	255	11.6	7.9	0.3	0.1	3.3	91.7	3.4
Colon	C18	1578	1315	83.3	263	16.7	9.2	0.2	0.1	7.2	90.6	8.4
Rectum	C19-20	1217	963	79.1	254	20.9	12.0	0.5	0.3	8.1	87.2	11.7
Anus	C21	220	164	74.5	56	25.5	14.1	0.0	0.9	10.5	85.0	12.2
Pancreas	C25	917	803	87.6	114	12.4	5.3	0.2	4.7	2.2	89.7	1.6
Larynx	C32	1880	1501	79.8	379	20.2	11.0	0.5	0.4	8.3	88.1	12.4
Lung	C33-34	3451	3102	89.9	349	10.1	6.4	0.3	0.5	2.9	92.8	3.0
Breast	C50	7294	5460	74.9	1834	25.1	12.2	0.3	0.3	12.3	87.2	30.9
Cervix	C53	4436	3290	74.2	1146	25.8	14.1	0.2	0.3	11.2	85.3	25.1
Ovary	C56	2029	1713	84.4	316	15.6	10.0	0.1	0.2	5.3	89.7	7.1
Penis	C60	327	234	71.6	93	28.4	15.9	1.8	0.6	10.1	81.7	20.3
Prostate	C61	1463	1194	81.6	269	18.4	13.4	0.1	0.2	4.7	86.3	13.2
Testis	C62	383	285	74.4	98	25.6	9.9	0.3	0.5	14.9	89.3	36.1
Kidney	C64	819	625	76.3	194	23.7	13.4	1.7	0.4	8.2	84.5	7.1
Urinary bladder	C67	1307	1000	76.5	307	23.5	13.6	1.1	0.8	8.0	84.5	16.5
Hodgkin lymphoma	C81	528	379	71.8	149	28.2	13.2	1.7	0.4	12.9	84.7	29.4
Non-Hodgkin lymphoma	C82-85+C96	2338	1906	81.5	432	18.5	9.9	0.4	0.7	7.5	89.0	5.9
Lymphoid leukaemia	C91	1099	947	86.2	152	13.8	8.8	1.0	0.5	3.5	89.7	1.5
Myeloid leukaemia	C92-94	1261	1124	89.1	137	10.9	7.7	0.7	0.3	2.2	91.4	1.0
Leukaemia unspecified	C95	345	312	90.4	33	9.6	6.2	1.4	0.6	1.4	91.9	0.3

*FU: follow-up; * non-random*

Table 3. Comparison of 1-, 3- and 5-year absolute and relative survival and 5-year age-standardized relative survival by site: Mumbai, India, 1992–1994 cases followed through 1999 and 1995–1999 cases followed-up until 2003

Site	ICD-10	Cases included	% Absolute survival			% Relative survival			% ASRS at 5-years	
			1-year	3-year	5-year	1-year	3-year	5-year	all ages	0-74 years
Lip	C00	161	78.8	62.7	55.8	80.9	67.7	63.6	63.4	61.3
Tongue	C01-02	2 106	56.5	31.2	25.3	58.3	34.2	29.3	27.8	29.7
Oral cavity	C03-06	2 769	60.5	39.4	32.3	62.2	42.8	37.0	35.0	36.0
Tonsil	C09	513	46.7	20.3	13.9	48.4	22.6	16.7	16.7	16.6
Oropharynx	C10	243	51.5	23.6	15.7	53.3	26.2	18.6	18.3	20.4
Nasopharynx	C11	243	57.3	28.7	22.9	58.6	30.8	25.5	20.3	24.7
Hypopharynx	C12-13	1 902	47.5	23.3	17.8	49.3	26.3	21.7	21.8	23.1
Oesophagus	C15	3 128	36.8	18.9	13.0	38.3	21.1	15.4	13.7	16.2
Stomach	C16	2 205	33.6	17.6	12.8	34.8	19.5	14.8	11.6	15.2
Colon	C18	1 578	52.5	35.1	27.4	54.5	38.8	32.3	25.4	30.3
Rectum	C19-20	1 217	59.7	37.2	28.6	61.9	41.2	33.6	26.1	31.1
Anus	C21	220	62.8	42.3	34.0	64.8	46.3	39.5	32.5	36.9
Pancreas	C25	917	22.9	15.7	12.5	23.8	17.4	14.6	13.2	15.2
Larynx	C32	1 880	59.9	37.2	28.6	62.3	41.8	34.6	32.8	36.0
Lung	C33-34	3 451	28.4	15.4	10.9	29.6	17.3	13.2	10.9	13.4
Breast	C50	7 294	77.9	56.6	46.0	79.7	60.4	51.4	48.2	51.6
Cervix	C53	4 436	75.2	53.6	42.2	76.6	56.6	46.1	43.8	46.4
Ovary	C56	2 029	49.7	29.1	22.8	50.7	30.7	24.6	21.0	22.9
Penis	C60	327	75.1	49.2	43.6	77.9	54.9	51.6	47.1	53.3
Prostate	C61	1 463	64.3	39.3	24.0	69.6	50.2	35.9	28.4	42.3
Testis	C62	383	69.3	58.0	53.0	70.0	59.5	55.2	55.1	56.2
Kidney	C64	819	53.0	38.2	31.2	54.8	41.8	36.0	32.1	35.2
Urinary bladder	C67	1 307	67.0	45.6	32.5	70.6	53.6	41.8	34.6	45.6
Hodgkin lymphoma	C81	528	70.0	58.5	48.8	71.0	60.8	51.7	50.6	52.2
Non-Hodgkin lymphoma	C82-85+C96	2 338	50.3	38.0	30.2	51.8	41.1	34.1	34.2	37.1
Lymphoid leukaemia	C91	1 099	34.8	22.0	15.2	35.4	22.9	16.3	14.8	15.5
Myeloid leukaemia	C92-94	1 261	31.2	20.6	13.7	31.8	21.5	14.6	12.8	15.2
Leukaemia unspecified	C95	345	18.7	10.3	6.1	19.2	10.9	6.7	5.9	7.1

ASRS: age-standardized relative survival

Table 4a. Site-wise number of cases, 5-year absolute and relative survival by sex: Mumbai, India, 1992–1994 cases followed through 1999 and 1995–1999 cases followed-up until 2003

Site	ICD-10	Cases included	Male % 5-year survival			Female % 5-year survival		
			No.	Abs	Rel	No.	Abs	Rel
Lip	C00	161	96	52.8	59.7	65	60.4	69.7
Tongue	C01-02	2 106	1 550	22.5	26.2	556	33.0	37.6
Oral cavity	C03-06	2 769	1 768	33.9	38.9	1 001	29.5	33.7
Tonsil	C09	513	453	11.7	14.0	60	30.8	37.9
Oropharynx	C10	243	220	15.3	18.0	23	19.1	24.3
Nasopharynx	C11	243	180	21.7	24.3	63	26.2	28.7
Hypopharynx	C12-13	1 902	1 522	17.1	21.2	380	20.7	23.7
Oesophagus	C15	3 128	1 866	13.5	16.3	1 262	12.3	14.1
Stomach	C16	2 205	1 507	13.1	15.4	698	12.1	13.7
Colon	C18	1 578	918	28.5	34.1	660	26.0	29.8
Rectum	C19-20	1 217	759	28.9	34.2	458	28.2	32.7
Anus	C21	220	127	32.3	37.9	93	36.3	41.6
Pancreas	C25	917	578	12.5	14.6	339	12.5	14.7
Larynx	C32	1 880	1 630	28.4	34.6	250	29.9	34.2
Lung	C33-34	3 451	2 705	11.0	13.5	746	10.5	12.0
Breast	C50	7 294				7 294	46.0	51.4
Cervix	C53	4 436				4 436	42.2	46.1
Ovary	C56	2 029				2 029	22.8	24.6
Penis	C60	327	327	43.6	51.6			
Prostate	C61	1 463	1 463	24.0	35.9			
Testis	C62	383	383	53.0	55.2			
Kidney	C64	819	569	30.1	35.3	250	33.7	37.4
Urinary bladder	C67	1 307	1 046	32.0	41.4	261	34.6	43.3
Hodgkin lymphoma	C81	528	370	53.3	56.5	158	38.9	41.1
Non-Hodgkin lymphoma	C82-85+C96	2 338	1 521	31.7	35.8	817	27.5	30.9
Lymphoid leukaemia	C91	1 099	725	14.6	15.5	374	16.4	17.7
Myeloid leukaemia	C92-94	1 261	755	14.7	15.8	506	12.2	13.0
Leukaemia unspecified	C95	345	195	5.8	6.3	150	6.6	7.2

Abs: absolute survival; Rel: relative survival

Table 4b. Site-wise number of cases and relative survival by age group: Mumbai, India, 1992–1994 cases followed through 1999 and 1995–1999 cases followed-up until 2003

Site	ICD-10	Cases included	Number of cases by age group					Relative survival by age group % 5-year survival				
			< 45	45-54	55-64	65-74	> 75	< 45	45-54	55-64	65-74	> 75
Lip	C00	161	32	56	42	22	9	66.7	62.2	67.1	50.7	86.1
Tongue	C01-02	2 106	415	553	567	419	152	42.1	32.2	26.2	19.8	7.0
Oral cavity	C03-06	2 769	669	744	708	463	185	45.7	38.5	33.8	25.7	28.1
Tonsil	C09	513	85	140	138	104	46	23.2	16.2	11.5	19.9	15.2
Oropharynx	C10	243	31	72	73	49	18	31.6	15.5	24.3	9.5	0.0
Nasopharynx	C11	243	106	43	48	34	12	34.4	23.7	16.9	17.5	0.0
Hypopharynx	C12-13	1 902	267	411	587	456	181	31.1	19.9	20.2	23.9	6.7
Oesophagus	C15	3 128	368	720	928	743	369	33.3	21.8	11.5	5.8	6.0
Stomach	C16	2 205	352	515	610	499	229	27.7	23.6	10.1	4.4	1.9
Colon	C18	1 578	325	357	380	329	187	44.1	42.5	27.9	18.8	17.6
Rectum	C19-20	1 217	279	271	279	268	120	43.2	41.9	32.5	16.2	16.0
Anus	C21	220	46	49	63	45	17	40.9	63.9	31.0	22.3	25.3
Pancreas	C25	917	128	209	249	236	95	28.6	16.9	9.1	12.3	8.9
Larynx	C32	1 880	240	416	561	484	179	47.8	39.0	35.9	24.0	17.8
Lung	C33-34	3 451	386	672	1 087	925	381	25.4	19.9	11.3	5.9	4.1
Breast	C50	7 294	2 179	2 038	1 647	1 023	407	57.6	52.7	47.9	43.8	29.8
Cervix	C53	4 436	1 333	1 358	1 018	569	158	61.1	48.6	32.7	24.0	20.9
Ovary	C56	2 029	672	538	462	260	97	40.9	23.7	12.3	5.7	9.5
Penis	C60	327	84	66	73	67	37	58.4	53.8	61.0	33.5	32.3
Prostate	C61	1 463	19	67	287	619	471	59.7	56.1	45.8	36.9	20.1
Testis	C62	383	300	37	26	15	5	56.8	55.8	55.0	33.0	0.0
Kidney	C64	819	230	157	199	170	63	49.6	39.0	34.6	17.3	21.8
Urinary bladder	C67	1 307	120	216	347	374	250	60.7	60.5	49.7	26.1	15.4
Hodgkin lymphoma	C81	528	341	71	61	40	15	60.9	50.0	22.0	24.2	18.5
Non-Hodgkin lymphoma	C82-85+C96	2 338	889	382	473	403	191	43.7	42.4	29.6	17.6	3.9
Lymphoid leukaemia	C91	1 099	803	70	93	70	63	17.6	14.3	10.4	13.1	12.2
Myeloid leukaemia	C92-94	1 261	691	203	179	125	63	18.4	13.3	5.6	13.9	0.0
Leukaemia unspecified	C95	345	200	33	41	44	27	7.2	5.6	9.3	8.5	0.0

Table 5. Proportion of cases and 5-year absolute survival by extent of disease and site: Mumbai, India, 1992–1999

Site	ICD-10	Cases included	% of cases by extent of disease				% 5-year absolute survival			
			Localized	Regional	Dist. met.	Unknown	Localized	Regional	Dist. met.	Unknown
Lip	C00	161	51.6	36.6	4.3	7.5	81.4	22.8	0.0	73.4
Tongue	C01-02	2 106	30.5	58.4	7.1	4.1	58.4	12.0	0.0	29.1
Oral cavity	C03-06	2 769	32.6	55.8	6.9	4.6	62.5	18.0	1.1	35.5
Colon	C18	1 578	38.7	26.7	25.9	8.7	51.8	19.1	1.6	27.5
Rectum	C19-20	1 217	46.2	26.0	20.3	7.5	46.5	19.8	1.6	32.4
Larynx	C32	1 880	33.2	51.1	9.7	6.1	57.1	16.5	0.5	23.2
Breast	C50	7 294	39.6	41.5	12.8	6.2	74.2	32.8	3.8	48.1
Cervix	C53	4 436	27.9	56.8	8.6	6.7	68.3	35.7	2.4	40.7
Ovary	C56	2 029	28.6	11.4	49.9	10.1	59.7	27.5	3.0	26.4

Dis. met.: distant metastasis

Table 6. Comparison of 5-year absolute and relative survival of cases diagnosed between 1982–1986 and 1992–1999

Site	ICD-10	% Complete FU at 5 years		% 5-year absolute survival		% 5-year relative survival	
		1982–1986	1992–1999	1982–1986	1992–1999	1982–1986	1992–1999
Breast	C50	75.2	87.2	51.1	46.0	55.1	51.4
Cervix	C53	73.3	85.3	47.7	42.2	50.7	46.1

FU: follow-up

Chapter 17

Cancer survival in South Karachi, Pakistan, 1995–1999

Bhurgri Y

Abstract

The Karachi cancer registry established in 1995 was the first population-based cancer registry in Pakistan. Cancer registration is done by active methods. The registry contributed data on survival for selected cancers of the head and neck registered during 1995–1999. Follow-up has been carried out predominantly by active methods with the median follow-up time ranging between 29–36 months for different cancers. The proportion of histologically verified diagnosis for various cancers ranged between 98–100%; there were no cases as death certificates only (DCOs); 86–93% of total registered cases were included for survival analysis. Five-year follow-up ranged between 67–76%. The 5-year age-standardized relative survival rates was the highest for cancer of the salivary gland (44%), followed by oral cavity (40%), tongue (39%) and tonsil (3%). Five-year relative survival by age group did not display any pattern or trend and was fluctuating. A majority of cases have been diagnosed with a regional spread of disease: tongue (51%), oral cavity (53%), salivary gland (46%) and tonsil (79%) and survival decreased with increasing extent of disease for these cancers.

Karachi cancer registry

The Karachi cancer registry was the first population-based cancer registry in Pakistan. It was established in 1995 at the Sindh Government Services Hospital by the government of Sindh, and contributed data to the quinquennial IARC publication *Cancer Incidence in Five Continents* for the first time in volume VIII [1]. Cancer registration is done by active methods [2]. Over 50 sources of registration, comprising hospitals in the government and private sectors and pathology laboratories, are visited for data collection on incident cancer cases from the medical records. The registry caters to a population of about 1.7 million in 1996 with a sex ratio of 856 females to 1000 males. The average annual age-standardized incidence rate is 139 per 100 000 among males and 169 per 100 000 among females with a lifetime cumulative risk of one in 6 of developing cancer for both sexes in the period 1995–1997 [2]. The top-ranking cancers among males are lung followed by oral cavity and larynx. Among females, the order is breast, ovary and oral cavity.

The registry has contributed data on survival from selected cancers of the head and neck registered during 1995–1999 for the first time in this volume of the IARC publication on *Cancer Survival in Africa, Asia, the Caribbean and Central America*.

Data quality indices (Table 1)

The proportion of cases with histologically verified cancer diagnosis in the series varied between 98–100%. No cases were registered on the basis of a death certificate only (DCO). The exclusion of cases owing to the non-availability of any follow-up information is 7%, ranging from 9% in cancer of the tonsil to 7% for oral cavity. Thus, 86–93% of the total cases registered are included in the estimation of the survival probability.

Outcome of follow-up (Table 2)

Follow-up has been carried out predominantly by active methods. These included abstraction of cancer mortality information from death certificates. The abstracted data are matched with the incident cancer database. Unmatched incident cases are then subjected to repeated scrutiny of records in the respective sources of registration and postal/ telephone enquiries to obtain the vital status information.

The closing date of follow-up was 31st December 2003. The median follow-up ranged from 29 months for cancer of the oral cavity to 36 months in tongue cancer. Complete follow-up information at five years from the incidence date ranged between 67–76%. The losses to follow-up are spread over all the time intervals from incidence date, from <1 year to >5 years. This minimizes the bias of estimation of survival probability in the respective years from the incidence date.

Survival statistics

All ages and both sexes together (Table 3)

The 5-year relative survival is the highest for cancer of the salivary gland (46%), followed in order by oral cavity (38%), tongue (37%) and tonsil (31%).

The 5-year age-standardized relative survival (ASRS) probability for all ages together was greater than the corresponding unadjusted one in cancers of the tongue, oral cavity and tonsil; this was reversed for cancer of the salivary gland. The 5-year ASRS (0–74 years of age) is less than the corresponding ASRS (all ages) for most cancers.

Sex
Male (Table 4a)

The 5-year relative survival was the highest for cancer of the salivary gland (45%), and the lowest was tongue cancer (25%). Survival from cancers of the oral cavity and tonsil is noticeably higher among males than females.

Female (Table 4a)

The top ranking cancer on 5-year relative survival was the tongue (52%), and the lowest in the ranking was tonsil (16%). Survival was markedly higher among females than males in cancer of the tongue.

Age group (Table 4b)

The 5-year relative survival by age group did not display any pattern or trend and was observed to fluctuate with increasing age groups.

Extent of disease (Table 5; Figure 1)

A majority of cases have been diagnosed with a regional spread of disease: tongue (51%), oral cavity (53%), salivary gland (46%) and tonsil (79%). Cases diagnosed with distant metastasis were negligible. Localized stage cancers are the least common among cancer of the tonsil (13%), while in the rest it ranged between 33-38%. The extent of disease was unknown in 8–22%. The 5-year absolute survival by extent of disease followed the expected pattern: highest for localized cases, followed by regional and distant metastasis cases among known categories of extent of disease.

References

1. Parkin DM, Whelan SL, Ferlay J and Storm H. *Cancer Incidence in Five Continents, Vol I to VIII: IARC Cancerbase No. 7*. IARCPress, Lyon, 2005.

2. Bhurgri Y, Bhurgri A, Hassan SH, Zaidi SH, Rahim A, Sankaranarayanan R, Parkin DM. Cancer incidence in Karachi, Pakistan: first results from Karachi Cancer Registry. *Int J Cancer*. 2000; 85(3): 325–329.

Figure 1. Absolute survival (%) from selected cancers by extent of disease, South Karachi, Pakistan

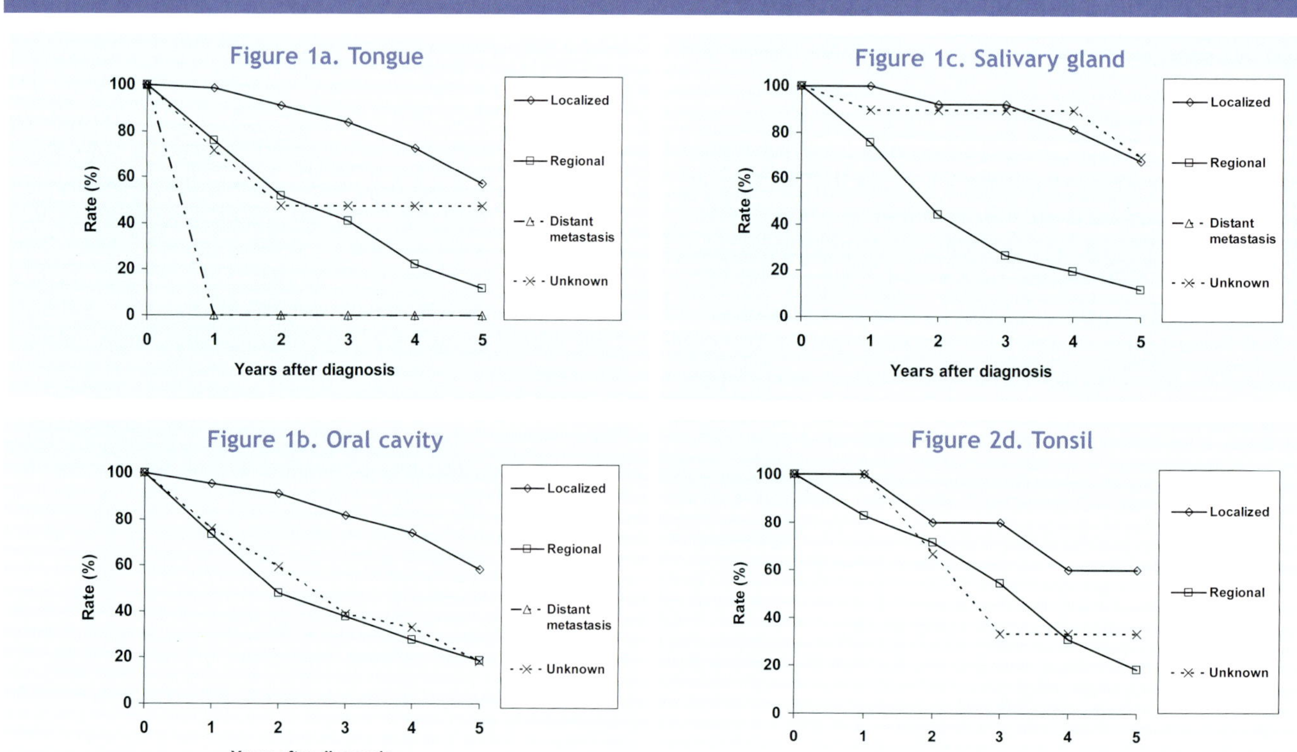

Table 1. Data quality indices - Proportion of histologically verified and death certificate only cases, number and proportion of included and excluded cases by site: South Karachi, Pakistan, 1995–1999 cases followed-up until 2003

Site	ICD-10	Total registered	%		Excluded cases					Included cases	
			HV	DCO	DCO	Follow-up	Others	Total	%	No.	%
Tongue	C01-02	196	99.5	0.0	0	16	0	16	8.2	180	91.8
Oral cavity	C03-06	443	98.4	0.0	0	30	0	30	6.8	413	93.2
Salivary gland	C07-08	51	98.0	0.0	0	3	2	5	9.8	46	90.2
Tonsil	C09	44	100.0	0.0	0	4	2	6	13.6	38	86.4

HV: histologically verified; DCO: death certificate only

Table 2. Number and proportion of cases with complete/incomplete follow-up (in years) and median follow-up (in months) by site: South Karachi, Pakistan, 1995–1999 cases followed-up until 2003

Site	ICD-10	Cases included	Complete FU		Incomplete FU: lost to FU						% with complete FU at 5 years	Median FU (in months)
			Alive/dead at end of FU				% lost to FU: years from diagnosis					
			No.	%	No.	%	< 1	1-3	3-5	> 5		
Tongue	C01-02	180	123	68.3	57	31.7	8.3	4.4	15.6	3.4	71.7	35.6
Oral cavity	C03-06	413	294	71.2	119	28.8	5.8	11.1	8.7	3.1	74.3	29.5
Salivary gland	C07-08	46	26	56.5	20	43.5	8.7	10.9	13.0	10.9	67.4	32.7
Tonsil	C09	38	29	76.3	9	23.7	5.3	10.5	7.9	0.0	76.3	35.5

FU: follow-up

Table 3. Comparison of 1-, 3- and 5-year absolute and relative survival and 5-year age-standardized relative survival by site: South Karachi, Pakistan, 1995–1999 cases followed-up until 2003

Site	ICD-10	Cases included	% Absolute survival			% Relative survival			% ASRS at 5-years	
			1-year	3-year	5-year	1-year	3-year	5-year	all ages	0-74 years
Tongue	C01-02	180	83.8	58.7	32.9	85.5	62.5	36.8	39.4	39.3
Oral cavity	C03-06	413	81.8	54.9	34.8	83.2	58.0	38.2	39.9	40.9
Salivary gland	C07-08	46	86.4	60.6	41.6	88.4	64.8	45.7	44.4	43.0
Tonsil	C09	38	86.5	56.4	26.9	88.9	61.2	31.0	33.6	32.3

ASRS: age-standardized relative survival

Table 4a. Site-wise number of cases, 5-year absolute and relative survival by sex: South Karachi, Pakistan, 1995–1999 cases followed-up until 2003

Site	ICD-10	Cases included	Male			Female		
			% 5-year survival			% 5-year survival		
			No.	Abs	Rel	No.	Abs	Rel
Tongue	C01-02	180	91	22.4	25.1	89	46.3	51.6
Oral cavity	C03-06	413	250	39.4	43.2	163	28.4	31.1
Salivary gland	C07-08	46	28	39.9	44.8	18	43.9	46.9
Tonsil	C09	38	27	29.7	33.9	11	12.9	15.5

Abs: absolute survival; Rel: relative survival

Table 4b. Site-wise number of cases and relative survival by age group: South Karachi, Pakistan, 1995–1999 cases followed-up until 2003

Site	ICD-10	Cases included	Number of cases by age group					Relative survival by age group % 5-year survival				
			< 45	45-54	55-64	65-74	> 75	< 45	45-54	55-64	65-74	> 75
Tongue	C01-02	180	53	32	46	40	9	25.4	48.9	40.6	36.9	43.7
Oral cavity	C03-06	413	136	114	76	64	23	29.5	44.9	48.8	34.1	32.5
Salivary gland	C07-08	46	16	10	7	11	2	43.5	80.1	19.2	45.7	
Tonsil	C09	38	7	6	12	8	5	34.1	50.3	0.0	51.2	45.2

Table 5. Proportion of cases and 5-year absolute survival by extent of disease and site: South Karachi, Pakistan, 1995–1999 cases followed-up until 2003

Site	ICD-10	Cases included	% of cases by extent of disease				% 5-year absolute survival			
			Localized	Regional	Dist. met.	Unknown	Localized	Regional	Dist. met.	Unknown
Tongue	C01-02	180	37.8	50.6	0.6	11.0	57.4	11.7	0.0	47.6
Oral cavity	C03-06	413	36.3	53.0	0.5	10.2	58.3	18.6		18.3
Salivary gland	C07-08	46	32.6	45.7	0.0	21.7	67.6	12.0		69.6
Tonsil	C09	38	13.2	78.9	0.0	7.9	60.0	18.5		33.3

Dis. met.: distant metastasis

Chapter 18

Cancer survival in Manila, Philippines, 1994–1995

Laudico A and Mapua C

Abstract

The population-based cancer registry in Manila, Philippines, called the Philippine Cancer Society-Manila Cancer Registry, was established in 1983. Cancer registration is pursued by active methods. The registry contributed survival data on a random sample of total incident cancers of breast (500), cervix (500), colon and rectum (300) registered in 1994–1995. Follow-up has been carried out by passive and active methods, with median follow-up ranging between 15–33 months for different cancers. The proportion of histologically verified diagnosis for various cancers ranged between 78–88%; 74–83% of the total submitted cases were included for survival analysis. Complete follow-up at five years was available in 75–82% of cases. Five-year age-standardized relative survival rates was the highest for cancer of the breast (52%) followed by colon (49%), cervix (36%) and rectum (31%). Five-year relative survival by age group did not display any pattern or trend and was fluctuating. A decreasing survival with increasing extent of disease was noted for all cancers.

Philippine cancer society - Manila cancer registry

The population-based cancer registry in Manila, called the Philippine Cancer Society-Manila Cancer Registry (PCS-MCR), was established in 1983 as an offshoot of the then ongoing cancer registration activity under the central tumour registry of the Philippines since 1968. PCS-MCR has been contributing data to the quinquennial IARC publication *Cancer Incidence in Five Continents* since volume VI [1]. Cancer registration is pursued by active methods [2]. The sources of registration, besides coordination with the Department of Health-Rizal Cancer Registry, include hospitals in the government and private sectors, consultants, pathology laboratories and imaging centres. Data are collected from hospital tumour registries and other records maintained at these places. The registry covers an area of 274.2 km^2 and caters to an entirely urban population of about 5.1 million in 1995 with a sex ratio of 1046 females to 1000 males. The average annual age-standardized incidence rate is 222 per 100 000 among males and 206 per 100 000 among females with a lifetime cumulative risk of one in 4 of developing cancer for both sexes in the period 1993–1997. The top ranking cancers among males are lung, liver and prostate. Among females, the order is breast, cervix and ovary.

The registry has contributed data on survival from cancers of the breast, cervix, colon and rectum for the first time in this volume of the IARC publication on *Cancer Survival in Africa, Asia, the Caribbean and Central America*. A random sample of 1300 cases out of the total incident cancers in 1994–1995 comprising about 500 cases each of female breast and cervix cancers (stratified by age) and 300 cases of colorectal cancers (stratified by age and sex) form the material for this study.

Data quality indices (Table 1)

The proportion of cases with histological confirmation of cancer diagnosis in this series ranges from 78% for colon cancer to 88% in rectal and breast cancers. No cases registered-based on a death certificate only (DCO) were included in the study. Cases without any follow-up information represent 21%, varying between 16–25% for different cancers. Thus, 74–83% of cases considered for the study are included in the estimation of the survival probability.

Outcome of follow-up (Table 2)

Follow-up has been carried out by passive and active methods. These included collection of cancer mortality information from the local civil registrar offices. The mortality data are first matched with the incident cancer database. The follow-up information for the unmatched incident cases is then obtained through the attending physicians, repeated scrutiny of records in the respective sources of registration, postal/telephone enquiries and house visits.

The closing date of follow-up was 31st December 2002. The median follow-up ranged from 15 months in cervix cancer to 33 months in breast cancer. Complete follow-up at five years from the incidence

The median follow-up was 6 months. Complete follow-up at five years from the incidence date was 30%. The losses to follow-up generally occurred in large numbers in the first year of follow-up and decreased through successive intervals of follow-up time. Though the losses to follow-up have been ascertained to be random, the high magnitude of incomplete follow-up at 5 years from diagnosis may introduce a bias in the estimation of survival probability.

Survival statistics

All ages and both sexes together (Table 3)

The relative survival probabilities of breast cancer at 1-, 3- and 5-year from the incidence date are 89%, 56% and 37%, respectively. The age-standardized relative survival for all ages together is 35%, while the corresponding figure for 0–74 years of age is 40%.

Age group (Table 4b)

The 5-year relative survival of breast cancer by age group did not display any pattern and was observed to be fluctuating with increasing age groups.

Extent of disease (Table 5)

A majority of breast cancer cases were diagnosed with a regional spread of disease (44%) followed by localized stage (17%). Distant metastasis accounted for 10%, while the extent of disease is unknown in 29%. The 5-year absolute survival rates by extent of disease were localized (65%), regional (35%), distant metastasis (12%) and unknown (35%).

Figure 1. Absolute survival (%) from breast cancer by extent of disease, Rizal, Philippines

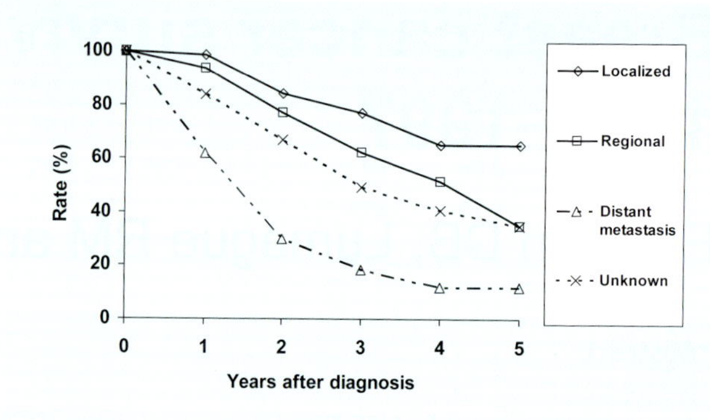

Survival trend (Table 6)

The data on trend in survival from breast cancer is available for two periods of time: 1987 [3] and 1996-1997. The 5-year relative survival in 1987 is 46% compared to 37% in 1996–1997.

References

1. Parkin DM, Whelan SL, Ferlay J and Storm H. *Cancer Incidence in Five Continents, Vol I to VIII: IARC Cancerbase No. 7*. IARCPress, Lyon, 2005.

2. Laudico AV, Esteban D and Parkin DM. *Cancer in the Philippines: IARC Technical Report No. 5*. IARCPress, Lyon, 1989.

3. Esteban D, Ngelangel C, Lacaya L, Robles E and Monson M. Cancer survival in Rizal, Philippines. In: *Cancer Survival in Developing Countries* (eds) R Sankaranarayanan, RJ Black and DM Parkin. IARC Scientific Publications No. 145. IARCPress, Lyon, 1998, pp 89–100.

Table 1. Data quality indices - Proportion of histologically verified and death certificate only cases, number and proportion of included and excluded cases by site: Rizal, Philippines, 1996–1997 cases followed-up until 2002

Site	ICD-10	Total registered	%		Excluded cases					Included cases	
			HV	DCO	DCO	Follow-up	Others	Total	%	No.	%
Breast	C50	1 570	90.3	5.9	93	174	4	271	17.3	1 299	82.7

HV: histologically verified; DCO: death certificate only

Table 2. Number and proportion of cases with complete/incomplete follow-up (in years) and median follow-up (in months) by site: Rizal, Philippines, 1996–1997 cases followed-up until 2002

Site	ICD-10	Cases included	Complete FU		Incomplete FU: lost to FU						% with complete FU at 5 years	Median FU (in months)
			Alive/dead at end of FU				% lost to FU: years from diagnosis					
			No.	%	No.	%	< 1	1-3	3-5	> 5		
Breast	C50	1 299	341	26.3	958	73.7	52.9	12.4	5.2	3.2	29.5	5.7

FU: follow-up

Table 3. Comparison of 1-, 3- and 5-year absolute and relative survival and 5-year age-standardized relative survival by site: Rizal, Philippines, 1996–1997 cases followed-up until 2002

Site	ICD-10	Cases included	% Absolute survival			% Relative survival			% ASRS at 5-years	
			1-year	3-year	5-year	1-year	3-year	5-year	all ages	0-74 years
Breast	C50	1 299	87.7	54.5	35.2	88.7	56.3	37.3	34.7	39.7

ASRS: age-standardized relative survival

Table 4a. Site-wise number of cases, 5-year absolute and relative survival by sex: Rizal, Philippines, 1996–1997 cases followed-up until 2002

Site	ICD-10	Cases included	Male			Female		
				% 5-year survival			% 5-year survival	
			No.	Abs	Rel	No.	Abs	Rel
Breast	C50	1 299	12	100.0	108.1	1 287	35.0	37.1

Abs: absolute survival; Rel: relative survival

Table 4b. Site-wise number of cases and relative survival by age group: Rizal, Philippines, 1996–1997 cases followed-up until 2002

Site	ICD-10	Cases included	Number of cases by age group					Relative survival by age group % 5-year survival				
			< 45	45-54	55-64	65-74	> 75	< 45	45-54	55-64	65-74	> 75
Breast	C50	1 299	441	415	259	126	58	40.6	28.8	46.7	43.2	0.0

Table 5. Proportion of cases and 5-year absolute survival by extent of disease and site: Rizal, Philippines, 1996–1997

Site	ICD-10	Cases included	% of cases by extent of disease				% 5-year absolute survival			
			Localized	Regional	Dist. met.	Unknown	Localized	Regional	Dist. met.	Unknown
Breast	C50	1 299	17.5	43.7	9.9	28.9	65.3	35.0	11.9	34.8

Dis. met.: distant metastasis

Table 6. Comparison of 5-year absolute and relative survival of cases diagnosed between 1987 and 1996–1997, Rizal, Philippines

Site	ICD-10	% 5-year absolute survival		% 5-year relative survival	
		1987	1996–1997	1987	1996–1997
Breast	C50	41.4	35.2	45.6	37.3

Chapter 20

Cancer survival in Busan, Republic of Korea, 1996–2001

Shin HR, Lee DH, Lee SY, Lee JT, Park HK, Rha SH, Whang IK, Jung KW, Won YJ and Kong HJ

Abstract

The Busan cancer registry was established in 1996; cancer registration is done by passive and active methods. The registry contributed survival data for 48 cancer sites or types registered during 1996–2001. Follow-up information has been gleaned predominantly by passive methods with median follow-up ranging between 1–57 months for various cancers. The proportion with histologically verified diagnosis for different cancers ranged between 20–100%; death certificates only (DCOs) comprised 0–53%; 47–100% of total registered cases were included for survival analysis. The top-ranking cancers on 5-year age-standardized relative survival rates were penis (94%), thyroid (91%), non-melanoma skin (89%), placenta (86%), breast (76%), Hodgkin lymphoma (75%) and testis (72%). Five-year relative survival by age group showed a decreasing trend with increasing age groups for cancers of the nasopharynx, gall bladder, lung, bone, soft tissue, breast, cervix, corpus uteri, thyroid, multiple myeloma, lymphoid leukaemia and myeloid leukaemia or was fluctuating for other cancers.

Busan cancer registry

The Busan cancer registry was established in 1996 in cooperation with the cancer centres in four university hospitals, supported by the Department of Public Health and Sanitation of Busan City and the medical association of Busan and funded by the Korean national cancer control programme. The registry contributed data to the quinquennial IARC publication *Cancer Incidence in Five Continents* for the first time in Vol VIII [1]. Cancer registration is done by passive and active methods. The principal source of information on 72% of cancer cases is the data file from the hospital-based Korean central cancer registry. The rest of the cases are registered by the active method of visiting more than 50 hospitals and perusing of records in the departments of anatomical pathology, diagnostic radiology and radiation oncology. The registry covers an area of 531.17 km^2 and caters to a population of about 3.9 million with a male female ratio of 1:1 in 1995. The average annual age-standardized incidence rate is 304 per 100 000 among males and 169 per 100 000 among females, with a lifetime cumulative risk of one in 4 of developing cancer in the period 1996–1997. The most common cancers among males are stomach, liver and lung. The rank order among females is stomach, cervix and breast [1].

The registry is contributing data on survival from 48 cancer sites or types registered during 1996–2001 for the first time in this volume of IARC publication on *Cancer Survival in Africa, Asia, the Caribbean and Central America*.

Data quality indices (Table 1)

The proportion of cases with histologically verified cancer diagnosis in the series is 69%, varying from 20% in liver cancer to 100% in cancer of the penis. The proportion of cases registered on the basis of death certificates only (DCO) is 8%, ranging between nil for a few cancers (tonsil, corpus uteri, placenta, penis, testis and ureter) and 53% for unspecified leukaemia. Cases excluded without any follow-up are negligible. Thus, 47–100% of the total cases registered are included in the estimation of the survival probability.

Outcome of follow-up (Table 2)

Follow-up information has been obtained predominantly by passive methods. These included obtaining of mortality information from the death certificates in the national statistical office. The mortality data are periodically matched with the incident cancer database. The vital status of the unmatched incident cases is also ascertained by scrutiny of hospital records. However, all incident cases for whom death information is not available were presumed to be alive on the last date of the year for which the mortality data are fully utilized for matching.

The closing date of follow-up was 31st December 2003. The median follow-up ranged from zero in case of unspecified leukaemia to 57 months for cancer of the placenta.

Survival statistics

All ages and both sexes together (Table 3)

The top-ranking cancers on 5-year relative survival are thyroid (93%), penis (89%), non-melanoma skin (89%) placenta (87%) and breast (82%). The lowest survival rate is encountered with pancreatic cancer (6%) preceded by unspecified leukaemia (8%), cancer of the liver (10%) and lung (12%), and multiple myeloma (12%). Salivary gland (71%) among other head and neck sites, colon and rectum (54-55%) among gastrointestinal sites and bladder (69%) among urinary system sites are the ones with higher survival than others. Hodgkin lymphoma had a better survival (65%) than non-Hodgkin (46%). The survival figures for leukaemias are 42% for lymphoid and 28% for myeloid.

Figure 1a. Top ten cancers (ranked by survival), Busan, Republic of Korea, 1996–2001

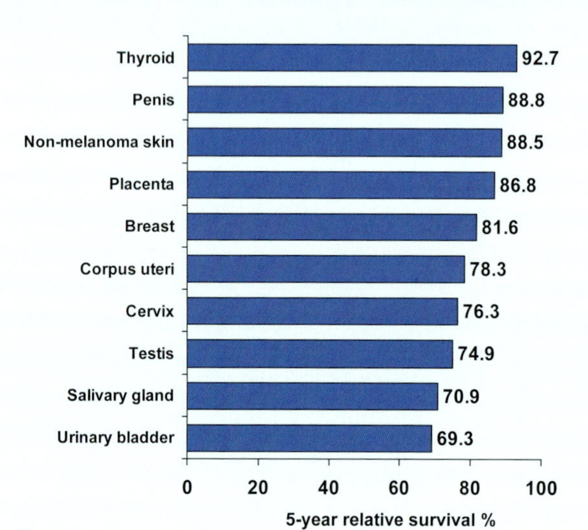

The 5-year age-standardized relative survival (ASRS) probability for all ages together is generally less than or similar to the corresponding unadjusted one for a majority of cancers. Also, the 5-year ASRS (0–74 years of age) is generally higher than or similar to the corresponding ASRS (all ages) for a majority of cancers.

Sex

Male (Table 4a)

The top-ranking site on 5-year relative survival is breast (89%). The survival figures for oropharynx including tonsil, larynx, bone, mesothelioma, ureter and unspecified leukaemia are noticeably higher among males than females.

Figure 1b. Top five cancers (ranked by survival), Male, Busan, Republic of Korea, 1996–2001

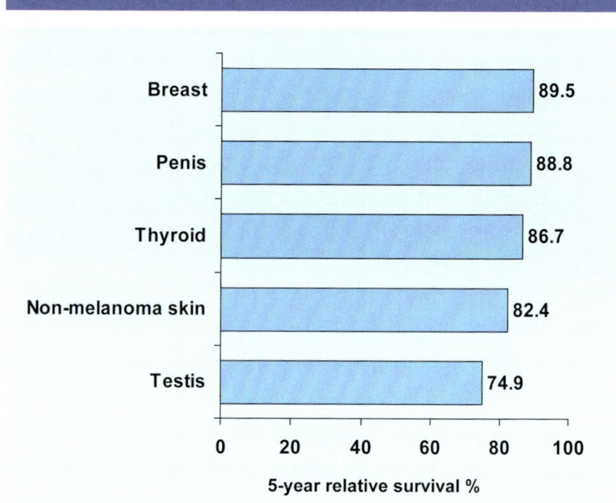

Female (Table 4a)

The top-ranking cancer in terms of 5-year relative survival is non-melanoma skin (94%). The survival estimates for cancers of the breast, cervix and ovary are 82%, 76% and 58%, respectively. Survival is distinctly higher among females than males for cancers of tongue, oral cavity, salivary gland, oesophagus, small intestine, non-melanoma skin, eye and adrenal/other endocrine glands.

Figure 1c. Top five cancers (ranked by survival), Female, Busan, Republic of Korea, 1996–2001

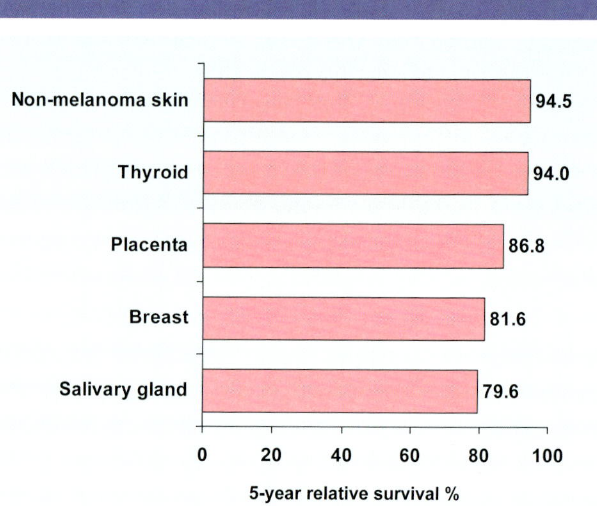

Age group (Table 4b)

The 5-year relative survival by age group reveals a decreasing survival with increasing age at diagnosis for cancers of the nasopharynx, gall bladder, lung, bone, soft tissue, breast, cervix, corpus uteri and thyroid, and multiple myeloma, lymphoid leukaemia and myeloid leukaemia. For all other cancers, the survival by age group did not display any pattern.

References

1. Parkin DM, Whelan SL, Ferlay J and Storm H. *Cancer Incidence in Five Continents, Vol I to VIII: IARC Cancerbase No. 7*. IARCPress, Lyon, 2005.

Table 3. Comparison of 1-, 3- and 5-year absolute and relative survival and 5-year age-standardized relative survival by site: Busan, Republic of Korea, 1996–2001 cases followed-up until 2003

Site	ICD-10	Cases included	% Absolute survival			% Relative survival			% ASRS at 5-years	
			1-year	3-year	5-year	1-year	3-year	5-year	all ages	0-74 years
Tongue	C01-02	144	72.9	50.1	46.9	74.2	52.5	51.0	52.3	52.8
Oral cavity	C03-06	156	69.9	52.2	41.1	71.6	55.7	45.5	45.4	48.4
Salivary gland	C07-08	86	90.7	75.2	66.9	91.9	78.0	70.9	65.0	70.3
Tonsil	C09	59	89.8	51.7	47.5	91.5	54.7	52.6	54.4	57.9
Oropharynx	C10	34	55.9	26.5	19.4	57.1	28.4	22.4	20.1	20.9
Nasopharynx	C11	134	85.1	57.5	49.9	86.0	59.3	52.7	46.6	53.2
Hypopharynx	C12-13	87	52.9	23.2	15.3	54.3	25.0	17.6	19.8	23.5
Oesophagus	C15	790	40.4	19.4	16.3	41.5	20.9	18.4	17.7	20.5
Stomach	C16	8 683	64.1	46.0	40.2	65.4	48.6	44.2	37.3	46.5
Small intestine	C17	141	49.6	30.5	18.7	50.8	32.3	20.7	21.0	24.2
Colon	C18	1 859	74.7	56.9	49.0	76.4	60.6	54.4	46.6	57.0
Rectum	C19-20	1 882	82.5	59.7	49.6	84.1	63.3	54.7	44.5	57.3
Anus	C21	60	80.0	53.1	45.9	82.1	57.0	51.6	40.0	61.7
Liver	C22	6 507	32.4	14.5	8.7	33.0	15.3	9.6	9.6	10.0
Gall bladder	C23-24	1 524	38.8	18.3	14.6	39.9	19.6	16.3	17.5	21.8
Pancreas	C25	1 011	21.9	7.5	5.5	22.4	8.1	6.3	6.5	7.4
Nose/Sinuses	C30-31	103	69.9	36.6	32.5	71.4	39.0	36.5	36.7	39.3
Larynx	C32	475	81.1	60.1	49.7	83.1	64.7	56.3	54.2	58.9
Lung	C33-34	4 796	34.7	14.2	10.5	35.7	15.3	11.9	11.6	13.7
Other thoracic organs	C37-38	148	60.1	37.3	32.5	61.1	38.9	34.5	25.0	34.1
Bone	C40-41	196	78.6	61.9	53.0	79.3	63.2	54.7	30.6	39.7
Melanoma of skin	C43	86	75.6	46.4	40.4	77.1	49.4	45.4	43.5	48.1
Other skin	C44	423	91.0	82.1	77.2	93.4	88.9	88.5	88.6	89.4
Mesothelioma	C45	30	33.3	16.2	16.2	33.8	16.8	17.1	12.4	17.0
Connective tissue	C47+C49	250	75.6	54.2	43.4	76.5	56.0	45.8	34.8	40.8
Breast	C50	2 642	95.8	85.8	79.6	96.3	87.0	81.6	75.5	80.6
Vulva	C51	25	96.0	79.0	62.1	97.6	83.0	67.2	53.4	72.7
Cervix	C53	2 264	91.5	80.0	74.1	92.1	81.4	76.3	69.5	75.8
Corpus uteri	C54	265	90.2	80.6	76.0	90.7	82.0	78.3	68.8	74.3
Ovary	C56	622	80.9	59.7	5.0	81.5	60.8	57.7	49.8	54.5
Placenta	C58	30	93.3	86.3	86.3	93.4	86.6	86.8	85.9	85.9
Penis	C60	29	96.6	82.5	73.5	99.4	91.4	88.8	94.3	73.0
Prostate	C61	430	84.9	56.7	41.9	89.2	66.0	54.5	47.0	59.5
Testis	C62	55	92.7	79.6	74.0	93.0	80.2	74.9	72.2	72.2
Kidney	C64	706	76.5	63.1	56.9	77.7	66.0	61.6	52.2	64.1
Renal pelvis	C65	74	75.7	51.7	44.3	77.5	55.7	50.4	46.0	54.6
Ureter	C66	77	68.8	56.5	48.0	70.8	61.3	55.4	62.7	68.1
Urinary bladder	C67	999	83.4	68.9	60.1	85.9	75.1	69.3	62.2	72.8
Eye	C69	36	80.6	66.7	60.1	81.8	68.7	62.4	44.2	59.3
Brain & nervous system	C70-72	520	63.3	44.5	37.3	63.9	45.5	38.5	36.0	37.5
Thyroid	C73	1 175	94.7	92.5	89.6	95.4	94.3	92.7	91.2	93.0
Adrenal gland, other	C74-75	56	67.9	58.6	51.6	68.2	59.1	52.4	32.3	32.3
Hodgkin lymphoma	C81	52	80.8	70.9	61.7	81.6	72.9	64.6	74.6	76.9
Non-Hodgkin lymphoma	C82-85+C96	785	66.9	50.3	43.2	67.8	52.3	46.2	46.6	49.0
Multiple myeloma	C90	182	53.8	21.4	11.2	54.9	22.5	12.2	12.4	14.5
Lymphoid leukaemia	C91	222	65.8	47.7	41.8	66.0	48.0	42.2	32.7	32.7
Myeloid leukaemia	C92-94	480	52.9	32.3	26.7	53.4	33.0	27.6	22.8	27.5
Leukaemia unspecified	C95	44	25.0	9.1	6.1	25.7	10.1	7.8	6.6	6.1

ASRS: age-standardized relative survival

Table 4a. Site-wise number of cases, 5-year absolute and relative survival by sex: Busan, Republic of Korea, 1996–2001 cases followed-up until 2003

Site	ICD-10	Cases included	Male % 5-year survival			Female % 5-year survival		
			No.	Abs	Rel	No.	Abs	Rel
Tongue	C01-02	144	97	41.6	45.9	47	57.7	61.5
Oral cavity	C03-06	156	108	34.3	38.7	48	55.4	59.3
Salivary gland	C07-08	86	48	59.2	63.9	38	76.6	79.6
Tonsil	C09	59	50	52.2	58.0	9	22.2	23.8
Oropharynx	C10	34	30	22.0	25.3	4	0.0	0.0
Nasopharynx	C11	134	87	47.9	51.5	47	54.8	55.9
Hypopharynx	C12-13	87	80	14.6	17.1	7	24.5	24.8
Oesophagus	C15	790	706	15.4	17.5	84	22.9	26.0
Stomach	C16	8 683	5 637	40.7	45.3	3 046	39.4	42.1
Small intestine	C17	141	91	13.0	14.9	50	30.9	32.3
Colon	C18	1 859	1 003	50.0	56.5	856	47.7	51.9
Rectum	C19-20	1 882	1 031	48.9	55.4	851	50.4	53.9
Anus	C21	60	27	46.2	54.5	33	45.5	49.0
Liver	C22	6 507	4 828	8.4	9.3	1 679	9.6	10.4
Gall bladder	C23-24	1 524	714	14.6	16.5	810	14.6	16.0
Pancreas	C25	1 011	600	4.3	5.1	411	7.2	8.0
Nose/Sinuses	C30-31	103	67	33.3	38.0	36	31.4	34.1
Larynx	C32	475	422	51.4	58.4	53	35.9	40.6
Lung	C33-34	4 796	3 518	9.9	11.3	1 278	12.0	13.4
Other thoracic organs	C37-38	148	101	30.3	32.1	47	37.0	39.4
Bone	C40-41	196	108	57.2	59.1	88	46.2	47.8
Melanoma of skin	C43	86	47	38.2	42.7	39	42.4	48.1
Other skin	C44	423	211	71.0	82.4	212	83.4	94.5
Mesothelioma	C45	30	15	20.0	21.7	15	11.4	11.7
Connective tissue	C47+C49	250	144	41.0	43.6	106	46.6	48.5
Breast	C50	2 642	19	69.7	89.5	2 623	79.7	81.6
Vulva	C51	25				25	62.1	67.2
Cervix	C53	2 264				2 264	74.1	76.3
Corpus uteri	C54	265				265	76.0	78.3
Ovary	C56	622				622	56.0	57.7
Placenta	C58	30				30	86.3	86.8
Penis	C60	29	29	73.5	88.8			
Prostate	C61	430	430	41.9	54.5			
Testis	C62	55	55	74.0	74.9			
Kidney	C64	706	477	55.1	60.2	229	60.9	64.5
Renal pelvis	C65	74	56	44.9	51.7	18	44.4	48.0
Ureter	C66	77	48	50.7	59.5	29	45.6	50.4
Urinary bladder	C67	999	800	60.8	70.4	199	56.4	64.0
Eye	C69	36	20	55.0	57.7	16	65.5	67.3
Brain & nervous system	C70-72	520	284	35.0	36.0	236	40.0	41.0
Thyroid	C73	1 175	206	81.3	86.7	969	91.3	94.0
Adrenal gland, other	C74-75	56	36	45.0	45.6	20	64.4	65.6
Hodgkin lymphoma	C81	52	32	59.7	63.3	20	65.7	67.7
Non-Hodgkin lymphoma	C82-85+C96	785	440	42.4	45.8	345	44.3	46.7
Multiple myeloma	C90	182	100	10.3	11.4	82	12.3	13.3
Lymphoid leukaemia	C91	222	142	37.4	37.7	80	49.7	50.1
Myeloid leukaemia	C92-94	480	273	25.6	26.8	207	28.1	28.8
Leukaemia unspecified	C95	44	22	13.6	17.7	22	0.0	0.0

Abs: absolute survival; Rel: relative survival

Table 4b. Site-wise number of cases and relative survival by age group: Busan, Republic of Korea, 1996–2001 cases followed-up until 2003

Site	ICD-10	Cases included	Number of cases by age group					Relative survival by age group % 5-year survival				
			< 45	45-54	55-64	65-74	> 75	< 45	45-54	55-64	65-74	> 75
Tongue	C01-02	144	28	27	57	23	9	55.7	72.8	41.5	44.7	48.1
Oral cavity	C03-06	156	26	23	47	43	17	85.4	42.5	54.4	15.4	28.6
Salivary gland	C07-08	86	31	13	24	14	4	88.9	94.9	53.9	47.6	
Tonsil	C09	59	6	13	20	18	2	85.5	78.7	42.8	30.3	73.1
Oropharynx	C10	34	2	7	13	10	2	0.0	29.7	25.4	25.3	0.0
Nasopharynx	C11	134	45	36	34	16	3	58.8	57.0	53.0	35.9	0.0
Hypopharynx	C12-13	87	5	18	34	21	9	20.2	53.5		14.6	0.0
Oesophagus	C15	790	23	130	310	240	87	22.1	28.5	18.8	14.4	9.9
Stomach	C16	8 683	1 348	1 686	2 701	2 077	871	53.1	55.9	48.1	34.3	14.8
Small intestine	C17	141	18	27	43	38	15	53.4	9.4	27.5	13.7	10.4
Colon	C18	1 859	261	325	550	457	266	60.6	67.4	58.8	48.5	30.9
Rectum	C19-20	1 882	270	414	536	456	206	53.7	59.8	63.4	53.0	23.4
Anus	C21	60	7	9	15	17	12	43.2	101.7	54.0	54.4	0.0
Liver	C22	6 507	797	1 711	2 096	1 400	503	12.6	10.6	9.6	6.0	8.0
Gall bladder	C23-24	1 524	79	223	440	509	273	32.3	29.3	18.9	10.2	5.4
Pancreas	C25	1 011	71	154	328	308	150	17.8	5.2	6.7	4.4	4.9
Nose/Sinuses	C30-31	103	13	19	35	26	10	53.9	20.1	32.9	45.0	31.4
Larynx	C32	475	22	95	172	142	44	61.0	65.9	63.0	45.9	38.2
Lung	C33-34	4 796	260	638	1 537	1 625	736	23.0	18.1	14.4	7.3	6.6
Other thoracic organs	C37-38	148	49	30	33	24	12	50.8	34.4	23.3	30.4	0.0
Bone	C40-41	196	123	21	27	17	8	68.5	43.0	38.1	17.8	0.0
Melanoma of skin	C43	86	21	14	23	17	11	37.1	55.0	42.7	67.7	27.5
Other skin	C44	423	64	65	109	110	75	93.3	95.3	86.7	84.6	86.5
Mesothelioma	C45	30	6	7	8	8	1	16.7	29.6	27.1	0.0	0.0
Connective tissue	C47+C49	250	104	46	54	35	11	56.2	54.8	39.1	23.4	17.7
Breast	C50	2 642	1 079	871	485	173	34	83.9	81.2	81.3	73.9	52.5
Vulva	C51	25	5	5	5	8	2	78.2	101.5	62.3	58.4	0.0
Cervix	C53	2 264	912	595	437	246	74	86.1	79.1	73.8	51.7	16.3
Corpus uteri	C54	265	76	87	72	28	2	91.1	79.5	71.0	61.0	
Ovary	C56	622	239	137	128	85	33	78.8	60.2	42.8	26.2	27.0
Placenta	C58	30	24	6	0	0	0	87.5	84.4			
Penis	C60	29	4	6	8	6	5	25.6	65.3	109.6	84.6	166.7
Prostate	C61	430	6	15	100	176	133	45.4	25.7	60.9	64.2	39.6
Testis	C62	55	49	3	3	0	0	78.5	34.6			
Kidney	C64	706	141	162	221	145	37	77.3	69.9	54.8	57.6	15.7
Renal pelvis	C65	74	8	10	29	21	6		62.5	56.7	39.2	
Ureter	C66	77	2	10	23	25	17	101.8	56.8	76.5	27.2	53.2
Urinary bladder	C67	999	89	152	304	290	164	81.9	89.1	74.4	60.4	46.2
Eye	C69	36	22	1	6	4	3	76.3	106.6	71.2	0.0	0.0
Brain & nervous system	C70-72	520	275	91	77	58	19	51.8	33.4	16.4	16.0	19.8
Thyroid	C73	1 175	554	265	199	122	35	98.1	96.2	92.7	77.8	32.6
Adrenal gland, other	C74-75	56	41	5	6	4	0	63.5	20.3	17.9	29.7	
Hodgkin lymphoma	C81	52	22	11	11	7	1	94.3	47.5	32.3	48.5	0.0
Non-Hodgkin lymphoma	C82-85+C96	785	245	147	200	135	58	56.9	47.3	48.9	27.5	27.3
Multiple myeloma	C90	182	10	35	68	58	11	27.6	18.3	15.5	5.7	0.0
Lymphoid leukaemia	C91	222	183	15	14	10	0	48.1	23.8	19.6	0.0	
Myeloid leukaemia	C92-94	480	270	60	85	50	15	36.0	29.9	16.8	6.8	0.0
Leukaemia unspecified	C95	44	13	4	5	13	9		0.0	0.0	9.5	16.7

Chapter 21

Cancer survival in Incheon, Republic of Korea, 1997–2001

Woo ZH, Hong YC, Kim WC and Pu YK

Abstract

The Incheon cancer registry was established in 1997. Cancer is not a notifiable disease, hence registration of cases is done by active methods. The registry contributed survival data for 42 cancer sites or types registered during 1997–2001. The follow-up information has been obtained predominantly by passive methods, with median follow-up ranging between 1–44 months for various cancers. The proportion with histologically verified diagnosis for different cancers ranged between 16–100%; death certificates only (DCOs) comprised 0–51%; 49–100% of total registered cases were included for the survival analysis. The top-ranking cancers on 5-year age-standardized relative survival rates were testis (98%), thyroid (90%), ureter (87%), adrenal gland (86%), non-melanoma skin (83%), corpus uteri (82%), Hodgkin lymphoma (81%), breast and cervix (74%). Five-year relative survival by age group showed a decreasing trend with increasing age groups for cancers of the stomach, small intestine, colon, gall bladder, larynx, lung, breast, cervix and ovary, and was fluctuating for other cancers.

Incheon cancer registry

The Incheon cancer registry was established in October 1997 at the College of Medicine, Inha University, Incheon. Data collection on incident cancer cases started retrospectively to include cases from the beginning of 1997. The registry is rather new, and its data were included in volume IX of the quinquennial IARC publication *Cancer Incidence in Five Continents*. [1] Cancer is not a notifiable disease, hence registration of cases is done by active methods. The principal sources of information on cancer cases are the records in more than 100 medical institutions, comprising hospitals in public and private sectors, pathology laboratories, radiation and imaging centres in and around Incheon. The registry covers an area of 986 km^2 and caters to an entirely urban population of about 2.6 million with a sex ratio of 980 females to 1000 males in 2004. The average annual age-standardized incidence rate (ASR) is 265 per 100 000 among males and 165 per 100 000 among females, with a lifetime cumulative risk of one in 4 of developing cancer in the period 1997–2002. The common age-standardized incidence rate of cancers among males are stomach (62), lung (50) and liver (37),and among females are breast (25), stomach (23) and cervix (20).

The registry is contributing data on survival from 42 cancer sites or types registered during 1997–2001 for the first time in this volume of IARC publication on *Cancer Survival in Africa, Asia, the Caribbean and Central America*.

Data quality indices (Table 1)

The proportion of cases with histologically verified cancer diagnosis in the series is 71%, varying from 16% (cancer of the uterus unspecified) to 100% (Hodgkin lymphoma). The frequency of cases registered on the basis of a death certificate only (DCOs) is 8%, ranging between nil in many cancers and 51% in uterus unspecified cancer. Cases excluded without any follow-up are negligible. Thus, 49–100% of the total cases registered are included in the estimation of the survival probability.

Outcome of follow-up (Table 2)

Follow-up information has been obtained predominantly by passive methods. These included obtaining cancer mortality information from the death certificates in vital statistics section. The mortality data are periodically matched with the incident cancer database using the national identity number. The vital status of the unmatched incident cases is also ascertained by review of medical charts. However, all incident cases for whom death information is not available were presumed to be alive on the last date of the year for which the mortality data are fully utilized for matching.

The closing date of follow-up was 31st December 2002. The median follow-up ranged from 1 month in unspecified uterus cancer to 44 months for Hodgkin lymphoma.

Survival statistics

All ages and both sexes together (Table 3)

The top-ranking cancers on 5-year relative survival are testis (98%), thyroid (92%), corpus uteri (84%), non-melanoma skin and ureter (83%). The lowest survival rate is encountered with pancreatic cancer (12%) preceded by unspecified uterus (15%), liver (16%), lung (18%) and gall bladder (20%). Salivary gland (69%) and nasopharynx (56%), among other head and neck cancers and colon and rectum (55%), among gastrointestinal cancers, have higher survival than others. Survival from cancers of the urinary system is 71% in urinary bladder and 67% for kidney. Hodgkin lymphoma had a better survival (83%) than non-Hodgkin (54%). The survival figures for leukaemias are 51% for lymphoid and 40% for myeloid.

Figure 1a. Top ten cancers (ranked by survival), Incheon, Republic of Korea, 1997–2001

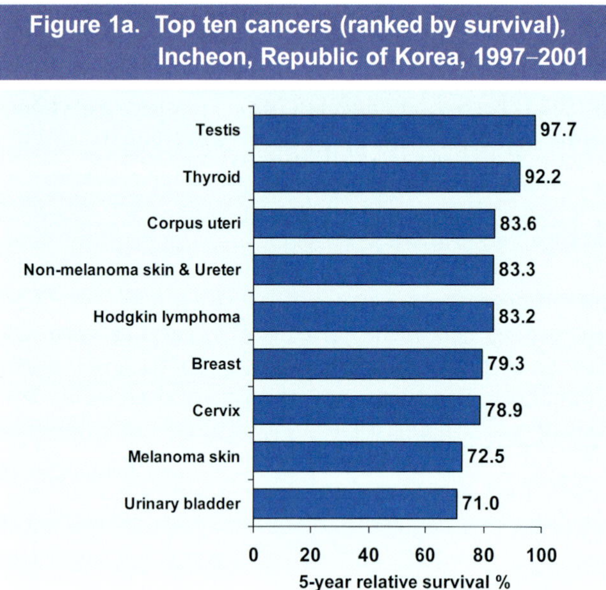

The 5-year age-standardized relative survival (ASRS) probability for all ages together is generally less than or similar to the corresponding unadjusted one for a majority of cancers. Also, the 5-year ASRS (0–74 years of age) is generally higher than or similar to the corresponding ASRS (all ages) for a majority of cancers.

Sex
Male (Table 4a)

The 5-year relative survival is distinctly higher in cancers of the tongue, other thoracic organs, non-melanoma skin, peritoneum, ureter, bladder and Hodgkin lymphoma among males than females.

Female (Table 4a)

The 5-year relative survival estimates for cancers of the breast, cervix and ovary are 79%, 79% and 60%, respectively. The survival is notably higher among females than males in cancers of the oral cavity, salivary gland, tonsil, nasopharynx, hypopharynx, small intestine, nose/sinuses, skin melanoma, adrenal gland, non-Hodgkin lymphoma, multiple myeloma and myeloid leukaemia.

Figure 1b. Top five cancers (ranked by survival), Male, Incheon, Republic of Korea, 1997–2001

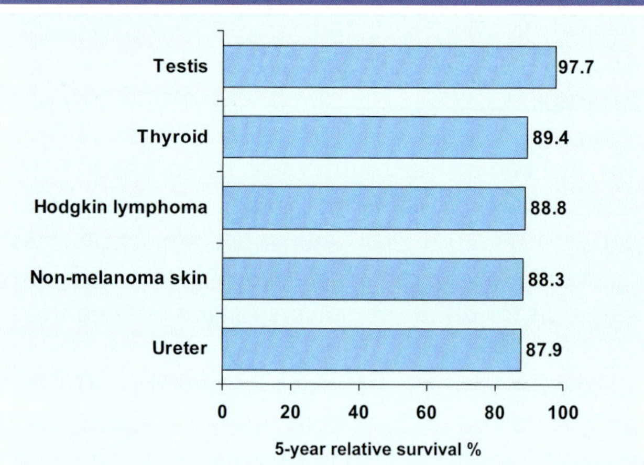

Figure 1c. Top five cancers (ranked by survival), Female, Busan, Republic of Korea, 1997–2001

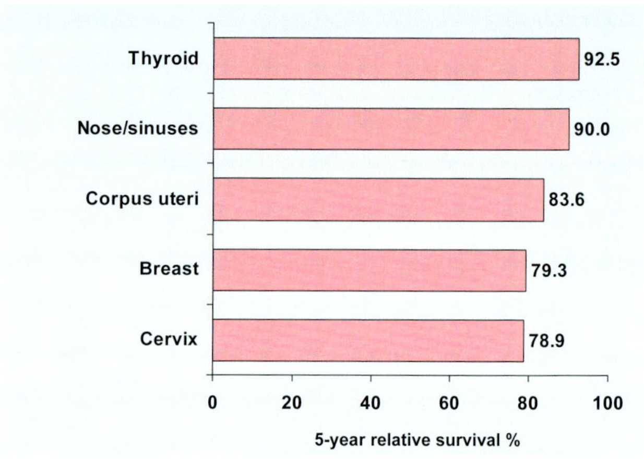

Age group (Table 4b)

The 5-year relative survival by age group reveals an inverse relationship: a decreasing survival with increasing age at diagnosis in cancers of the stomach, small intestine, colon, gall bladder, larynx, lung, breast, cervix and ovary. For other cancers, no pattern on the survival by age group is forthcoming.

References

1. Curado MP, Edwards B, Shin HR, Storm H, Ferlay J, Heanue M and Boyle P. *Cancer Incidence in Five Continents, Vol. IX : IARC Scientific Publications No. 160.* IARCPress, Lyon, IARC.

Table 1. Data quality indices - Proportion of histologically verified and death certificate only cases, number and proportion of included and excluded cases by site: Incheon, Republic of Korea, 1997–2001 cases followed-up until 2002

Site	ICD-10	Total registered	%		Excluded cases					Included cases	
			HV	DCO	DCO	Follow-up	Others	Total	%	No.	%
Tongue	C01-02	52	86.5	3.8	2	0	0	2	3.8	50	96.2
Oral cavity	C03-06	76	78.9	15.8	12	0	0	12	15.8	64	84.2
Salivary gland	C07-08	51	78.4	3.9	2	0	0	2	3.9	49	96.1
Tonsil	C09	27	85.2	0.0	0	0	0	0	0.0	27	100.0
Nasopharynx	C11	74	91.9	0.0	0	0	0	0	0.0	74	100.0
Hypopharynx	C12-13	51	78.4	0.0	0	0	0	0	0.0	51	100.0
Oesophagus	C15	347	75.2	12.1	42	1	0	43	12.4	304	87.6
Stomach	C16	4 693	81.2	8.3	389	2	9	400	8.5	4 293	91.5
Small intestine	C17	86	86.0	4.7	4	0	1	5	5.8	81	94.2
Colon	C18	1 215	80.1	7.7	94	1	0	95	7.8	1 120	92.2
Rectum	C19-20	1 168	86.7	3.9	45	0	1	46	3.9	1 122	96.1
Liver	C22	2 672	20.9	12.7	339	1	4	344	12.9	2 328	87.1
Gall bladder	C23-24	580	51.6	12.8	74	0	0	74	12.8	506	87.2
Pancreas	C25	625	32.8	17.1	107	0	0	107	17.1	518	82.9
Nose/Sinuses	C30-31	52	86.5	3.8	2	0	0	2	3.8	50	96.2
Larynx	C32	247	76.9	10.1	25	0	0	25	10.1	222	89.9
Lung	C33-34	2 974	63.8	13.6	405	0	3	408	13.7	2 566	86.3
Other thoracic organs	C37-38	66	66.7	13.6	9	1	0	10	15.2	56	84.8
Bone	C40-41	115	71.3	7.8	9	0	2	11	9.6	104	90.4
Melanoma of skin	C43	45	95.6	0.0	0	0	0	0	0.0	45	100.0
Other skin	C44	276	89.1	4.3	12	0	0	12	4.3	264	95.7
Connective tissue	C47+C49	138	88.4	2.2	3	0	0	3	2.2	135	97.8
Peritoneum	C48	57	63.2	5.3	3	0	0	3	5.3	54	94.7
Breast	C50	1 505	90.8	3.9	59	1	0	60	4.0	1 445	96.0
Cervix	C53	1 334	90.4	2.3	31	1	4	36	2.7	1 298	97.3
Corpus uteri	C54	140	95.0	0.0	0	0	0	0	0.0	140	100.0
Uterus unspecified	C55	67	16.4	50.7	34	0	0	34	50.7	33	49.3
Ovary	C56	420	79.3	7.1	30	0	0	30	7.1	390	92.9
Prostate	C61	309	83.8	8.7	27	0	0	27	8.7	282	91.3
Testis	C62	29	89.7	0.0	0	0	0	0	0.0	29	100.0
Kidney	C64	292	72.3	4.5	13	0	0	13	4.5	279	95.5
Renal pelvis	C65	34	91.2	0.0	0	0	0	0	0.0	34	100.0
Ureter	C66	34	88.2	2.9	1	0	0	1	2.9	33	97.1
Urinary bladder	C67	508	81.1	8.1	41	0	0	41	8.1	467	91.9
Brain & nervous system	C70-72	386	57.3	13.5	52	0	1	53	13.7	333	86.3
Thyroid	C73	729	90.1	2.3	17	0	0	17	2.3	712	97.7
Adrenal gland	C74	32	71.9	6.3	2	0	0	2	6.3	30	93.8
Hodgkin lymphoma	C81	28	100.0	0.0	0	0	0	0	0.0	28	100.0
Non-Hodgkin lymphoma	C82-85+C96	488	98.6	0.0	0	0	5	5	1.0	483	99.0
Multiple myeloma	C90	89	95.5	0.0	0	0	0	0	0.0	89	100.0
Lymphoid leukaemia	C91	125	98.4	0.0	0	0	0	0	0.0	125	100.0
Myeloid leukaemia	C92-94	251	98.0	0.0	0	0	1	1	0.4	250	99.6

HV: histologically verified; DCO: death certificate only

Table 2. Number and proportion of cases by vital status and median follow-up (in months) by site: Incheon, Republic of Korea, 1997–2001 cases followed-up until 2002

Site	ICD-10	Cases included	Dead		Alive		Complete FU		Median FU (in months)
			No.	%	No.	%	No.	%	
Tongue	C01-02	50	26	52.0	24	48.0	50	100.0	23.2
Oral cavity	C03-06	64	26	40.6	38	59.4	64	100.0	24.4
Salivary gland	C07-08	49	15	30.6	34	69.4	49	100.0	37.6
Tonsil	C09	27	14	51.9	13	48.1	27	100.0	18.9
Nasopharynx	C11	74	32	43.2	42	56.8	74	100.0	24.7
Hypopharynx	C12-13	51	33	64.7	18	35.3	51	100.0	18.5
Oesophagus	C15	304	226	74.3	78	25.7	304	100.0	10.4
Stomach	C16	4 293	2 099	48.9	2 194	51.1	4 293	100.0	19.9
Small intestine	C17	81	47	58.0	34	42.0	81	100.0	14.1
Colon	C18	1 120	448	40.0	672	60.0	1 120	100.0	24.2
Rectum	C19-20	1 122	434	38.7	688	61.3	1 122	100.0	24.9
Liver	C22	2 328	1 816	78.0	512	22.0	2 328	100.0	5.6
Gall bladder	C23-24	506	377	74.5	129	25.5	506	100.0	9.4
Pancreas	C25	518	440	84.9	78	15.1	518	100.0	4.1
Nose/Sinuses	C30-31	50	17	34.0	33	66.0	50	100.0	31.2
Larynx	C32	222	91	41.0	131	59.0	222	100.0	23.9
Lung	C33-34	2 566	2 002	78.0	564	22.0	2 566	100.0	7.5
Other thoracic organs	C37-38	56	29	51.8	27	48.2	56	100.0	18.3
Bone	C40-41	104	33	31.7	71	68.3	104	100.0	35.8
Melanoma of skin	C43	45	15	33.3	30	66.7	45	100.0	21.5
Other skin	C44	264	58	22.0	206	78.0	264	100.0	32.2
Connective tissue	C47+C49	135	46	34.1	89	65.9	135	100.0	28.9
Peritoneum	C48	54	36	66.7	18	33.3	54	100.0	19.3
Breast	C50	1 445	201	13.9	1 244	86.1	1 445	100.0	34.3
Cervix	C53	1 298	234	18.0	1 064	82.0	1 298	100.0	38.4
Corpus uteri	C54	140	23	16.4	117	83.6	140	100.0	34.5
Uterus unspecified	C55	33	23	69.7	10	30.3	33	100.0	0.9
Ovary	C56	390	119	30.5	271	69.5	390	100.0	32.8
Prostate	C61	282	96	34.0	186	66.0	282	100.0	25.1
Testis	C62	29	1	3.4	28	96.6	29	100.0	39.5
Kidney	C64	279	86	30.8	193	69.2	279	100.0	27.5
Renal pelvis	C65	34	12	35.3	22	64.7	34	100.0	25.5
Ureter	C66	33	9	27.3	24	72.7	33	100.0	26.3
Urinary bladder	C67	467	134	28.7	333	71.3	467	100.0	30.2
Brain & nervous system	C70-72	333	171	51.4	162	48.6	333	100.0	19.6
Thyroid	C73	712	49	6.9	663	93.1	712	100.0	41.0
Adrenal gland	C74	30	11	36.7	19	63.3	30	100.0	25.3
Hodgkin lymphoma	C81	28	5	17.9	23	82.1	28	100.0	43.9
Non-Hodgkin lymphoma	C82-85+C96	483	220	45.5	263	54.5	483	100.0	22.5
Multiple myeloma	C90	89	57	64.0	32	36.0	89	100.0	15.4
Lymphoid leukaemia	C91	125	58	46.4	67	53.6	125	100.0	20.4
Myeloid leukaemia	C92-94	250	143	57.2	107	42.8	250	100.0	18.0

FU: follow-up

Table 3. Comparison of 1-, 3- and 5-year absolute and relative survival and 5-year age-standardized relative survival by site: Incheon, Republic of Korea, 1997–2001 cases followed-up until 2002

Site	ICD-10	Cases included	% Absolute survival			% Relative survival			% ASRS at 5-years	
			1-year	3-year	5-year	1-year	3-year	5-year	all ages	0-74 years
Tongue	C01-02	50	61.5	47.1	40.6	63.0	49.8	44.2	44.7	52.0
Oral cavity	C03-06	64	61.8	48.7	45.5	63.5	52.4	50.7	51.3	54.4
Salivary gland	C07-08	49	86.3	70.5	63.3	87.9	74.4	69.3	66.9	69.7
Tonsil	C09	27	74.1	47.9	40.5	75.8	50.9	44.5	42.3	48.4
Nasopharynx	C11	74	77.0	56.5	53.5	77.7	57.9	55.9	45.2	53.6
Hypopharynx	C12-13	51	60.8	41.8	29.1	62.5	45.0	32.7	37.1	38.3
Oesophagus	C15	304	39.9	20.4	17.7	41.1	22.4	21.3	21.7	25.9
Stomach	C16	4 293	61.2	46.7	41.9	62.7	49.9	47.0	42.9	50.0
Small intestine	C17	81	51.2	40.8	34.1	52.5	43.4	37.5	34.6	47.7
Colon	C18	1 120	69.6	54.7	48.7	71.4	58.6	54.5	49.5	57.4
Rectum	C19-20	1 122	77.7	58.7	49.6	79.4	62.6	55.4	46.7	57.6
Liver	C22	2 328	32.4	18.6	14.9	33.0	19.6	16.3	16.0	16.8
Gall bladder	C23-24	506	39.3	21.7	17.5	40.5	23.7	20.3	22.5	25.3
Pancreas	C25	518	21.9	11.9	11.0	22.5	12.7	12.3	11.3	14.2
Nose/Sinuses	C30-31	50	76.9	63.1	56.5	78.6	67.4	62.6	73.9	63.4
Larynx	C32	222	65.2	53.5	48.1	67.0	58.0	55.2	55.5	61.6
Lung	C33-34	2 566	34.0	17.5	15.5	35.2	19.1	18.3	18.4	20.6
Other thoracic organs	C37-38	56	54.5	38.3	30.7	55.7	41.0	34.2	31.2	32.5
Bone	C40-41	104	73.9	67.2	59.9	74.9	69.1	63.0	43.2	46.9
Melanoma of skin	C43	45	80.0	64.0	64.0	81.6	68.3	72.5	71.0	71.5
Other skin	C44	264	85.9	74.0	69.7	88.8	81.7	83.3	83.0	85.4
Connective tissue	C47+C49	135	80.4	67.4	55.1	81.4	69.6	58.5	53.5	55.6
Peritoneum	C48	54	54.4	35.7	30.0	55.7	37.8	33.4	31.1	28.4
Breast	C50	1 445	91.3	82.6	77.3	91.8	83.9	79.3	74.3	78.5
Cervix	C53	1 298	90.1	81.5	76.3	90.8	83.1	78.9	73.8	79.5
Corpus uteri	C54	140	89.3	85.0	80.2	90.0	87.0	83.6	82.2	72.3
Uterus unspecified	C55	33	14.9	14.9	14.9	15.2	15.3	15.4	19.1	26.2
Ovary	C56	390	78.3	65.7	58.0	79.1	67.2	60.3	52.7	58.7
Prostate	C61	282	78.6	58.1	50.4	82.9	67.9	65.5	63.5	69.4
Testis	C62	29	100.0	96.1	96.1	100.3	97.1	97.7	98.3	98.3
Kidney	C64	279	74.7	65.1	61.1	76.2	68.7	66.9	64.4	67.9
Renal pelvis	C65	34	82.4	63.9	47.9	84.1	68.0	53.2	61.4	72.3
Ureter	C66	33	76.5	69.8	69.8	79.0	77.2	83.3	87.2	91.0
Urinary bladder	C67	467	78.0	65.5	60.1	80.7	72.1	71.0	65.9	76.1
Brain & nervous system	C70-72	333	56.5	43.7	38.5	57.2	44.9	40.0	39.6	41.0
Thyroid	C73	712	93.8	91.5	89.4	94.5	93.3	92.2	90.0	92.6
Adrenal gland	C74	30	75.0	54.8	54.8	75.4	55.5	56.1	86.1	78.4
Hodgkin lymphoma	C81	28	85.7	81.3	81.3	86.3	82.6	83.2	81.1	82.8
Non-Hodgkin lymphoma	C82-85+C96	483	70.3	53.0	50.9	71.4	55.2	54.2	53.8	57.4
Multiple myeloma	C90	89	56.2	33.7	25.3	57.3	35.9	28.4	27.2	29.0
Lymphoid leukaemia	C91	125	67.2	50.2	50.2	67.5	50.7	50.8	38.1	40.3
Myeloid leukaemia	C92-94	250	62.6	42.4	38.3	63.1	43.4	39.9	38.8	36.0

ASRS: age-standardized relative survival

Table 4a. Site-wise number of cases, 5-year absolute and relative survival by sex: Incheon, Republic of Korea, 1997–2001 cases followed-up until 2002

Site	ICD-10	Cases included	Male % 5-year survival			Female % 5-year survival		
			No.	Abs	Rel	No.	Abs	Rel
Tongue	C01-02	50	34	41.2	45.8	16	0.0	0.0
Oral cavity	C03-06	64	44	37.6	43.2	20	67.1	71.5
Salivary gland	C07-08	49	26	54.7	64.7	23	73.9	75.5
Tonsil	C09	27	19	31.3	34.3	8	61.4	67.8
Nasopharynx	C11	74	52	46.4	49.5	22	70.1	71.3
Hypopharynx	C12-13	51	49	25.8	28.8	2	100.0	121.7
Oesophagus	C15	304	268	18.0	21.9	36	15.1	16.4
Stomach	C16	4 293	2 896	42.1	48.0	1 397	41.5	45.0
Small intestine	C17	81	55	24.7	27.7	26	47.3	50.5
Colon	C18	1 120	593	49.0	56.1	527	48.3	52.8
Rectum	C19-20	1 122	622	44.7	51.4	500	55.4	59.9
Liver	C22	2 328	1 717	14.2	15.7	611	16.8	17.8
Gall bladder	C23-24	506	265	15.7	18.5	241	19.5	22.4
Pancreas	C25	518	313	10.7	12.0	205	11.5	12.6
Nose/Sinuses	C30-31	50	36	48.4	53.2	14	79.4	90.0
Larynx	C32	222	197	48.5	56.1	25	44.8	49.4
Lung	C33-34	2 566	1 884	14.1	16.8	682	19.4	22.1
Other thoracic organs	C37-38	56	29	37.9	41.1	27	0.0	0.0
Bone	C40-41	104	58	60.1	63.6	46	61.7	64.1
Melanoma of skin	C43	45	25	55.7	66.5	20	73.7	78.0
Other skin	C44	264	136	73.6	88.3	128	66.1	78.6
Connective tissue	C47+C49	135	73	57.2	60.4	62	55.6	59.8
Peritoneum	C48	54	25	36.0	41.8	29	22.6	23.5
Breast	C50	1 445	10	70.7	83.0	1 435	77.4	79.3
Cervix	C53	1 298				1 298	76.3	78.9
Corpus uteri	C54	140				140	80.2	83.6
Uterus unspecified	C55	33				33	14.9	15.4
Ovary	C56	390				390	58.0	60.3
Prostate	C61	282	282	50.4	65.5			
Testis	C62	29	29	96.1	97.7			
Kidney	C64	279	184	59.3	65.9	95	64.6	68.9
Renal pelvis	C65	34	24	50.0	55.9	10		
Ureter	C66	33	23	73.5	87.9	10	60.0	71.3
Urinary bladder	C67	467	376	62.0	73.6	91	53.0	60.6
Brain & nervous system	C70-72	333	152	34.6	36.1	181	41.5	43.1
Thyroid	C73	712	93	84.0	89.4	619	90.2	92.5
Adrenal gland	C74	30	16	47.8	48.4	14	62.2	64.1
Hodgkin lymphoma	C81	28	22	86.4	88.8	6	62.5	62.8
Non-Hodgkin lymphoma	C82-85+C96	483	289	45.5	49.1	194	59.1	61.6
Multiple myeloma	C90	89	48	12.3	14.3	41	37.3	40.7
Lymphoid leukaemia	C91	125	62	49.3	49.7	63	51.0	51.8
Myeloid leukaemia	C92-94	250	139	32.7	34.2	111	45.6	47.4

Abs: absolute survival; Rel: relative survival

Table 4b. Site-wise number of cases and relative survival by age group: Incheon, Republic of Korea, 1997–2001 cases followed-up until 2002

Site	ICD-10	Cases included	Number of cases by age group					Relative survival by age group % 5-year survival				
			< 45	45-54	55-64	65-74	> 75	< 45	45-54	55-64	65-74	> 75
Tongue	C01-02	50	11	11	10	11	7	55.1	40.0	52.8	50.6	0.0
Oral cavity	C03-06	64	8	14	22	15	5	78.5	38.9	44.6		27.9
Salivary gland	C07-08	49	17	10	9	8	5	81.0	61.9	80.6	57.5	52.2
Tonsil	C09	27	5	8	4	5	5		55.7	26.9	90.3	0.0
Nasopharynx	C11	74	34	17	15	6	2	64.7	51.1	57.1	29.7	0.0
Hypopharynx	C12-13	51	1	5	26	15	4	102.0	14.1	39.1		33.3
Oesophagus	C15	304	7	33	115	107	42		23.9	21.6	23.7	13.8
Stomach	C16	4 293	741	750	1 162	1 113	527	56.0	54.8	51.2	42.1	26.4
Small intestine	C17	81	12	11	24	23	11	75.9	65.9	36.0	33.0	0.0
Colon	C18	1 120	161	181	297	315	166	68.2	63.8	56.5	50.1	38.1
Rectum	C19-20	1 122	157	192	354	273	146	53.7	58.9	67.3	50.1	28.0
Liver	C22	2 328	366	589	762	419	192	20.0	16.6	17.8	12.7	14.3
Gall bladder	C23-24	506	39	71	139	153	104	41.9	28.4	19.4	16.5	15.6
Pancreas	C25	518	43	90	154	145	86	24.7	14.8	19.2	5.3	5.7
Nose/Sinuses	C30-31	50	7	12	10	14	7	86.5	28.6	70.1	64.6	120.5
Larynx	C32	222	11	31	91	65	24	84.9	61.6	57.8	53.3	35.6
Lung	C33-34	2 566	171	312	700	895	488	28.1	28.0	18.7	16.0	13.2
Other thoracic organs	C37-38	56	21	9	10	10	6	47.7	0.0	28.0	45.2	
Bone	C40-41	104	70	8	9	6	11	78.4	65.9	40.6	21.8	30.4
Melanoma of skin	C43	45	11	5	13	11	5	82.3	58.8	90.4		62.0
Other skin	C44	264	44	31	50	69	70	96.9	77.6	81.3	86.4	77.0
Connective tissue	C47+C49	135	65	26	21	12	11	67.4	63.8	36.6	71.4	45.0
Peritoneum	C48	54	15	10	10	10	9	47.1	38.5	0.0		38.0
Breast	C50	1 445	642	420	250	104	29	81.2	80.1	78.9	71.0	60.3
Cervix	C53	1 298	555	284	260	147	52	88.3	78.0	76.5	68.4	30.1
Corpus uteri	C54	140	41	42	30	22	5	100.6	99.2	68.1	36.2	136.8
Uterus unspecified	C55	33	6	6	4	14	3	75.5	25.4	9.4		0.0
Ovary	C56	390	171	73	69	53	24	77.8	60.0	48.2	42.7	18.6
Prostate	C61	282	1	16	58	114	93	100.2	91.3	60.9	69.2	62.9
Testis	C62	29	26	2	1	0	0	96.5	105.3			
Kidney	C64	279	67	40	82	63	27	83.9	82.4	67.9	44.5	60.3
Renal pelvis	C65	34	2	1	18	10	3	101.5		60.0	31.1	
Ureter	C66	33	0	1	12	13	7			66.2	101.8	81.6
Urinary bladder	C67	467	39	71	117	156	84	73.7	87.8	79.3	69.1	50.6
Brain & nervous system	C70-72	333	170	46	61	38	18	49.9	32.7	38.3	26.3	23.6
Thyroid	C73	712	365	133	127	63	24	100.0	94.3	95.6	70.3	
Adrenal gland	C74	30	22	3	3	1	1	45.1	102.7		107.3	
Hodgkin lymphoma	C81	28	18	5	3	2	0	88.3	83.9			
Non-Hodgkin lymphoma	C82-85+C96	483	185	84	98	78	38	65.1	67.4	50.4	32.9	
Multiple myeloma	C90	89	10	21	28	19	11	32.3	28.2	37.7	19.9	21.8
Lymphoid leukaemia	C91	125	100	7	9	6	3	57.8		47.1	0.0	
Myeloid leukaemia	C92-94	250	136	52	31	16	15	47.9	38.8		0.0	51.6

The closing date of follow-up was 31st December 2001. The median follow-up ranged from 5 months for cancer of the pancreas to 82 months for cancer of the placenta.

Survival statistics

All ages and both sexes together (Table 3)

The top-ranking cancers on 5-year relative survival are thyroid (95%), testis (94%), placenta and non-melanoma skin (93%) and corpus uteri (85%). The lowest survival rate is encountered with pancreatic cancer and unspecified leukaemia (15%) preceded by lung, liver and oesophagus (19%). Larynx (72%) and salivary gland (69%), among other head and neck cancers, and colon (64%) and rectum (61%), among gastrointestinal cancers, have higher survival than others. Survival from cancers of the urinary system ranged between 76% for urinary bladder and 43% for unspecified category. Hodgkin lymphoma had a better survival (74%) than non-Hodgkin (57%). The survival figures for leukaemias are 43% for lymphoid and 27% for myeloid.

Figure 1a. Top ten cancers (ranked by survival), Seoul, Republic of Korea, 1993–1997

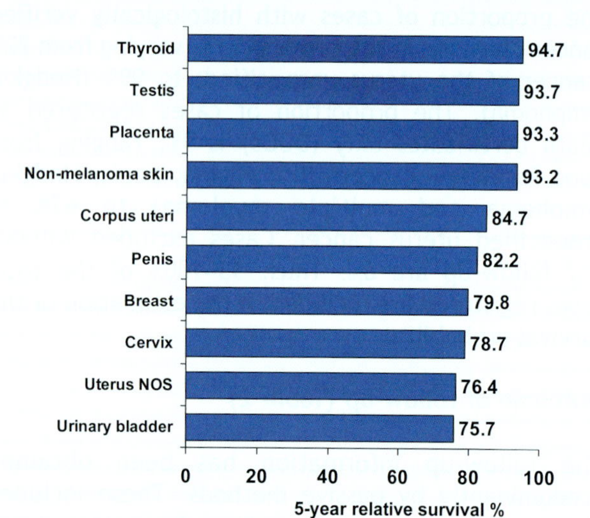

The 5-year age-standardized relative survival (ASRS) probability for all ages together is generally less than or similar to the corresponding unadjusted one for a majority of cancers. Also, the 5-year ASRS (0–74 years of age) is generally higher than or similar to the corresponding ASRS (all ages) for a majority of cancers.

Sex

Male (Table 4a)

The 5-year relative survival probabilities for lip, larynx, renal pelvis, bladder and unspecified urinary system cancers are noticeably higher among males than females.

Figure 1b. Top five cancers (ranked by survival), Male, Seoul, Republic of Korea, 1993–1997

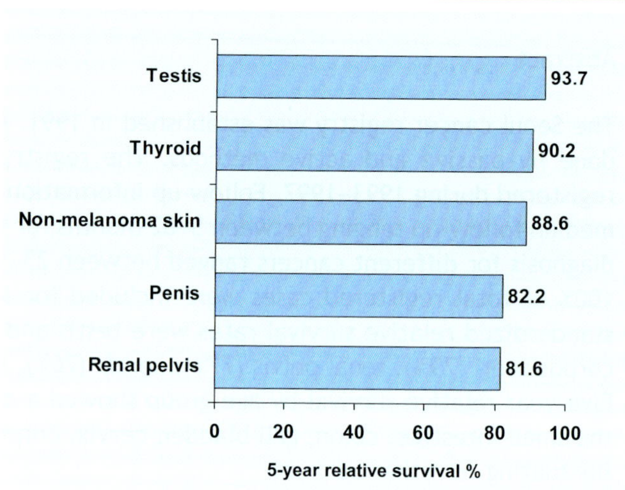

Female (Table 4a)

The 5-year relative survival estimates for cancers of the breast, cervix and ovary are 80%, 79% and 66%, respectively. Survival is distinctly higher among females than males for cancers of the oral cavity, salivary gland, nasopharynx, nose/sinuses, other thoracic organs, skin melanoma and non-melanoma, mesothelioma, Hodgkin lymphoma and lymphoid leukaemia.

Figure 1c. Top five cancers (ranked by survival), Female, Seoul, Republic of Korea, 1993–1997

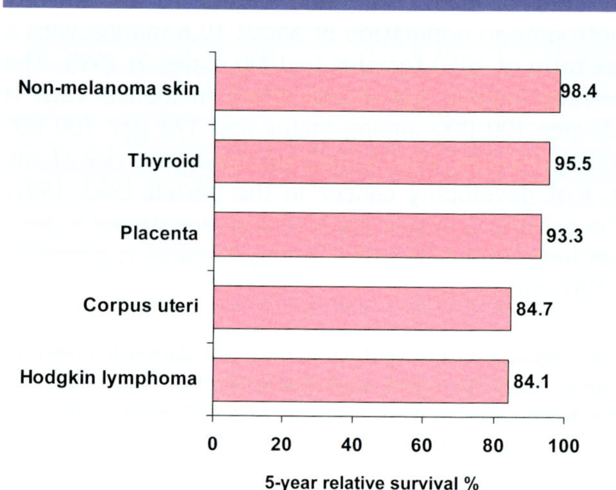

Age group (Table 4b)

The 5-year relative survival by age group reveals an inverse relationship: a decreasing survival with increasing age at diagnosis for cancers of the small intestine, colon, gall bladder, cervix, corpus uteri, ovary, kidney, urinary bladder and thyroid. For all other cancers, the survival by age group did not display any pattern.

References

1. Parkin DM, Whelan SL, Ferlay J and Storm H. *Cancer Incidence in Five Continents, Vol I to VIII: IARC Cancerbase No. 7.* IARCPress, Lyon, 2005.

Table 1. Data quality indices - Proportion of histologically verified and death certificate only cases, number and proportion of included and excluded cases by site: Seoul, Republic of Korea, 1993–1997 cases followed-up until 2001

Site	ICD-10	Total registered	%		Excluded cases					Included cases	
			HV	DCO	DCO	Follow-up	Others	Total	%	No.	%
Lip	C00	26	88.5	0.0	0	0	0	0	0.0	26	100.0
Tongue	C01-02	268	83.6	6.0	16	9	0	25	9.3	243	90.7
Oral cavity	C03-06	344	80.2	8.4	29	12	0	41	11.9	303	88.1
Salivary gland	C07-08	204	89.7	1.0	2	8	0	10	4.9	194	95.1
Tonsil	C09	98	86.7	1.0	1	5	0	6	6.1	92	93.9
Oropharynx	C10	57	75.4	3.5	2	3	0	5	8.8	52	91.2
Nasopharynx	C11	295	81.7	0.7	2	15	0	17	5.8	278	94.2
Hypopharynx	C12-13	180	86.1	3.9	7	3	0	10	5.6	170	94.4
Oesophagus	C15	1 353	72.8	10.6	143	76	0	219	16.2	1 134	83.8
Stomach	C16	18 914	77.9	9.0	1710	1021	3	2734	14.5	16 180	85.5
Small intestine	C17	284	75.4	7.7	22	20	0	42	14.8	242	85.2
Colon	C18	4 277	79.1	7.3	314	243	0	557	13.0	3 720	87.0
Rectum	C19-20	4 071	87.9	2.8	112	243	1	356	8.7	3 715	91.3
Anus	C21	420	37.1	21.2	89	18	0	107	25.5	313	74.5
Liver	C22	12 120	24.3	13.3	1611	635	2	2248	18.5	9 872	81.5
Gall bladder	C23-24	2 751	51.9	11.7	321	137	0	458	16.6	2 293	83.4
Pancreas	C25	2 284	38.2	15.6	356	121	0	477	20.9	1 807	79.1
Gastrointestinal tract	C26	174	10.3	65.5	114	2	0	116	66.7	58	33.3
Nose/Sinuses	C30-31	246	85.4	4.5	11	11	0	22	8.9	224	91.1
Larynx	C32	956	75.5	12.7	121	44	0	165	17.3	791	82.7
Lung	C33-34	10 294	67.8	12.7	1311	499	2	1812	17.6	8 482	82.4
Other thoracic organs	C37-38	265	74.3	10.6	28	11	0	39	14.7	226	85.3
Bone	C40-41	424	74.5	11.3	48	27	6	81	19.1	343	80.9
Melanoma of skin	C43	199	93.0	2.5	5	15	0	20	10.1	179	89.9
Other skin	C44	719	89.7	5.7	41	59	1	101	14.0	618	86.0
Mesothelioma	C45	56	87.5	1.8	1	3	0	4	7.1	52	92.9
Connective tissue	C47+C49	542	86.9	4.6	25	32	1	58	10.7	484	89.3
Peritoneum	C48	180	76.7	5.6	10	10	0	20	11.1	160	88.9
Breast	C50	5 907	88.3	3.3	196	356	0	552	9.3	5 355	90.7
Vulva	C51	59	93.2	1.7	1	3	0	4	6.8	55	93.2
Vagina	C52	53	94.3	0.0	0	7	0	7	13.2	46	86.8
Cervix	C53	5 861	88.2	2.0	119	381	4	504	8.6	5 357	91.4
Corpus uteri	C54	571	94.7	0.5	3	46	0	49	8.6	522	91.4
Uterus unspecified	C55	267	22.8	66.7	178	2	0	180	67.4	87	32.6
Ovary	C56	1 451	87.3	2.8	40	104	2	146	10.1	1 305	89.9
Other female genital org.	C57	119	39.5	26.1	31	3	0	34	28.6	85	71.4
Placenta	C58	121	40.5	2.5	3	5	0	8	6.6	113	93.4
Penis	C60	47	97.9	0.0	0	4	0	4	8.5	43	91.5
Prostate	C61	1 051	81.3	4.7	49	54	0	103	9.8	948	90.2
Testis	C62	121	91.7	3.3	4	10	1	15	12.4	106	87.6
Kidney	C64	1 302	81.6	4.5	59	66	0	125	9.6	1 177	90.4
Renal pelvis	C65	155	94.2	0.6	1	7	0	8	5.2	147	94.8
Ureter	C66	117	91.5	1.7	2	11	0	13	11.1	104	88.9
Urinary bladder	C67	2 153	85.6	5.2	112	110	1	223	10.4	1 930	89.6
Other urinary organs	C68	104	34.6	33.7	35	5	0	40	38.5	64	61.5
Eye	C69	104	73.1	5.8	6	5	0	11	10.6	93	89.4
Brain & nervous system	C70-72	1 570	57.8	19.4	304	103	0	407	25.9	1 163	74.1
Thyroid	C73	2 883	93.8	1.5	43	183	0	226	7.8	2 657	92.2
Adrenal gland	C74	103	65.0	10.7	11	5	0	16	15.5	87	84.5
Other endocrine	C75	107	44.9	20.6	22	7	0	29	27.1	78	72.9
Hodgkin lymphoma	C81	144	99.3	0.0	0	11	0	11	7.6	133	92.4
Non-Hodgkin lymphoma	C82-85+C96	1 872	92.7	4.2	79	113	0	192	10.3	1 680	89.7
Multiple myeloma	C90	375	93.9	0.0	0	28	0	28	7.5	347	92.5
Lymphoid leukaemia	C91	641	98.6	1.2	8	38	0	46	7.2	595	92.8
Myeloid leukaemia	C92-94	1 336	96.6	2.8	38	79	0	117	8.8	1 219	91.2
Leukaemia unspecified	C95	166	42.2	45.8	76	10	0	86	51.8	80	48.2

HV: histologically verified; DCO: death certificate only

Table 2. Number and proportion of cases by vital status and median follow-up (in months) by site: Seoul, Republic of Korea, 1993–1997 cases followed-up until 2001

Site	ICD-10	Cases included	Dead		Alive		Complete FU		Median FU (in months)
			No.	%	No.	%	No.	%	
Lip	C00	26	13	50.0	13	50.0	26	100.0	46.0
Tongue	C01-02	243	115	47.3	128	52.7	243	100.0	54.4
Oral cavity	C03-06	303	169	55.8	134	44.2	303	100.0	36.2
Salivary gland	C07-08	194	71	36.6	123	63.4	194	100.0	62.5
Tonsil	C09	92	47	51.1	45	48.9	92	100.0	52.4
Oropharynx	C10	52	36	69.2	16	30.8	52	100.0	21.9
Nasopharynx	C11	278	164	59.0	114	41.0	278	100.0	40.4
Hypopharynx	C12-13	170	129	75.9	41	24.1	170	100.0	15.1
Oesophagus	C15	1 134	947	83.5	187	16.5	1 134	100.0	9.2
Stomach	C16	16 180	9 354	57.8	6 826	42.2	16 180	100.0	28.3
Small intestine	C17	242	172	71.1	70	28.9	242	100.0	15.6
Colon	C18	3 720	1 641	44.1	2 079	55.9	3 720	100.0	54.5
Rectum	C19-20	3 715	1 743	46.9	1 972	53.1	3 715	100.0	53.2
Anus	C21	313	233	74.4	80	25.6	313	100.0	16.2
Liver	C22	9 872	8 208	83.1	1 664	16.9	9 872	100.0	6.2
Gall bladder	C23-24	2 293	1 779	77.6	514	22.4	2 293	100.0	9.1
Pancreas	C25	1 807	1 572	87.0	235	13.0	1 807	100.0	4.8
Gastrointestinal tract	C26	58	47	81.0	11	19.0	58	100.0	4.6
Nose/Sinuses	C30-31	224	126	56.3	98	43.8	224	100.0	47.9
Larynx	C32	791	320	40.5	471	59.5	791	100.0	58.5
Lung	C33-34	8 482	7 166	84.5	1 316	15.5	8 482	100.0	8.3
Other thoracic organs	C37-38	226	122	54.0	104	46.0	226	100.0	34.0
Bone	C40-41	343	186	54.2	157	45.8	343	100.0	44.9
Melanoma of skin	C43	179	96	53.6	83	46.4	179	100.0	50.6
Other skin	C44	618	131	21.2	487	78.8	618	100.0	68.7
Mesothelioma	C45	52	33	63.5	19	36.5	52	100.0	23.4
Connective tissue	C47+C49	484	228	47.1	256	52.9	484	100.0	53.7
Peritoneum	C48	160	102	63.8	58	36.3	160	100.0	28.3
Breast	C50	5 355	1 298	24.2	4 057	75.8	5 355	100.0	66.5
Vulva	C51	55	22	40.0	33	60.0	55	100.0	52.8
Vagina	C52	46	16	34.8	30	65.2	46	100.0	65.8
Cervix	C53	5 357	1 342	25.1	4 015	74.9	5 357	100.0	67.5
Corpus uteri	C54	522	99	19.0	423	81.0	522	100.0	72.2
Uterus unspecified	C55	87	26	29.9	61	70.1	87	100.0	67.2
Ovary	C56	1 305	483	37.0	822	63.0	1 305	100.0	58.3
Other female genital org.	C57	85	51	60.0	34	40.0	85	100.0	22.9
Placenta	C58	113	8	7.1	105	92.9	113	100.0	81.5
Penis	C60	43	16	37.2	27	62.8	43	100.0	61.0
Prostate	C61	948	460	48.5	488	51.5	948	100.0	53.6
Testis	C62	106	11	10.4	95	89.6	106	100.0	75.9
Kidney	C64	1 177	444	37.7	733	62.3	1 177	100.0	59.4
Renal pelvis	C65	147	53	36.1	94	63.9	147	100.0	61.4
Ureter	C66	104	51	49.0	53	51.0	104	100.0	55.8
Urinary bladder	C67	1 930	712	36.9	1 218	63.1	1 930	100.0	60.4
Other urinary organs	C68	64	42	65.6	22	34.4	64	100.0	19.3
Eye	C69	93	31	33.3	62	66.7	93	100.0	65.9
Brain & nervous system	C70-72	1 163	721	62.0	442	38.0	1 163	100.0	21.2
Thyroid	C73	2 657	229	8.6	2 428	91.4	2 657	100.0	72.0
Adrenal gland	C74	87	54	62.1	33	37.9	87	100.0	32.7
Other endocrine	C75	78	29	37.2	49	62.8	78	100.0	60.6
Hodgkin lymphoma	C81	133	40	30.1	93	69.9	133	100.0	63.6
Non-Hodgkin lymphoma	C82-85+C96	1 680	799	47.6	881	52.4	1 680	100.0	52.7
Multiple myeloma	C90	347	257	74.1	90	25.9	347	100.0	24.1
Lymphoid leukaemia	C91	595	352	59.2	243	40.8	595	100.0	27.6
Myeloid leukaemia	C92-94	1 219	915	75.1	304	24.9	1 219	100.0	13.6
Leukaemia unspecified	C95	80	68	85.0	12	15.0	80	100.0	5.7

FU: follow-up

Table 3. Comparison of 1-, 3- and 5-year absolute and relative survival and 5-year age-standardized relative survival by site: Seoul, Republic of Korea, 1993–1997 cases followed-up until 2001

Site	ICD-10	Cases included	% Absolute survival			% Relative survival			% ASRS at 5-years	
			1-year	3-year	5-year	1-year	3-year	5-year	all ages	0-74 years
Lip	C00	26	76.9	53.8	50.0	80.3	61.1	61.8	65.5	71.6
Tongue	C01-02	243	79.0	59.7	54.4	80.8	63.7	61.0	60.8	59.6
Oral cavity	C03-06	303	73.3	50.2	45.7	74.9	53.4	50.6	49.9	51.6
Salivary gland	C07-08	194	89.2	70.6	64.3	90.4	73.6	68.7	62.7	64.4
Tonsil	C09	92	77.2	56.5	51.9	78.6	59.6	56.6	55.0	58.3
Oropharynx	C10	52	67.3	40.4	32.7	68.9	42.8	35.7	37.0	42.8
Nasopharynx	C11	278	81.7	52.5	43.7	82.7	54.4	46.3	41.3	47.1
Hypopharynx	C12-13	170	56.5	28.2	25.1	58.0	30.7	29.3	31.3	31.3
Oesophagus	C15	1 134	42.3	20.4	16.8	43.6	22.1	19.2	20.0	22.8
Stomach	C16	16 180	64.2	47.3	42.9	65.6	50.2	47.6	43.3	49.2
Small intestine	C17	242	55.4	36.4	30.0	56.5	38.3	32.8	29.6	34.5
Colon	C18	3 720	77.1	62.2	56.8	78.9	66.7	64.1	59.8	65.7
Rectum	C19-20	3 715	82.5	61.8	54.3	84.2	65.8	60.6	57.5	61.5
Anus	C21	313	56.2	34.2	28.0	57.8	37.3	32.4	31.5	33.8
Liver	C22	9 872	38.7	21.9	17.5	39.4	23.1	19.2	18.9	20.3
Gall bladder	C23-24	2 293	44.3	27.3	23.0	45.5	29.5	26.4	27.9	30.3
Pancreas	C25	1 807	26.1	14.4	13.1	26.8	15.6	15.0	15.6	17.1
Gastrointestinal tract	C26	58	41.4	27.6	22.3	42.7	30.3	26.2	26.2	27.0
Nose/Sinuses	C30-31	224	74.1	54.0	45.9	75.3	56.9	50.4	53.1	50.9
Larynx	C32	791	83.1	65.7	61.5	85.5	71.8	71.8	71.0	75.6
Lung	C33-34	8 482	40.2	18.6	15.9	41.4	20.3	18.5	18.1	19.7
Other thoracic organs	C37-38	226	67.3	49.6	46.3	68.3	51.6	49.4	39.1	47.1
Bone	C40-41	343	73.5	53.6	46.3	74.1	54.9	48.1	39.2	39.8
Melanoma of skin	C43	179	81.0	56.4	48.1	82.4	59.6	52.8	52.6	49.5
Other skin	C44	618	91.3	83.2	80.0	93.9	90.8	93.2	93.4	92.6
Mesothelioma	C45	52	61.5	44.2	40.4	62.5	46.0	43.4	43.8	40.8
Connective tissue	C47+C49	484	79.5	61.0	53.8	80.6	63.2	57.2	50.8	55.7
Peritoneum	C48	160	65.6	46.3	38.4	66.5	47.7	40.4	30.4	41.2
Breast	C50	5 355	94.0	82.7	77.7	94.5	84.0	79.8	74.4	78.6
Vulva	C51	55	90.9	65.5	60.0	92.4	69.2	66.4	67.8	69.3
Vagina	C52	46	82.6	71.7	67.2	83.8	74.3	71.1	62.5	75.6
Cervix	C53	5 357	91.3	79.6	75.7	92.0	81.4	78.7	76.2	79.2
Corpus uteri	C54	522	93.9	85.2	81.8	94.5	87.0	84.7	78.8	81.7
Uterus unspecified	C55	87	86.2	77.0	73.6	87.0	78.7	76.4	68.7	77.8
Ovary	C56	1 305	84.3	69.3	64.2	84.9	70.7	66.2	57.8	62.2
Other female genital org.	C57	85	57.6	45.9	41.2	58.2	47.3	43.2	38.9	40.1
Placenta	C58	113	96.5	94.7	92.8	96.6	95.0	93.3	95.3	95.3
Penis	C60	43	88.4	76.7	64.9	92.0	87.9	82.2	85.8	77.5
Prostate	C61	948	85.4	64.0	53.5	90.3	76.3	72.8	74.4	70.2
Testis	C62	106	96.2	92.5	91.5	96.6	93.7	93.7	94.9	93.9
Kidney	C64	1 177	80.6	67.9	63.0	82.1	71.6	68.9	63.5	70.3
Renal pelvis	C65	147	84.4	70.7	65.1	86.3	76.4	74.9	77.4	71.1
Ureter	C66	104	85.6	60.6	54.4	87.8	65.7	63.1	57.5	57.5
Urinary bladder	C67	1 930	85.5	70.7	64.2	88.3	77.9	75.7	70.9	79.5
Other urinary organs	C68	64	54.7	40.6	34.1	57.1	46.7	42.8	42.1	44.3
Eye	C69	93	86.0	72.0	67.7	86.7	73.8	70.5	62.2	58.1
Brain & nervous system	C70-72	1 163	62.9	42.5	39.2	63.4	43.3	40.4	37.1	38.9
Thyroid	C73	2 657	95.7	93.7	91.6	96.4	95.6	94.7	92.8	94.4
Adrenal gland	C74	87	67.8	46.0	40.8	68.2	46.6	41.7	23.1	31.6
Other endocrine	C75	78	80.8	64.1	62.7	81.7	65.6	64.7	37.7	50.4
Hodgkin lymphoma	C81	133	85.7	75.2	71.2	86.5	77.1	74.4	75.3	76.3
Non-Hodgkin lymphoma	C82-85+C96	1 680	71.3	57.4	53.5	72.3	59.6	57.0	56.7	58.0
Multiple myeloma	C90	347	65.1	38.3	27.4	66.4	40.6	30.1	29.4	32.0
Lymphoid leukaemia	C91	595	67.1	46.4	41.8	67.4	46.8	42.5	33.8	38.5
Myeloid leukaemia	C92-94	1 219	54.5	31.8	25.8	54.9	32.5	26.6	22.7	26.3
Leukaemia unspecified	C95	80	28.8	17.5	14.8	29.2	18.1	15.3	13.8	16.8

ASRS: age-standardized relative survival

Table 4a. Site-wise number of cases, 5-year absolute and relative survival by sex: Seoul, Republic of Korea, 1993–1997 cases followed-up until 2001

Site	ICD-10	Cases included	Male	% 5-year survival		Female	% 5-year survival	
			No.	Abs	Rel	No.	Abs	Rel
Lip	C00	26	14	50.0	65.0	12	50.0	58.8
Tongue	C01-02	243	163	52.5	59.8	80	58.3	63.4
Oral cavity	C03-06	303	221	38.8	44.1	82	64.2	67.7
Salivary gland	C07-08	194	109	54.9	60.2	85	76.3	79.4
Tonsil	C09	92	74	50.0	55.1	18	60.7	63.9
Oropharynx	C10	52	42	33.3	36.4	10	30.0	32.6
Nasopharynx	C11	278	204	37.5	40.4	74	60.8	62.4
Hypopharynx	C12-13	170	159	24.3	28.7	11	36.4	37.8
Oesophagus	C15	1 134	995	15.5	17.8	139	25.9	28.9
Stomach	C16	16 180	10 439	43.1	48.5	5 741	42.7	45.9
Small intestine	C17	242	143	27.9	31.2	99	33.0	35.2
Colon	C18	3 720	1 985	59.4	68.5	1 735	53.8	59.1
Rectum	C19-20	3 715	2 091	52.9	60.3	1 624	56.0	60.9
Anus	C21	313	138	21.5	26.1	175	33.1	37.2
Liver	C22	9 872	7 553	16.9	18.7	2 319	19.4	20.8
Gall bladder	C23-24	2 293	1 127	24.3	28.5	1 166	21.8	24.4
Pancreas	C25	1 807	993	11.8	13.8	814	14.7	16.3
Gastrointestinal tract	C26	58	35	16.9	20.1	23	30.4	35.4
Nose/Sinuses	C30-31	224	142	40.8	45.3	82	54.6	59.0
Larynx	C32	791	717	62.5	73.0	74	52.3	59.9
Lung	C33-34	8 482	6 197	15.4	18.1	2 285	17.5	19.5
Other thoracic organs	C37-38	226	138	42.6	45.6	88	52.1	55.3
Bone	C40-41	343	200	43.7	45.7	143	49.9	51.3
Melanoma of skin	C43	179	87	40.7	45.1	92	55.0	60.0
Other skin	C44	618	328	75.8	88.6	290	84.8	98.4
Mesothelioma	C45	52	32	37.5	39.9	20	45.0	49.0
Connective tissue	C47+C49	484	261	50.6	54.5	223	57.6	60.3
Peritoneum	C48	160	82	42.1	44.5	78	34.5	35.9
Breast	C50	5 355	35	60.0	68.7	5 320	77.8	79.9
Vulva	C51	55				55	60.0	66.4
Vagina	C52	46				46	67.2	71.1
Cervix	C53	5 357				5 357	75.7	78.7
Corpus uteri	C54	522				522	81.8	84.7
Uterus unspecified	C55	87				87	73.6	76.4
Ovary	C56	1 305				1 305	64.2	66.2
Other female genital org.	C57	85				85	41.2	43.2
Placenta	C58	113				113	92.8	93.3
Penis	C60	43	43	64.9	82.2			
Prostate	C61	948	948	53.5	72.8			
Testis	C62	106	106	91.5	93.7			
Kidney	C64	1 177	781	61.2	68.0	396	66.5	70.6
Renal pelvis	C65	147	103	70.6	81.6	44	52.3	59.5
Ureter	C66	104	70	52.1	62.0	34	58.8	64.8
Urinary bladder	C67	1 930	1 595	65.4	77.6	335	58.6	66.8
Other urinary organs	C68	64	33	36.1	49.0	31	32.3	36.4
Eye	C69	93	58	69.0	72.1	35	65.7	67.8
Brain & nervous system	C70-72	1 163	643	37.5	38.9	520	41.3	42.2
Thyroid	C73	2 657	416	84.2	90.2	2 241	93.0	95.5
Adrenal gland	C74	87	50	41.0	42.2	37	40.4	40.8
Other endocrine	C75	78	56	62.5	64.9	22	63.3	64.3
Hodgkin lymphoma	C81	133	75	63.6	66.9	58	81.0	84.1
Non-Hodgkin lymphoma	C82-85+C96	1 680	986	50.8	54.9	694	57.2	60.0
Multiple myeloma	C90	347	196	24.7	28.0	151	31.0	32.7
Lymphoid leukaemia	C91	595	343	37.4	38.1	252	47.9	48.4
Myeloid leukaemia	C92-94	1 219	671	26.8	27.9	548	24.5	25.0
Leukaemia unspecified	C95	80	40	12.5	13.2	40	16.9	17.2

Abs: absolute survival; Rel: relative survival

Table 4b. Site-wise number of cases and relative survival by age group: Seoul, Republic of Korea, 1993–1997 cases followed-up until 2001

Site	ICD-10	Cases included	Number of cases by age group					Relative survival by age group % 5-year survival				
			< 45	45-54	55-64	65-74	> 75	< 45	45-54	55-64	65-74	> 75
Lip	C00	26	2	3	4	6	11	100.5	33.9	82.3	78.5	44.3
Tongue	C01-02	243	39	53	74	49	28	83.1	60.4	55.7	45.5	77.0
Oral cavity	C03-06	303	50	59	97	64	33	83.0	43.5	47.0	42.9	38.3
Salivary gland	C07-08	194	62	54	42	23	13	84.4	63.0	72.0	35.2	64.5
Tonsil	C09	92	13	25	29	19	6	85.8	58.3	59.2	31.5	51.3
Oropharynx	C10	52	8	13	11	13	7	63.3	32.0	49.0	28.1	0.0
Nasopharynx	C11	278	98	72	64	32	12	57.7	54.4	23.2	41.6	37.1
Hypopharynx	C12-13	170	5	33	59	57	16	40.8	35.0	24.2	29.0	38.2
Oesophagus	C15	1 134	24	169	448	336	157	42.2	19.7	23.0	15.1	12.5
Stomach	C16	16 180	2 728	3 154	4 715	3 769	1 814	52.7	55.5	50.9	41.0	29.7
Small intestine	C17	242	45	44	70	55	28	42.8	37.6	36.7	24.2	16.0
Colon	C18	3 720	478	702	1 059	948	533	69.5	67.3	67.4	62.2	51.0
Rectum	C19-20	3 715	495	774	1 119	895	432	59.8	63.0	62.9	60.6	52.0
Anus	C21	313	39	60	73	68	73	20.7	37.4	35.0	36.4	27.5
Liver	C22	9 872	1 309	2 918	3 159	1 802	684	25.3	18.8	18.8	18.3	13.1
Gall bladder	C23-24	2 293	151	346	662	668	466	42.9	30.0	26.5	23.9	22.0
Pancreas	C25	1 807	138	273	544	521	331	32.7	17.1	10.7	14.9	13.4
Gastrointestinal tract	C26	58	7	6	14	18	13	14.4	48.9	15.6	32.9	24.4
Nose/Sinuses	C30-31	224	53	60	55	37	19	46.7	49.9	44.9	60.4	61.4
Larynx	C32	791	33	131	302	214	111	80.0	79.9	71.6	74.4	53.8
Lung	C33-34	8 482	482	1 218	2 504	2 788	1 490	23.5	23.6	20.1	15.8	14.9
Other thoracic organs	C37-38	226	86	38	41	44	17	64.3	54.7	37.0	37.4	16.6
Bone	C40-41	343	227	30	42	27	17	52.0	58.5	47.9	9.0	38.1
Melanoma of skin	C43	179	42	40	49	28	20	37.2	56.6	60.9	50.0	66.5
Other skin	C44	618	113	94	131	149	131	86.8	90.1	93.7	98.7	97.0
Mesothelioma	C45	52	13	14	12	8	5	46.8	44.4	44.2	30.2	53.7
Connective tissue	C47+C49	484	227	78	77	64	38	61.5	65.9	54.2	45.1	35.5
Peritoneum	C48	160	61	34	35	20	10	50.7	32.9	40.0	41.4	0.0
Breast	C50	5 355	2 107	1 814	922	387	125	81.6	82.0	77.7	71.3	56.5
Vulva	C51	55	10	8	11	19	7	60.4	63.5	84.7	59.1	68.0
Vagina	C52	46	10	11	11	9	5	80.4	72.8	85.3	64.0	26.7
Cervix	C53	5 357	1 794	1 373	1 262	711	217	87.1	79.4	75.4	68.3	52.9
Corpus uteri	C54	522	158	169	126	51	18	90.9	88.3	78.9	72.4	71.4
Uterus unspecified	C55	87	35	21	13	12	6	77.6	82.2	95.9	57.0	45.5
Ovary	C56	1 305	572	287	242	139	65	81.5	64.1	52.2	44.1	35.5
Other female genital org.	C57	85	26	22	17	15	5	54.2	46.2	42.7	21.8	33.1
Placenta	C58	113	99	13	1	0	0	94.2	85.9	102.7		
Penis	C60	43	4	6	11	11	11	101.8	69.4	50.4	89.7	112.2
Prostate	C61	948	9	25	193	365	356	33.7	57.7	74.0	71.2	77.3
Testis	C62	106	90	8	3	4	1	91.8	104.5	109.9	91.9	150.5
Kidney	C64	1 177	240	258	353	229	97	80.9	75.8	68.7	58.3	42.6
Renal pelvis	C65	147	10	29	44	51	13	61.0	64.5	81.4	73.8	96.8
Ureter	C66	104	3	21	29	36	15	34.1	44.2	74.8	69.6	57.2
Urinary bladder	C67	1 930	184	302	541	516	387	92.7	84.9	76.8	75.0	57.3
Other urinary organs	C68	64	3	7	16	14	24	33.6	59.0	40.4	50.4	35.8
Eye	C69	93	62	12	12	3	4	69.7	60.4	98.6	0.0	79.5
Brain & nervous system	C70-72	1 163	651	169	205	106	32	51.9	34.7	25.0	14.3	14.0
Thyroid	C73	2 657	1 348	560	424	234	91	99.6	97.1	93.1	79.9	44.7
Adrenal gland	C74	87	62	10	11	3	1	43.0	51.8	39.7	0.0	0.0
Other endocrine	C75	78	53	6	10	4	5	73.7	86.4	54.4	0.0	0.0
Hodgkin lymphoma	C81	133	76	20	17	17	3	83.3	72.4	50.7	62.8	57.3
Non-Hodgkin lymphoma	C82-85+C96	1 680	608	335	378	264	95	62.6	58.8	56.0	46.4	49.5
Multiple myeloma	C90	347	39	71	111	95	31	56.7	27.1	30.1	27.4	7.6
Lymphoid leukaemia	C91	595	483	34	33	36	9	46.1	18.1	25.2	39.2	14.2
Myeloid leukaemia	C92-94	1 219	701	187	178	113	40	33.1	20.9	20.9	10.4	7.2
Leukaemia unspecified	C95	80	41	10	10	10	9	29.4	0.0	0.0	0.0	0.0

Chapter 23

Breast cancer survival in Riyadh, Saudi Arabia, 1994–1996

Hamdan NA, Ravichandran K and Dyab AR

Abstract

The national cancer registry in Saudi Arabia has functioned since 1994, collecting population-based incidence data on malignant and in situ tumours. Cancer registration is carried out by both passive and active methods. The registry contributed data on survival from cancer of the breast registered in 1994–1996 from Riyadh province. Follow-up was carried out predominantly by active methods, and the median follow-up was 57 months. The proportion of cases with a histological confirmation of breast cancer diagnosis was almost 100%; there were no cases registered based on death certificate only (DCO); 93% of total cases registered were included in the survival analysis. Complete follow-up at five years was 80%. Relative survival rates at one, three and five years were 96%, 83% and 65%, respectively. Five-year age-standardized relative survival was 65%. Five-year relative survival by age group did not show any pattern and was fluctuating. Five-year absolute survival by extent of disease was localized (70%), regional (56%), distant metastasis (57%) and unknown (62%).

National cancer registry

The national cancer registry in Saudi Arabia has functioned since 1994, collecting population-based incidence data on malignant and in situ tumours. It is based at Gulf Centre for Cancer registration, King Faisal Specialist Hospital, Riyadh. Cancer registration is carried out by both passive and active methods. Cancer care services are provided predominantly by the Ministry of Health, which includes cancer centres with all diagnostic and treatment facilities and other hospitals with some participation from private sector. Data are collected from all these sources by scrutiny of records or linkage with data in computer systems maintained at these places. The registry covers an area of 3 855 000 km^2 and caters to a mixed urban and rural estimated population of about 20.7 million in 1998 with a sex ratio of 1264 males to 1000 females; the corresponding Saudi population is 15.1 million with 1020 males to 1000 females. The average annual age-standardized incidence rate among Saudis was 65 per 100 000 among males and 68 per 100 000 among females, with a lifetime cumulative risk of one in 13 of developing cancer for both sexes in the period 1997–1998. The top-ranking cancers among males are liver, followed by non-Hodgkin lymphoma and leukaemia. Among females, the order is breast, thyroid and leukaemia [1].

The registry contributed data on survival from cancer of the breast registered in 1994–1996 from Riyadh province in this volume of the IARC puplication on *Cancer Survival in Africa, Asia, the Caribbean and Central America.*

Data quality indices (Table 1)

The proportion of cases with histological confirmation of breast cancer diagnosis in this series was almost 100%, and there were no cases registered based on death certificate only (DCO). Cases without any follow-up information made up 6% and other inconsistencies in data constituted 1%. Thus, 298 (93%) of 321 cases registered were included in the estimation of survival probability.

Outcome of follow-up (Table 2)

Follow-up was carried out predominantly by active methods, since no centralized mortality registration system existed. The methods included postal and telephone enquiries, repeated scrutiny of records or data linkage with computer systems at source hospitals [2].

The closing date of follow-up was 31st December 2001. The median follow-up was 57 months. Complete follow-up at five years from the incidence date was 80%. The majority of losses to follow-up occurred in the first year of follow-up and decreased through successive intervals of follow-up time. The losses to follow-up have been ascertained to be random.

Survival statistics

All ages and both sexes together (Table 3)

The relative survival probabilities at one, three and five years from the incidence date were 96%, 83% and 65%, respectively. The 5-year age-standardized relative survival for all ages together was 65%, while the corresponding figure for 0–74 years of age was 65%.

Age group (Table 4b)

The 5-year relative survival by age group does not display any pattern and was observed to be fluctuating.

Extent of disease (Table 5)

There was not much of a difference in proportion of cases diagnosed with localized (31%) or regional spread of disease (33%). Distant metastasis accounted for 21%, while the extent of disease was unknown in 15%. The 5-year absolute survival by extent of disease was localized (70%), regional (56%), distant metastasis (57%) and unknown (62%).

Figure 1. 5- year Absolute survival (%) from breast cancer by extent of disease, Riyadh, Saudi Arabia

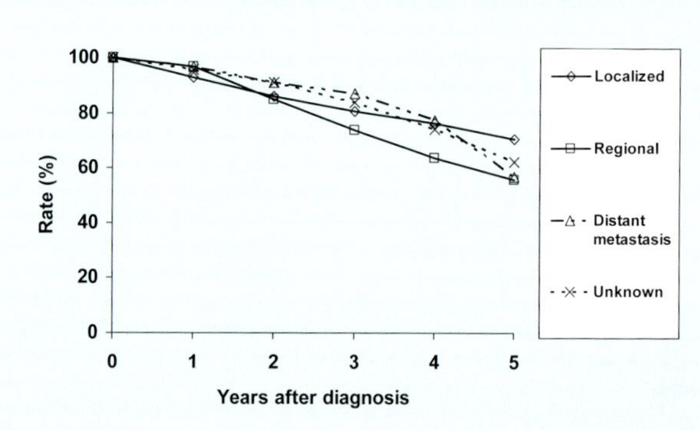

References

1. National Cancer Registry. *Cancer incidence report, Saudi Arabia: 1997–1998*. Ministry of Health, Kingdom of Saudi Arabia, 2001.

2. Ravichandran K, Hamdan AH, Dyab AR. Population-based survival of female breast cancer cases in Riyadh region, Saudi Arabia. *Asian Pacific J Cancer Prev*. 2005; 6: 72–76.

Table 1. Data quality indices - Proportion of histologically verified and death certificate only cases, number and proportion of included and excluded cases by site: Riyadh, Saudi Arabia, 1994–1996 cases followed-up until 2001

Site	ICD-10	Total registered	%		Excluded cases					Included cases	
			HV	DCO	DCO	Follow-up	Others	Total	%	No.	%
Breast	C50	321	99.7	0.0	0	18	5	23	7.2	298	92.8

HV: histologically verified; DCO: death certificate only

Table 2. Number and proportion of cases with complete/incomplete follow-up (in years) and median follow-up (in months) by site: Riyadh, Saudi Arabia, 1994–1996 cases followed-up until 2001

Site	ICD-10	Cases included	Complete FU Alive/dead at end of FU		Incomplete FU: lost to FU		% lost to FU: years from diagnosis				% with complete FU at 5 years	Median FU (in months)
			No.	%	No.	%	< 1	1-3	3-5	> 5		
Breast	C50	298	233	78.2	65	21.8	12.7	4.4	3.0	1.7	79.9	57.4

FU: follow-up

Table 3. Comparison of 1-, 3- and 5-year absolute and relative survival and 5-year age-standardized relative survival by site: Riyadh, Saudi Arabia, 1994–1996 cases followed-up until 2001

Site	ICD-10	Cases included	% Absolute survival			% Relative survival			% ASRS at 5-years	
			1-year	3-year	5-year	1-year	3-year	5-year	all ages	0-74 years
Breast	C50	298	95.3	80.2	61.3	96.3	82.7	64.5	65.3	64.5

ASRS: age-standardized relative survival

Table 4a. Site-wise number of cases, 5-year absolute and relative survival by sex: Riyadh, Saudi Arabia, 1994–1996 cases followed-up until 2001

Site	ICD-10	Cases included	Male % 5-year survival			Female % 5-year survival		
			No.	Abs	Rel	No.	Abs	Rel
Breast	C50	298				298	61.3	64.5

Abs: absolute survival; Rel: relative survival

Table 4b. Site-wise number of cases and relative survival by age group: Riyadh, Saudi Arabia, 1994–1996 cases followed-up until 2001

Site	ICD-10	Cases included	Number of cases by age group					Relative survival by age group % 5-year survival				
			< 45	45-54	55-64	65-74	> 75	< 45	45-54	55-64	65-74	> 75
Breast	C50	298	145	62	56	20	15	62.8	68.7	64.4	61.5	71.1

Table 5. Proportion of cases and 5-year absolute survival by extent of disease and site: Riyadh, Saudi Arabia, 1994–1996

Site	ICD-10	Cases included	% of cases by extent of disease				% 5-year absolute survival			
			Localized	Regional	Dist. met.	Unknown	Localized	Regional	Dist. met.	Unknown
Breast	C50	298	30.9	32.6	20.8	15.7	70.4	55.7	56.7	62.3

Dis. met.: distant metastasis

Chapter 24

Cancer survival in Singapore, 1993–1997

Chia KS

Abstract

The Singapore cancer registry is a national registry established in 1968. Cancer registration is done by passive methods. The registry contributed survival data on 45 cancer sites or types registered during 1993–1997. Data on 34 cancers registered during 1968–1997 were utilized for survival trend by period and cohort approaches. Follow-up was done by passive methods, with median follow-up ranging between 2–72 months for different cancers. The proportion with histologically verified diagnosis for various cancers ranged between 27–100%; death certificates only (DCOs) comprised 0–7%; 76–100% of total registered cases were included for the survival analysis. The top-ranking cancers on 5-year age-standardized relative survival rates were non-melanoma skin (96%), thyroid (90%), testis (88%), corpus uteri (77%), breast (74%), Hodgkin lymphoma (73%) and penis (70%). Five-year relative survival by age group showed either a decreasing trend with increasing age groups or was fluctuating. Localized stage of disease ranged between 18–65% for various cancers and survival decreased with increasing extent of disease. Period survival closely predicted survival experience of cancers diagnosed in that period, and an increasing trend in period survival over different periods indicated an improved prognosis for cancers diagnosed in those calendar periods.

Singapore cancer registry

The Singapore cancer registry is a national registry established in 1968 to obtain information on cancer patterns in the entire country. The registry has been contributing data to the quinquennial IARC publication *Cancer Incidence in Five Continents* since volume III [1]. Cancer notification is voluntary, and registration of cases is predominantly by passive methods with no personal contact with cases. The principal sources of information on incident cancer cases are the notification forms from all sections of the medical profession, pathology and hospital records [2]. The registry caters to a population of about 4.1 million with a sex ratio of 986 females to 1000 males in 2002, comprising major ethnic groups of Chinese, Malays and Indians. The average annual age-standardized incidence rate of all cancers and ethnic populations together is 235 per 100 000 among males and 200 per 100 000 among females in 1998–1999 [3].

The registry contributed data on survival from 45 cancer sites or types for the first time in this volume of the IARC publication on *Cancer Survival in Africa, Asia, the Caribbean and Central America*. In the present volume, the main tables pertain to the period 1993–1997. The data on survival for the years 1968–1992 are also utilized to elicit the trend in cancer survival using different approaches.

Data quality indices (Table 1)

The proportion of cases with histologically verified cancer diagnosis in the series varied from 100% for many cancers to 27% in liver cancer. The frequency of cases registered based on a death certificate only (DCO) range between nil among many cancers to 7% in unspecified leukaemia. Cases excluded from the study, due to lack of follow-up and other basic information, are in the range of 0% for mesothelioma and 24% for bone cancers. Thus, 76–100% of the total cases registered are included in the estimation of the survival probability.

Outcome of follow-up (Table 2)

The follow-up of cases has been completely carried out by passive methods. Since certification of death is virtually complete, the cancer mortality information received from the death certificate is matched with the incident cancer database. The vital status of the unmatched incident case is then collected by scrutiny of hospital records, and all such cases are presumed to be alive until the end of the calendar year for which the mortality data are fully available.

The closing date of follow-up was 31st December 2001. The median follow-up ranged from 2 months for liver cancer and unspecified leukaemia to 72 months for testicular cancer. The completeness of follow-up at 5 years from the incidence date was 100% for all cancers as there are no losses to follow-up.

Survival statistics

All ages and both sexes together (Table 3)

The top-ranking cancers on 5-year relative survival are non-melanoma skin (96%), thyroid (90%), testis (87%), corpus uteri (81%) and breast (76%). The lowest survival rate is encountered with cancer of the pancreas (4%), preceded by cancer of the liver (5%), oesophagus (6%) and lung (7%) and mesothelioma (9%). Salivary gland (69%) among other head and neck cancers and colon and rectum (50%) among gastrointestinal cancers have a higher survival rate than others in the category. Hodgkin lymphoma has a better survival rate than non-Hodgkin. The survival figures for haematopoietic malignancies are as follows: multiple myeloma (19%), lymphoid leukaemia (46%), myeloid leukaemia (18%) and unspecified leukaemia (9%).

Figure 1a. Top ten cancers (ranked by survival), Singapore, 1993–1997

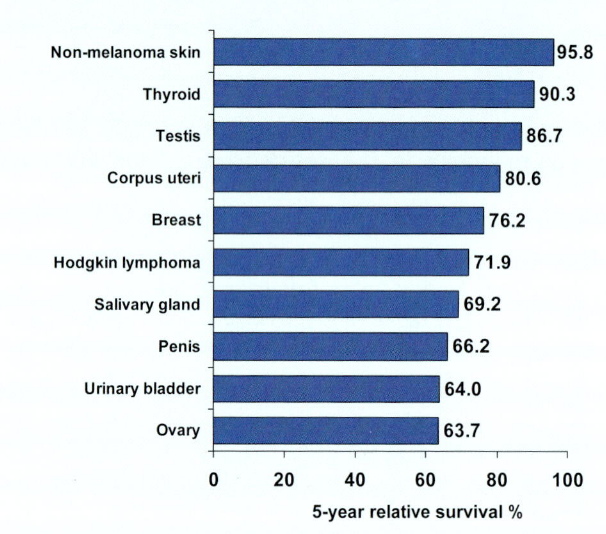

The 5-year age-standardized relative survival (ASRS) probability for all ages together is observed to be less than or similar to the corresponding unadjusted one for a majority of cancers. Also, the 5-year ASRS (0–74 years of age) is generally higher than or similar to the corresponding ASRS (all ages) for a majority of cancers.

Sex

Male (Table 4a)

The 5-year relative survival of cancer of the testis is 87%, prostate is 63% and penis is 66%. Cancers of the hypopharynx, breast, small intestine and urinary bladder have a notably higher survival among males than females.

Figure 1b. Top five cancers (ranked by survival), Male, Singapore, 1993–1997

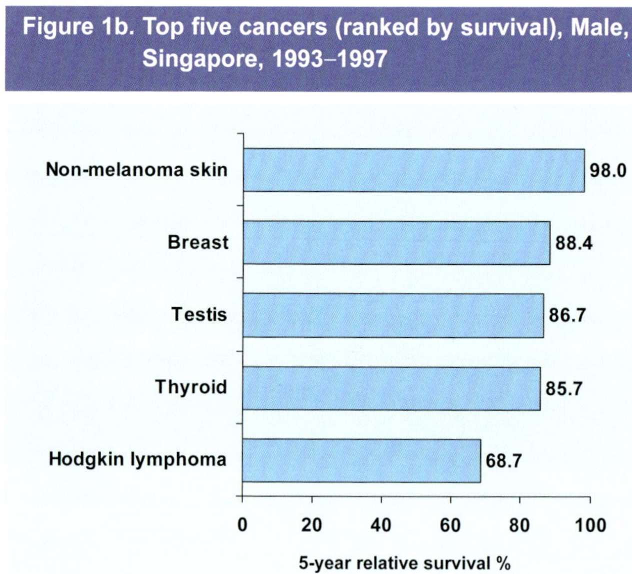

Female (Table 4a)

The 5-year relative survival from cancers of the breast, uterine cervix, ovary and vulva are 76%, 64%, 64% and 62%, respectively. Survival is markedly higher among females than males in most cancers of the head and neck, rectum, anus, other thoracic organs, melanoma and non-melanoma skin, renal pelvis, Hodgkin and non-Hodgkin lymphoma and lymphoid leukaemia.

Figure 1c. Top five cancers (ranked by survival), Female, Singapore, 1993–1997

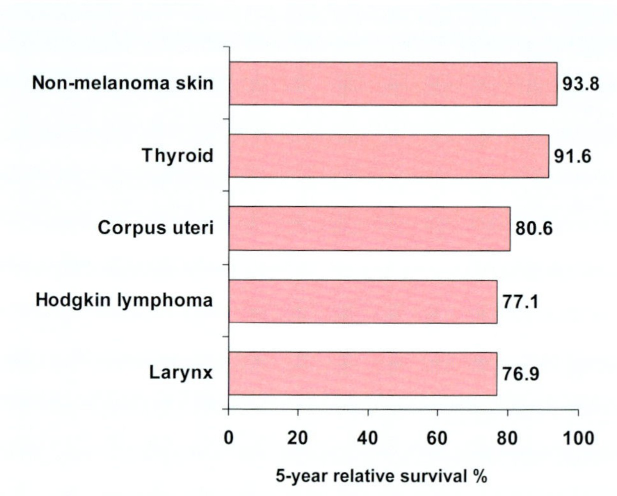

Age group (Table 4b)

The 5-year relative survival by age group reveals no distinct pattern or trend, and fluctuates with increasing age groups for most cancers. However, an inverse relationship between age group and survival was observed for cancers of the salivary gland, gall bladder, larynx, other thoracic organs, mesothelioma, corpus uteri, ovary, brain, thyroid and myeloid leukaemia.

Extent of disease (Table 5; Figure 2)

The information on the clinical extent of disease is analysed for selected cancer sites. Most of the cancers have been diagnosed at a localized stage ranging between 18–65% for various cancers. Nasopharyngeal cancer is an exception wherein a majority (36%) have regional spread of disease at diagnosis. Distant metastasis at diagnosis vary from 20% for ovarian cancer to 1% in cancer of the oral cavity. The unknown category is substantial, ranging between 24–50%. Survival is the highest among localized cancers, followed by regional and distant metastasis cases among the known categories.

Survival trend (Table 6)

The trend of survival data, estimated by the same method of semi-complete analytic approach as in the previous tables, is available for 34 cancer sites or types spanning 10 years in two time periods, 1988–1992 and 1993–1997. An increasing trend with an absolute difference of 8–10% and more between the two calendar periods is observed in cancers of the colon, rectum, larynx, non-melanoma skin, prostate and urinary bladder. The survival was similar for a majority of other cancers in successive calendar periods.

Trend of survival by period and cohort approaches (Tables 7-9; Figure 3)

The availability of data on registration and follow-up together for both a long (from the calendar year 1968) and up to a recent period (year 1997) of calendar time led to the possibility of estimating up-to-date survival and trend by period approach. Survival is also estimated by cohort approach for comparison.

The 5-, 10- and 15-year relative survival estimates by cohort and period approaches are estimated for the different 5-year calendar periods from 1973–1977 to 1993–1997. A distinct correspondence between the two approaches is forthcoming. The period survival estimates at 5, 10 and 15 years of follow-up in a calendar period are seen to resemble the cohort survival estimates of the succeeding calendar periods after 5, 10 and 15 years respectively for most cancers. Thus, period survival closely predicts the survival experience of cancer cases diagnosed in that period. An increasing trend of period survival estimates over the different calendar periods is an indicator for improved prognosis for cancers diagnosed in those calendar periods.

References

1. Parkin DM, Whelan SL, Ferlay J and Storm H. *Cancer Incidence in Five Continents, Vol I to VIII: IARC Cancerbase No. 7.* IARCPress, Lyon, 2005.

2. Lee HP, Day NE and Shanmugaratnam K. *Cancer incidence in Singapore 1968–1982: IARC Scientific Publications No. 91.* National University of Singapore, Singapore, 1988.

3. Chia KS, Lee JJ, Wong JL, Gao W, Lee HP, Shanmugaratnam K. Cancer incidence in Singapore, 1998 to 1999. *Ann Acad Med Singapore.* 2002; 31(6): 745–750.

Figure 2. Absolute survival (%) from selected cancers by extent of disease, Singapore, 1993–1997

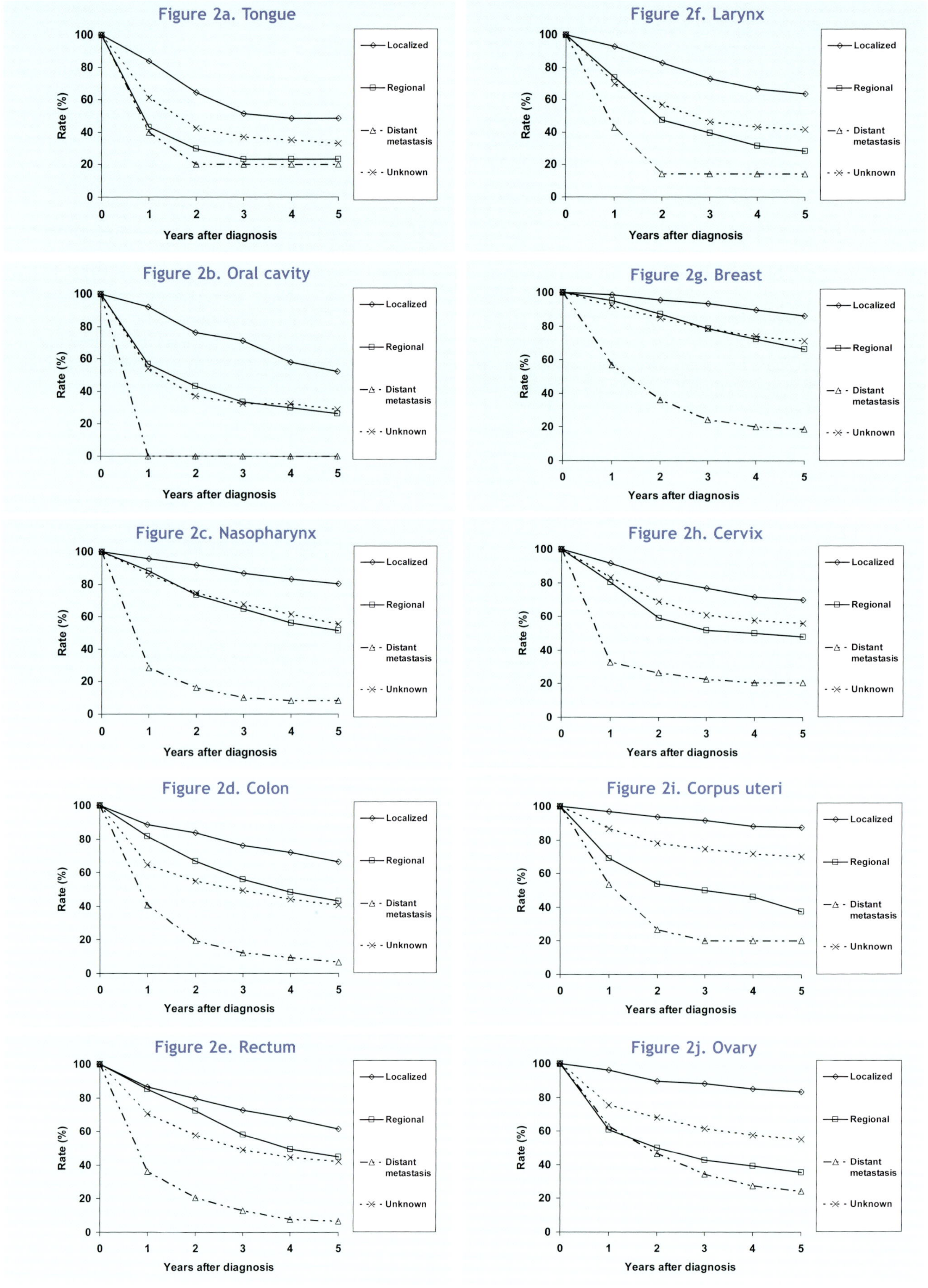

Figure 2a. Tongue

Figure 2f. Larynx

Figure 2b. Oral cavity

Figure 2g. Breast

Figure 2c. Nasopharynx

Figure 2h. Cervix

Figure 2d. Colon

Figure 2i. Corpus uteri

Figure 2e. Rectum

Figure 2j. Ovary

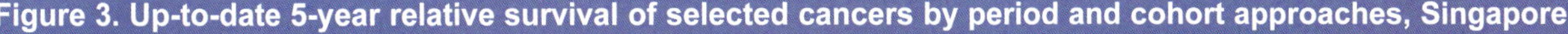

Figure 3. Up-to-date 5-year relative survival of selected cancers by period and cohort approaches, Singapore

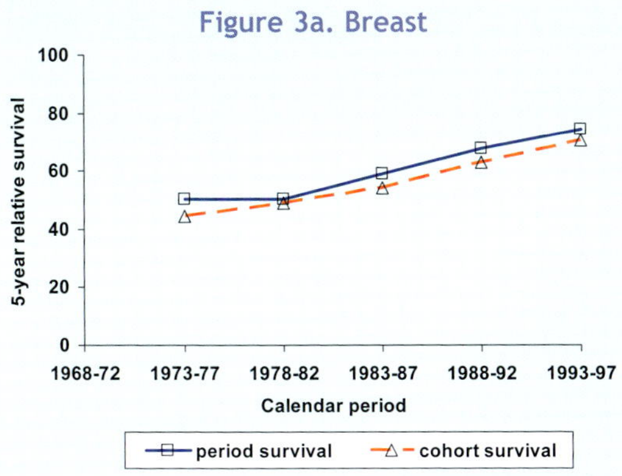

Figure 3a. Breast

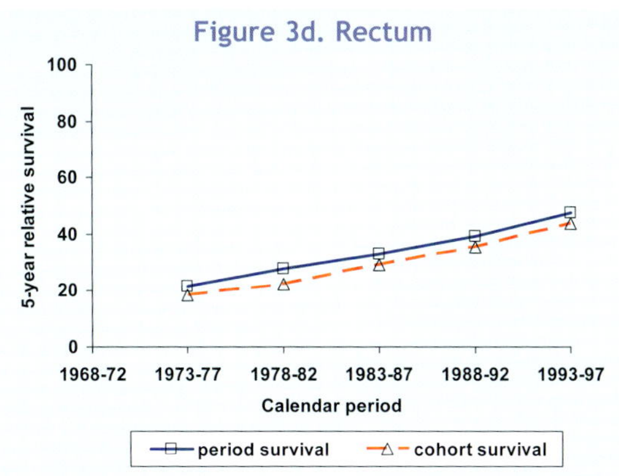

Figure 3d. Rectum

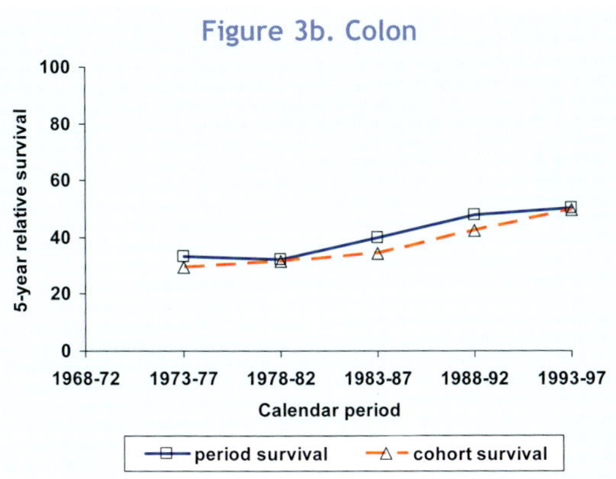

Figure 3b. Colon

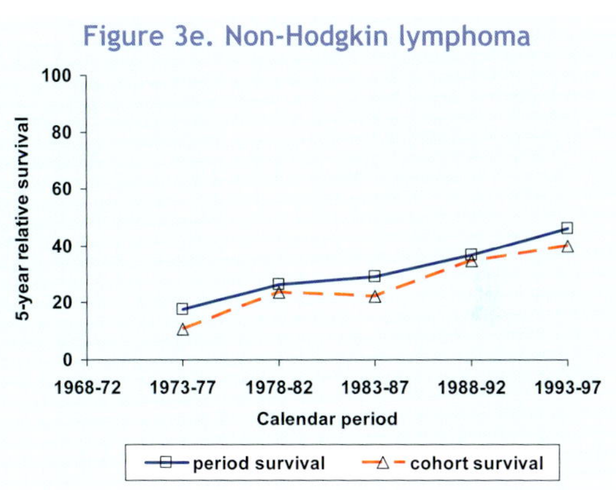

Figure 3e. Non-Hodgkin lymphoma

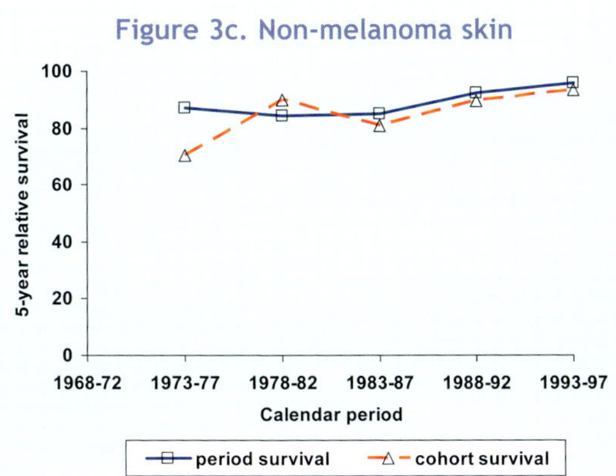

Figure 3c. Non-melanoma skin

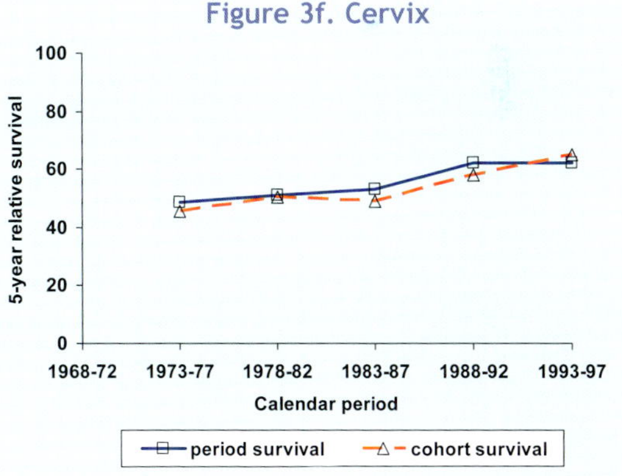

Figure 3f. Cervix

Table 1. Data quality indices - Proportion of histologically verified and death certificate only cases, number and proportion of included and excluded cases by site: Singapore, 1993–1997 cases followed-up until 2001

Site	ICD-10	Total registered	%		Excluded cases					Included cases	
			HV	DCO	DCO	Follow-up	Others	Total	%	No.	%
Tongue	C01-02	124	100.0	0.0	0	4	0	4	3.2	120	96.8
Oral cavity	C03-06	138	97.8	0.0	0	3	0	3	2.2	135	97.8
Salivary gland	C07-08	95	98.9	0.0	0	2	6	8	8.4	87	91.6
Tonsil	C09	40	97.5	0.0	0	2	0	2	5.0	38	95.0
Nasopharynx	C11	1 459	98.8	0.0	0	53	2	55	3.8	1 404	96.2
Hypopharynx	C12-13	92	98.9	0.0	0	2	0	2	2.2	90	97.8
Oesophagus	C15	459	92.4	1.5	7	5	1	13	2.8	446	97.2
Stomach	C16	2 191	94.0	1.1	25	41	25	91	4.2	2 100	95.8
Small intestine	C17	88	94.3	0.0	0	3	5	8	9.1	80	90.9
Colon	C18	2 628	93.3	0.8	20	79	28	127	4.8	2 501	95.2
Rectum	C19-20	1 831	97.2	0.2	3	66	9	78	4.3	1 753	95.7
Anus	C21	53	98.1	0.0	0	0	0	0	0.0	53	100.0
Liver	C22	1 655	26.8	5.2	86	19	0	105	6.3	1 550	93.7
Gall bladder	C23-24	299	73.9	1.7	5	5	0	10	3.3	289	96.7
Pancreas	C25	536	41.8	3.4	18	3	3	24	4.5	512	95.5
Nose/Sinuses	C30-31	73	98.6	0.0	0	1	1	2	2.7	71	97.3
Larynx	C32	326	96.9	0.0	0	14	1	15	4.6	311	95.4
Lung	C33-34	4 386	82.4	1.7	74	56	3	133	3.0	4 253	97.0
Other thoracic organs	C37-38	65	89.2	1.5	1	1	0	2	3.1	63	96.9
Bone	C40-41	80	96.3	1.3	1	2	16	19	23.8	61	76.3
Melanoma of skin	C43	66	100.0	0.0	0	6	0	6	9.1	60	90.9
Other skin	C44	1 163	99.5	0.1	1	124	1	126	10.8	1 037	89.2
Mesothelioma	C45	34	100.0	0.0	0	0	0	0	0.0	34	100.0
Connective tissue	C47+C49	185	94.6	1.1	2	7	10	19	10.3	166	89.7
Peritoneum	C48	44	86.4	0.0	0	1	3	4	9.1	40	90.9
Breast	C50	3 395	98.9	0.2	7	147	37	191	5.6	3 204	94.4
Vulva	C51	38	100.0	0.0	0	3	0	3	7.9	35	92.1
Cervix	C53	1 037	98.7	0.3	3	50	0	53	5.1	984	94.9
Corpus uteri	C54	532	97.7	1.1	6	32	11	49	9.2	483	90.8
Ovary	C56	787	96.6	0.6	5	35	29	69	8.8	718	91.2
Penis	C60	42	100.0	0.0	0	1	0	1	2.4	41	97.6
Prostate	C61	796	95.1	0.5	4	39	1	44	5.5	752	94.5
Testis	C62	87	95.4	0.0	0	6	6	12	13.8	75	86.2
Kidney	C64	387	81.7	1.3	5	12	1	18	4.7	369	95.3
Renal pelvis	C65	45	95.6	0.0	0	1	0	1	2.2	44	97.8
Urinary bladder	C67	520	96.2	0.0	0	20	4	24	4.6	496	95.4
Brain & nervous system	C70-72	314	81.5	4.1	13	3	8	24	7.6	290	92.4
Thyroid	C73	588	97.6	0.0	0	33	1	34	5.8	554	94.2
Adrenal gland	C74	32	81.3	3.1	1	1	2	4	12.5	28	87.5
Hodgkin lymphoma	C81	79	100.0	0.0	0	6	0	6	7.6	73	92.4
Non-Hodgkin lymphoma	C82-85+C96	834	100.0	0.7	6	38	0	44	5.3	790	94.7
Multiple myeloma	C90	167	100.0	3.6	6	2	0	8	4.8	159	95.2
Lymphoid leukaemia	C91	209	100.0	0.5	1	3	0	4	1.9	205	98.1
Myeloid leukaemia	C92-94	408	100.0	0.7	3	15	0	18	4.4	390	95.6
Leukaemia unspecified	C95	80	100.0	7.5	6	2	0	8	10.0	72	90.0

HV: histologically verified; DCO: death certificate only

Table 2. Number and proportion of cases by vital status and median follow-up (in months) by site: Singapore, 1993–1997 cases followed-up until 2001

Site	ICD-10	Cases included	Dead		Alive		Complete FU		Median FU (in months)
			No.	%	No.	%	No.	%	
Tongue	C01-02	120	81	67.5	39	32.5	120	100.0	18.7
Oral cavity	C03-06	135	93	68.9	42	31.1	135	100.0	17.9
Salivary gland	C07-08	87	30	34.5	57	65.5	87	100.0	62.9
Tonsil	C09	38	25	65.8	13	34.2	38	100.0	34.4
Nasopharynx	C11	1 404	659	46.9	745	53.1	1 404	100.0	56.9
Hypopharynx	C12-13	90	84	93.3	6	6.7	90	100.0	10.0
Oesophagus	C15	446	424	95.1	22	4.9	446	100.0	5.3
Stomach	C16	2 100	1 727	82.2	373	17.8	2 100	100.0	8.5
Small intestine	C17	80	63	78.8	17	21.3	80	100.0	12.9
Colon	C18	2 501	1 540	61.6	961	38.4	2 501	100.0	37.8
Rectum	C19-20	1 753	1 064	60.7	689	39.3	1 753	100.0	41.1
Anus	C21	53	39	73.6	14	26.4	53	100.0	22.6
Liver	C22	1 550	1 490	96.1	60	3.9	1 550	100.0	2.2
Gall bladder	C23-24	289	261	90.3	28	9.7	289	100.0	5.2
Pancreas	C25	512	495	96.7	17	3.3	512	100.0	2.6
Nose/Sinuses	C30-31	71	45	63.4	26	36.6	71	100.0	34.9
Larynx	C32	311	174	55.9	137	44.1	311	100.0	45.9
Lung	C33-34	4 253	4 031	94.8	222	5.2	4 253	100.0	5.4
Other thoracic organs	C37-38	63	37	58.7	26	41.3	63	100.0	39.1
Bone	C40-41	61	39	63.9	22	36.1	61	100.0	29.5
Melanoma of skin	C43	60	41	68.3	19	31.7	60	100.0	31.6
Other skin	C44	1 037	311	30.0	726	70.0	1 037	100.0	67.2
Mesothelioma	C45	34	31	91.2	3	8.8	34	100.0	6.3
Connective tissue	C47+C49	166	84	50.6	82	49.4	166	100.0	49.7
Peritoneum	C48	40	30	75.0	10	25.0	40	100.0	18.9
Breast	C50	3 204	1 018	31.8	2 186	68.2	3 204	100.0	64.1
Vulva	C51	35	16	45.7	19	54.3	35	100.0	56.1
Cervix	C53	984	416	42.3	568	57.7	984	100.0	58.4
Corpus uteri	C54	483	124	25.7	359	74.3	483	100.0	63.6
Ovary	C56	718	293	40.8	425	59.2	718	100.0	59.0
Penis	C60	41	19	46.3	22	53.7	41	100.0	55.0
Prostate	C61	752	459	61.0	293	39.0	752	100.0	48.9
Testis	C62	75	11	14.7	64	85.3	75	100.0	71.8
Kidney	C64	369	211	57.2	158	42.8	369	100.0	34.6
Renal pelvis	C65	44	31	70.5	13	29.5	44	100.0	11.0
Urinary bladder	C67	496	252	50.8	244	49.2	496	100.0	52.2
Brain & nervous system	C70-72	290	211	72.8	79	27.2	290	100.0	15.0
Thyroid	C73	554	83	15.0	471	85.0	554	100.0	72.5
Adrenal gland	C74	28	18	64.3	10	35.7	28	100.0	22.6
Hodgkin lymphoma	C81	73	23	31.5	50	68.5	73	100.0	69.4
Non-Hodgkin lymphoma	C82-85+C96	790	472	59.7	318	40.3	790	100.0	23.3
Multiple myeloma	C90	159	138	86.8	21	13.2	159	100.0	16.1
Lymphoid leukaemia	C91	205	119	58.0	86	42.0	205	100.0	36.4
Myeloid leukaemia	C92-94	390	327	83.8	63	16.2	390	100.0	7.7
Leukaemia unspecified	C95	72	66	91.7	6	8.3	72	100.0	2.3

FU: follow-up

Table 3. Comparison of 1-, 3- and 5-year absolute and relative survival and 5-year age-standardized relative survival by site: Singapore, 1993–1997 cases followed-up until 2001

Site	ICD-10	Cases included	% Absolute survival			% Relative survival			% ASRS at 5-years	
			1-year	3-year	5-year	1-year	3-year	5-year	all ages	0-74 years
Tongue	C01-02	120	61.7	36.7	34.0	63.5	39.8	39.0	40.8	44.3
Oral cavity	C03-06	135	64.4	43.0	34.5	66.9	47.6	40.6	45.4	49.2
Salivary gland	C07-08	87	85.1	75.9	65.0	86.6	79.0	69.2	63.0	70.1
Tonsil	C09	38	65.8	47.4	36.1	67.3	49.9	39.2	38.3	44.7
Nasopharynx	C11	1 404	86.6	68.1	56.7	87.5	70.1	59.5	53.6	59.2
Hypopharynx	C12-13	90	43.3	17.8	8.7	45.1	20.0	10.6	11.0	11.9
Oesophagus	C15	446	25.1	8.3	5.3	26.4	9.2	6.2	9.3	12.1
Stomach	C16	2 100	43.1	24.2	19.4	45.0	27.1	23.3	23.9	27.4
Small intestine	C17	80	51.3	35.0	22.4	52.8	38.1	25.8	25.4	28.5
Colon	C18	2 501	70.3	51.0	41.8	73.0	56.9	50.2	49.5	52.5
Rectum	C19-20	1 753	73.5	52.5	42.7	76.1	58.0	50.4	49.0	52.1
Anus	C21	53	60.4	37.7	31.8	63.9	44.3	41.9	39.5	40.4
Liver	C22	1 550	18.3	6.8	4.4	19.0	7.5	5.1	6.0	6.5
Gall bladder	C23-24	289	34.9	17.0	11.9	36.3	18.8	14.0	15.0	18.3
Pancreas	C25	512	11.5	5.3	3.4	12.0	5.8	4.0	4.1	4.8
Nose/Sinuses	C30-31	71	71.8	49.3	40.8	73.9	53.1	45.9	44.3	50.4
Larynx	C32	311	77.8	54.3	47.3	81.0	61.0	57.1	61.0	65.7
Lung	C33-34	4 253	28.9	9.0	6.0	30.2	10.1	7.2	7.7	9.3
Other thoracic organs	C37-38	63	68.3	50.8	44.2	69.0	52.3	46.2	33.8	41.0
Bone	C40-41	61	67.2	47.5	37.2	67.7	48.7	38.5	41.8	38.5
Melanoma of skin	C43	60	71.7	45.0	34.7	73.9	48.7	39.4	39.9	44.5
Other skin	C44	1 037	93.1	82.7	75.2	97.7	95.6	95.8	95.6	95.2
Mesothelioma	C45	34	23.5	11.8	8.4	24.0	12.2	8.8	8.3	11.4
Connective tissue	C47+C49	166	72.3	54.2	51.2	73.6	56.9	55.1	48.2	57.1
Peritoneum	C48	40	60.0	32.5	24.9	60.8	33.3	25.8	19.2	26.2
Breast	C50	3 204	93.0	80.6	72.1	94.0	83.2	76.2	73.9	76.4
Vulva	C51	35	80.0	57.1	54.3	82.5	61.7	62.0	67.0	66.4
Cervix	C53	984	84.2	65.5	59.9	85.3	67.9	63.5	63.2	65.7
Corpus uteri	C54	483	90.3	81.0	76.4	91.3	83.6	80.6	76.5	79.6
Ovary	C56	718	81.8	67.5	61.2	82.7	69.3	63.7	56.2	62.4
Penis	C60	41	82.9	70.7	55.5	85.7	78.5	66.2	70.3	74.8
Prostate	C61	752	82.4	57.7	44.6	88.2	70.8	63.0	61.3	64.3
Testis	C62	75	92.0	89.3	85.1	92.4	90.3	86.7	88.2	88.2
Kidney	C64	369	66.4	49.9	45.3	68.2	53.4	50.7	47.2	55.0
Renal pelvis	C65	44	47.7	34.1	31.5	49.3	37.0	36.1	32.4	43.9
Urinary bladder	C67	496	76.6	58.9	51.8	80.2	67.0	64.0	62.7	71.9
Brain & nervous system	C70-72	290	56.9	35.2	30.2	57.5	35.8	30.9	27.6	29.6
Thyroid	C73	554	92.1	88.8	86.3	93.2	91.4	90.3	89.5	91.2
Adrenal gland	C74	28	60.7	42.9	39.3	61.4	43.4	39.9	23.5	32.1
Hodgkin lymphoma	C81	73	87.7	76.7	69.6	88.4	78.3	71.9	73.1	75.4
Non-Hodgkin lymphoma	C82-85+C96	790	59.5	45.9	42.5	61.1	49.0	47.1	49.2	52.0
Multiple myeloma	C90	159	54.7	28.3	17.2	56.6	30.8	19.4	22.3	26.0
Lymphoid leukaemia	C91	205	68.3	50.2	44.8	68.8	51.1	45.9	35.9	42.9
Myeloid leukaemia	C92-94	390	42.1	22.6	16.7	43.1	23.6	17.7	19.3	22.6
Leukaemia unspecified	C95	72	22.2	12.5	8.3	22.9	13.4	9.0	10.7	12.9

ASRS: age-standardized relative survival

Table 4a. Site-wise number of cases, 5-year absolute and relative survival by sex: Singapore, 1993–1997 cases followed-up until 2001

Site	ICD-10	Cases included	Male % 5-year survival			Female % 5-year survival		
			No.	Abs	Rel	No.	Abs	Rel
Tongue	C01-02	120	73	24.4	28.2	47	48.9	55.8
Oral cavity	C03-06	135	91	31.3	37.7	44	40.9	46.3
Salivary gland	C07-08	87	50	61.4	66.7	37	69.9	72.5
Tonsil	C09	38	27	32.6	35.4	11	45.5	49.4
Nasopharynx	C11	1 404	1 046	54.1	56.9	358	64.6	67.1
Hypopharynx	C12-13	90	84	9.4	11.4	6	0.0	0.0
Oesophagus	C15	446	342	4.9	5.8	104	6.5	7.7
Stomach	C16	2 100	1 289	19.0	23.3	811	20.0	23.2
Small intestine	C17	80	43	25.4	30.1	37	18.9	21.3
Colon	C18	2 501	1 270	41.9	51.3	1 231	41.6	49.2
Rectum	C19-20	1 753	1 006	40.3	48.2	747	46.0	53.4
Anus	C21	53	22	22.7	31.3	31	38.6	49.9
Liver	C22	1 550	1 204	4.6	5.4	346	3.6	4.2
Gall bladder	C23-24	289	132	12.8	15.3	157	11.2	13.0
Pancreas	C25	512	290	3.2	3.8	222	3.6	4.1
Nose/Sinuses	C30-31	71	49	30.5	34.9	22	63.6	69.6
Larynx	C32	311	284	45.5	55.2	27	66.7	76.9
Lung	C33-34	4 253	2 941	5.8	7.1	1 312	6.3	7.2
Other thoracic organs	C37-38	63	42	40.3	42.5	21	52.4	53.8
Bone	C40-41	61	33	36.4	36.9	28	37.6	39.8
Melanoma of skin	C43	60	28	28.6	34.1	32	40.3	44.1
Other skin	C44	1 037	490	76.5	98.0	547	74.1	93.8
Mesothelioma	C45	34	26	6.9	7.3	8	12.5	13.1
Connective tissue	C47+C49	166	96	53.1	57.2	70	48.6	52.1
Peritoneum	C48	40	12	16.7	17.6	28	28.4	29.3
Breast	C50	3 204	13	76.2	88.4	3 191	72.1	76.1
Vulva	C51	35				35	54.3	62.0
Cervix	C53	984				984	59.9	63.5
Corpus uteri	C54	483				483	76.4	80.6
Ovary	C56	718				718	61.2	63.7
Penis	C60	41	41	55.5	66.2			
Prostate	C61	752	752	44.6	63.0			
Testis	C62	75	75	85.1	86.7			
Kidney	C64	369	253	44.1	50.2	116	48.0	51.5
Renal pelvis	C65	44	31	25.6	29.7	13	46.2	51.8
Urinary bladder	C67	496	390	53.1	65.6	106	47.0	58.2
Brain & nervous system	C70-72	290	163	31.7	32.6	127	28.3	28.8
Thyroid	C73	554	123	79.6	85.7	431	88.2	91.6
Adrenal gland	C74	28	14	35.7	36.3	14	42.9	43.4
Hodgkin lymphoma	C81	73	44	65.7	68.7	29	75.9	77.1
Non-Hodgkin lymphoma	C82-85+C96	790	476	37.9	42.4	314	49.5	54.0
Multiple myeloma	C90	159	82	20.2	22.9	77	14.1	15.7
Lymphoid leukaemia	C91	205	127	41.6	42.8	78	50.0	51.0
Myeloid leukaemia	C92-94	390	224	16.2	17.3	166	17.3	18.2
Leukaemia unspecified	C95	72	37	8.1	8.9	35	8.6	9.0

Abs: absolute survival; Rel: relative survival

Table 4b. Site-wise number of cases and relative survival by age group: Singapore, 1993–1997 cases followed-up until 2001

Site	ICD-10	Cases included	Number of cases by age group					Relative survival by age group % 5-year survival				
			< 45	45-54	55-64	65-74	> 75	< 45	45-54	55-64	65-74	> 75
Tongue	C01-02	120	23	17	34	20	26	30.6	54.3	34.8	56.7	28.2
Oral cavity	C03-06	135	12	16	39	36	32	92.3	44.7	30.1	47.3	21.0
Salivary gland	C07-08	87	33	17	14	14	9	84.7	77.9	67.7	51.7	20.7
Tonsil	C09	38	5	8	13	9	3	80.6	38.7	48.1	13.0	0.0
Nasopharynx	C11	1 404	547	407	281	110	59	67.1	60.7	50.6	51.2	32.7
Hypopharynx	C12-13	90	3	16	20	28	23		12.9	21.5	4.5	6.9
Oesophagus	C15	446	8	45	97	148	148	38.0	9.1	4.5	9.8	0.7
Stomach	C16	2 100	145	211	450	623	671	28.9	29.0	31.6	21.5	15.3
Small intestine	C17	80	15	12	15	24	14	26.9	42.7	28.5	19.3	13.8
Colon	C18	2 501	196	303	551	747	704	55.4	56.0	54.6	47.8	45.6
Rectum	C19-20	1 753	162	245	433	499	414	54.0	52.4	57.0	47.3	44.5
Anus	C21	53	1	4	11	11	26	0.0	76.3	48.2	32.6	38.8
Liver	C22	1 550	157	191	363	469	370	10.9	6.9	4.3	3.7	4.1
Gall bladder	C23-24	289	20	42	58	91	78	25.2	18.8	16.6	14.3	4.3
Pancreas	C25	512	25	64	115	164	144	8.1	3.2	6.4	2.9	3.0
Nose/Sinuses	C30-31	71	11	10	22	17	11	45.8	71.5	39.6	50.3	27.3
Larynx	C32	311	10	37	88	99	77	80.9	78.2	57.0	56.9	42.7
Lung	C33-34	4 253	195	374	918	1 520	1 246	9.8	13.6	10.0	5.9	3.7
Other thoracic organs	C37-38	63	31	10	16	4	2	54.9	51.0	33.9	29.4	0.0
Bone	C40-41	61	44	6	6	2	3	40.7	11.3	35.5	56.5	50.4
Melanoma of skin	C43	60	19	6	6	13	16	47.6	48.6	35.6	45.1	21.2
Other skin	C44	1 037	113	114	193	230	387	96.3	95.3	92.9	96.4	97.5
Mesothelioma	C45	34	4	6	11	9	4	25.2	17.2	9.5	0.0	0.0
Connective tissue	C47+C49	166	74	21	30	24	17	58.4	53.7	75.3	40.4	20.2
Peritoneum	C48	40	12	9	7	10	2	33.4	34.1	30.5	11.2	0.0
Breast	C50	3 204	936	1 025	645	369	229	77.8	78.9	75.8	72.0	63.0
Vulva	C51	35	3	7	7	6	12	100.6	43.7	60.0	77.7	58.3
Cervix	C53	984	273	273	214	128	96	77.6	61.3	58.7	59.2	43.0
Corpus uteri	C54	483	96	140	142	75	30	87.8	86.8	79.0	68.1	65.5
Ovary	C56	718	270	189	116	89	54	83.6	60.5	52.0	45.9	24.8
Penis	C60	41	2	7	10	16	6	101.3	59.2	76.9	60.6	58.6
Prostate	C61	752	4	7	98	283	360	50.5	42.6	67.0	66.2	59.8
Testis	C62	75	57	9	7	2	0	91.9	91.3	58.9	0.0	
Kidney	C64	369	58	76	87	92	56	60.8	64.5	53.4	45.1	22.3
Renal pelvis	C65	44	2	6	15	14	7	50.5	34.6	21.9	68.8	0.0
Urinary bladder	C67	496	34	52	100	147	163	77.2	81.1	82.8	57.3	47.9
Brain & nervous system	C70-72	290	171	32	36	34	17	43.8	28.8	9.0	3.7	0.0
Thyroid	C73	554	287	93	74	56	44	99.8	95.4	90.1	66.2	41.5
Adrenal gland	C74	28	20	1	3	1	3	50.1	101.9	0.0	0.0	0.0
Hodgkin lymphoma	C81	73	42	15	6	8	2	86.1	54.2	51.4	60.9	0.0
Non-Hodgkin lymphoma	C82-85+C96	790	231	122	159	144	134	54.0	64.0	46.5	39.4	25.5
Multiple myeloma	C90	159	11	29	37	42	40	45.9	49.6	20.3	1.7	3.9
Lymphoid leukaemia	C91	205	155	11	14	18	7	51.6	37.1	23.5	33.5	0.0
Myeloid leukaemia	C92-94	390	152	42	57	75	64	32.2	14.4	10.8	4.4	4.5
Leukaemia unspecified	C95	72	27	4	8	16	17	22.3	0.0	0.0	0.0	0.0

Table 5. Proportion of cases and 5-year absolute survival by extent of disease and site: Singapore, 1993–1997

Site	ICD-10	Cases included	% of cases by extent of disease				% 5-year absolute survival			
			Localized	Regional	Dist. met.	Unknown	Localized	Regional	Dist. met.	Unknown
Tongue	C01-02	120	25.8	25.0	4.2	45.0	48.4	23.3	20.0	33.1
Oral cavity	C03-06	135	28.1	22.2	1.5	48.2	52.2	26.3	0.0	28.9
Nasopharynx	C11	1 404	18.2	36.3	3.5	42.0	80.1	51.3	8.2	55.3
Colon	C18	2 501	27.0	22.4	18.8	31.8	66.5	43.2	6.6	40.6
Rectum	C19-20	1 753	30.3	27.0	16.8	25.9	61.6	44.9	6.6	41.9
Larynx	C32	311	35.7	12.2	2.3	49.8	63.6	28.6	14.3	41.8
Breast	C50	3 204	30.6	22.5	4.8	42.1	85.9	66.3	18.8	71.2
Cervix	C53	984	45.5	5.7	5.0	43.8	69.7	48.0	20.4	55.7
Corpus uteri	C54	483	64.8	5.4	6.2	23.6	87.4	37.4	20.0	70.0
Ovary	C56	718	45.7	3.9	19.8	30.6	83.3	35.4	24.5	55.2

Dis. met.: distant metastasis

Table 6. Comparison of 5-year absolute and relative survival of cases diagnosed between 1988–1992 and 1993–1997, Singapore

Site	ICD-10	% 5-year absolute survival		% 5-year relative survival	
		1988–1992	1993–1997	1988–1992	1993–1997
Tongue	C01-02	35.9	34.0	39.8	39.0
Oral cavity	C03-06	37.7	34.5	43.1	40.6
Salivary gland	C07-08	67.6	65.0	71.9	69.2
Tonsil	C09	21.2	36.1	24.2	39.2
Nasopharynx	C11	50.5	56.7	52.8	59.5
Hypopharynx	C12-13	15.0	8.7	17.7	10.6
Oesophagus	C15	3.3	5.3	4.0	6.2
Stomach	C16	16.6	19.4	19.8	23.3
Colon	C18	41.1	41.8	48.8	50.2
Rectum	C19-20	37.0	42.7	43.4	50.4
Liver	C22	2.3	4.4	2.7	5.1
Gall bladder	C23-24	12.1	11.9	14.5	14.0
Pancreas	C25	5.6	3.4	6.4	4.0
Nose/Sinuses	C30-31	34.7	40.8	37.1	45.9
Larynx	C32	40.0	47.3	47.1	57.1
Lung	C33-34	5.3	6.0	6.2	7.2
Bone	C40-41	52.9	37.2	54.5	38.5
Other skin	C44	76.1	75.2	93.7	95.8
Connective tissue	C47+C49	47.8	51.2	51.3	55.1
Breast	C50	66.3	72.1	70.1	76.2
Cervix	C53	61.2	59.9	64.6	63.5
Corpus uteri	C54	71.3	76.4	74.7	80.6
Ovary	C56	63.4	61.2	66.1	63.7
Prostate	C61	37.3	44.6	52.3	63.0
Testis	C62	83.0	85.1	84.6	86.7
Kidney	C64	38.1	45.3	42.7	50.7
Urinary bladder	C67	48.4	51.8	60.6	64.0
Brain & nervous system	C70-72	22.5	30.2	23.3	30.9
Thyroid	C73	83.5	86.3	86.8	90.3
Hodgkin lymphoma	C81	52.7	69.6	55.0	71.9
Non-Hodgkin lymphoma	C82-85+C96	35.5	42.5	38.6	47.1
Multiple myeloma	C90	16.3	17.2	18.9	19.4
Lymphoid leukaemia	C91	15.6	44.8	16.6	45.9
Myeloid leukaemia	C92-94	15.0	16.7	15.8	17.7

Table 7. Number of cases by cancer site and calendar period, Singapore Cancer Registry, 1968–1997

Site	ICD-10	Number of cases						Total
		1968–72	1973–77	1978–82	1983–87	1988–92	1993–97	1968-97
Tongue	C01-02	69	75	90	103	103	120	560
Oral cavity	C03-06	83	82	106	112	130	135	648
Salivary gland	C07-08	25	45	51	66	74	87	348
Tonsil	C09	34	40	57	36	52	38	257
Nasopharynx	C11	670	850	933	1 118	1 413	1 404	6 388
Hypopharynx	C12-13	30	41	55	49	80	90	345
Oesophagus	C15	505	509	509	469	488	446	2 926
Stomach	C16	1 355	1 551	1 619	1 846	1 966	2 100	10 437
Colon	C18	475	708	1 045	1 474	2 176	2 501	8 379
Rectum	C19-20	392	595	796	999	1 301	1 753	5 836
Liver	C22	886	951	1 125	1 042	1 069	1 550	6 623
Gall bladder	C23-24	47	95	114	143	198	289	886
Pancreas	C25	113	158	218	306	355	512	1 662
Nose/Sinuses	C30-31	37	63	69	66	72	71	378
Larynx	C32	181	200	247	254	295	311	1 488
Lung	C33-34	1 547	2 228	2 841	3 314	3 634	4 253	17 817
Bone	C40-41	51	70	91	89	104	61	466
Other skin	C44	244	338	529	609	848	1 037	3 605
Connective tissue	C47+C49	61	106	94	163	136	166	726
Breast	C50	574	749	1 110	1 550	2 436	3 204	9 623
Cervix	C53	512	599	683	817	920	984	4 515
Corpus uteri	C54	115	115	183	266	376	483	1 538
Ovary	C56	173	215	353	428	604	718	2 491
Prostate	C61	77	112	200	296	459	752	1 896
Testis	C62	31	31	42	53	53	75	285
Kidney	C64	77	85	125	176	244	369	1 076
Urinary bladder	C67	164	217	305	369	444	496	1 995
Brain & nervous system	C70-72	67	87	126	173	213	290	956
Thyroid	C73	149	181	254	431	502	554	2 071
Hodgkin lymphoma	C81	34	46	46	44	55	73	298
Non-Hodgkin lymphoma	C82-85+C96	151	212	329	465	574	790	2 521
Multiple myeloma	C90	30	39	56	111	129	159	524
Lymphoid leukaemia	C91	112	92	106	133	147	205	795
Myeloid leukaemia	C92-94	181	195	228	261	320	390	1 575

Table 9 (Continued).

Site	ICD-10	% 15-year relative survival					
		Period approach			Cohort approach		
		1983–87	1988–92	1993–97	1983–87	1988–92	1993–97
Tongue	C01-02	23.6	28.6	35.4	27.3	22.8	24.4
Oral cavity	C03-06	28.8	32.9	32.3	24.2	14.8	22.9
Salivary gland	C07-08	84.5	57.7	55.1	57.0	44.8	62.6
Tonsil	C09	24.3	24.3	31.7	17.4	20.5	25.5
Nasopharynx	C11	22.1	33.7	39.2	17.9	17.3	26.1
Hypopharynx	C12-13	0.0	7.4	16.2	0.0	0.0	4.0
Oesophagus	C15	7.9	4.7	3.9	3.5	4.4	6.2
Stomach	C16	11.8	17.4	18.4	5.8	3.3	11.8
Colon	C18	36.3	45.8	45.8	27.7	24.6	33.4
Rectum	C19-20	24.7	36.2	40.4	17.6	14.8	22.6
Liver	C22	2.1	1.4	3.4	1.3	2.5	2.9
Gall bladder	C23-24	8.3	15.3	9.6	4.2	7.3	8.5
Pancreas	C25	8.9	3.4	5.3	5.6	6.2	3.6
Nose/Sinuses	C30-31	22.3	35.1	19.9	15.4	13.5	26.3
Larynx	C32	27.1	33.8	44.3	17.5	18.0	23.7
Lung	C33-34	4.8	4.6	5.3	3.5	2.5	4.9
Bone	C40-41	38.5	51.9	42.8	25.4	29.7	45.9
Other skin	C44	70.2	86.3	90.7	83.5	56.1	73.0
Connective tissue	C47+C49	51.1	42.2	45.3	38.1	37.7	37.3
Breast	C50	39.6	52.8	58.6	34.1	31.3	39.8
Cervix	C53	48.6	54.4	56.6	44.3	40.3	44.5
Corpus uteri	C54	63.2	70.5	79.5	47.5	43.2	57.2
Ovary	C56	51.3	63.1	60.1	40.6	36.5	51.3
Prostate	C61	29.4	16.6	24.2	19.7	14.9	10.7
Testis	C62	78.2	70.5	80.2	32.1	54.6	52.0
Kidney	C64	15.5	47.5	40.0	20.1	13.8	30.1
Urinary bladder	C67	29.2	63.1	59.3	24.6	24.9	45.3
Brain & nervous system	C70-72	19.1	20.8	21.9	16.7	9.9	24.0
Thyroid	C73	92.0	90.1	92.6	73.4	71.3	81.3
Hodgkin lymphoma	C81	33.0	36.4	59.2	29.5	20.0	39.8
Non-Hodgkin lymphoma	C82-85+C9	24.5	28.0	43.5	14.8	8.2	17.2
Multiple myeloma	C90	15.6	9.4	7.6	17.6	16.8	12.9
Lymphoid leukaemia	C91	5.1	9.6	17.4	9.3	1.0	12.6
Myeloid leukaemia	C92-94	3.7	3.5	9.1	1.2	0.0	1.7

Chapter 25

Cancer survival in Chiang Mai, Thailand, 1993–1997

Sumitsawan Y, Srisukho S, Sastraruji A, Chaisaengkhum U, Maneesai P and Waisri N

Abstract

The Chiang Mai tumour registry was established in 1978 as a hospital-based cancer registry, and population-based cancer registration started in 1986, with retrospective data collection on cancer incidence and mortality since 1983. Registration of cases is done by active methods. Data on survival for 36 cancer sites or types registered during 1993–1997 are reported here. Follow-up has been carried out predominantly by active methods, with median follow-up ranging between 1–39 months for different cancers. The proportion of histologically verified diagnosis for various cancers ranged between 28–100%; death certificate only (DCO) cases comprised 0–56%; 33–92% of total registered cases were included for survival analysis. Complete follow-up at five years ranged from 59–100% for different cancers. The 5-year age-standardized relative survival rates was the highest for Hodgkin lymphoma (70%) followed by thyroid (65%), cervix (57%), breast (56%) and corpus uteri (49%). The 5-year relative survival by age group showed either an inverse relationship or was fluctuating. An overwhelmingly high proportion of cases were diagnosed with a regional spread of disease, ranging between 44–82% for different cancers and survival decreased with increasing extent of disease for all cancers studied.

Chiang Mai tumour registry

The Chiang Mai tumour registry was established in 1978 as a hospital-based cancer registry in The Maharaj Nakorn Chiang Mai Hospital and is fully supported by the Faculty of Medicine, Chiang Mai University. Population-based cancer registration started in 1986, with retrospective data collection on cancer incidence and mortality since 1983. The registry has been contributing data to the quinquennial IARC publication Cancer Incidence in Five Continents since volume VI [1]. Cancer registration is done by active methods. The principal sources of information on cancer cases are the hospital and pathology records. The registry caters to a mixed urban and rural population of about 1.4 million with a sex ratio of 995 females to 1000 males in 1995. The average annual age-standardized incidence rate is 145 per 100 000 among males and 151 per 100 000 among females with a lifetime cumulative risk of one in 6 of developing cancer for both sexes in the period 1993–1997. The top-ranking cancers among males are lung followed by liver and stomach. Among females, the order is cervix, lung and breast.

The registry contributed data on survival from 37 cancer sites or types for the first volume of the IARC publication on *Cancer Survival in Developing Countries* [2]. Data on survival from 36 cancer sites or types registered during 1993–1997 are reported in this second volume.

Data quality indices (Table 1)

The proportion of cases with histologically verified cancer diagnosis in our series is 77%, varying between 28–100%. The proportion of cases registered as death certificate only (DCO) is 5.5%, ranging between nil for many cancers and 56% for unspecified cancer. Cases excluded without any follow-up constitute 16%. The exclusion of cases from the survival analysis is the greatest among the gastrointestinal cancer of the gall bladder (67%) and the least among lymphoid leukaemia (8%). Thus, 33–92% of the total cases registered are included in the estimation of the survival probability.

Outcome of follow-up (Table 2)

Follow-up has been carried out predominantly by active methods. These included abstraction of cancer mortality information from the Chiang Mai public health service records. The abstracted data are matched with the incident cancer database. Unmatched incident cases are then subjected to one or more of the following to obtain the vital status information: repeated scrutiny of records in the respective sources of registration, postal enquiry and house visits.

The closing date of follow-up was 31st December 2000. The median follow-up (in months) ranged between 1.4 months for unspecified leukaemia to 39 months for breast and corpus uteri cancers. Complete follow-up information at five years from the incidence date ranged from 100% for unspecified leukaemia to 59% for non-melanoma skin cancer. The proportion of cases lost to follow-up was generally the highest within 3 years from the incidence date.

Survival statistics

All ages and both sexes together (Table 3)

The 5-year relative survival is the highest for corpus uteri cancer (68%) followed by thyroid (67%), breast (62%), cervix (60%) and Hodgkin lymphoma (53%). The lowest survival rate is encountered with liver cancer, with a figure of 3%. Nasopharynx (37%), among other head and neck cancers, and colon (31%), among gastrointestinal cancers, have the highest survival. Survival from cancers of the urinary system is 31% for urinary bladder and 19% for kidney. Hodgkin lymphoma had a better survival (53%) than non-Hodgkin (26%). The survival figures for leukaemias are 20% for lymphoid, 11% for myeloid and 10% for unspecified.

Figure 1a. Top ten cancers (ranked by survival), Chiang Mai, Thailand, 1993–1997

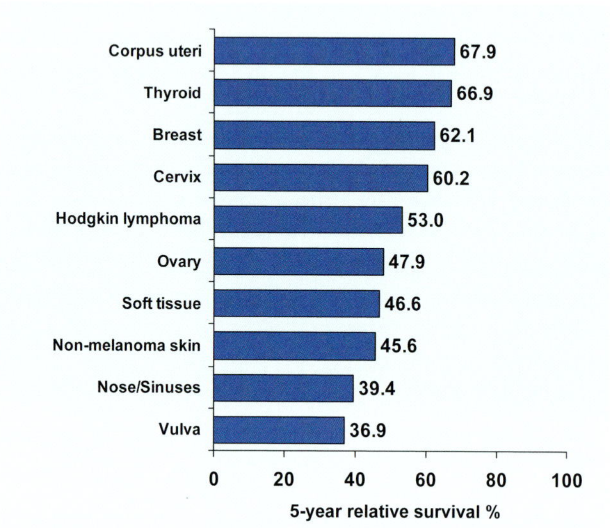

The 5-year age-standardized relative survival (ASRS) probability for all ages together was generally less than or similar to the corresponding unadjusted one for most cancers. Also, the 5-year ASRS (0–74 years of age) was generally higher than or similar to the corresponding ASRS (all ages) for a majority of cancers.

Sex

Male (Table 4a)

The top five cancers ranked on the 5-year relative survival were Hodgkin disease (59%), thyroid (49%), soft tissue (47%), non-melanoma skin (39%) and prostate (35%). Survival from Hodgkin lymphoma and laryngeal cancer was noticeably higher among males than females.

Figure 1b. Top five cancers (ranked by survival), Male, Chiang Mai, Thailand, 1993–1997

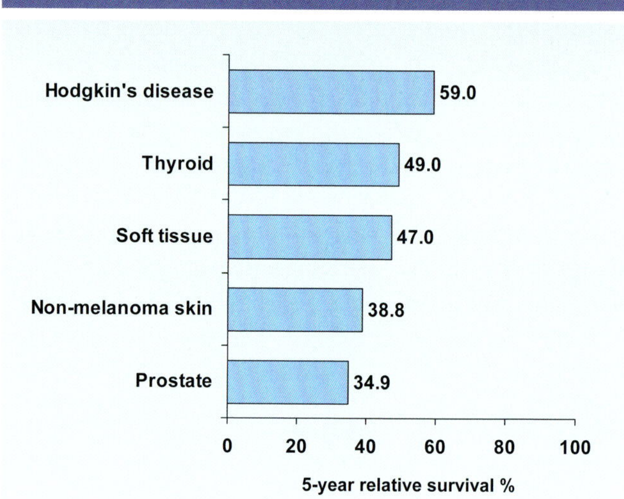

Female (Table 4a)

The top-ranking cancers in terms of 5-year relative survival are thyroid (73%), corpus uteri (68%), breast

Figure 1c. Top five cancers (ranked by survival), Female, Chiang Mai, Thailand, 1993–1997

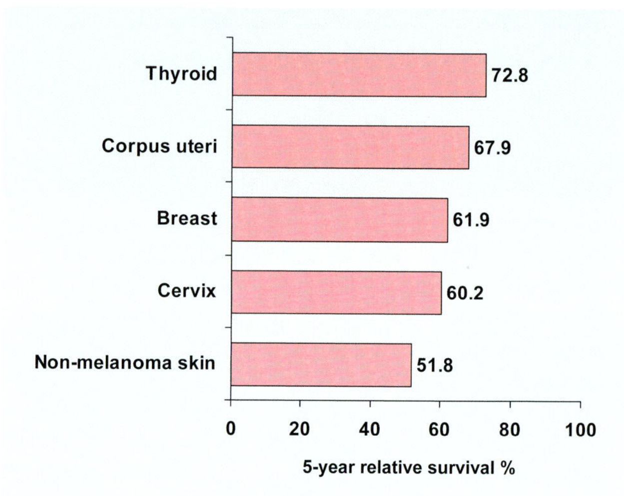

(62%), cervix (60%) and non-melanoma skin (52%). Survival was distinctly higher among females than males for cancers of the oral cavity, nasopharynx, oesophagus, gall bladder, bone, non-melanoma skin, brain and thyroid, and non-Hodgkin lymphoma and unspecified leukaemia.

Age group (Table 4b)

The 5-year relative survival by age group reveals an inverse relationship: a decreasing survival with increasing age at diagnosis for cancers of the cervix and body uterus. In the rest, it is observed to be fluctuating.

Extent of disease (Table 5; Figure 2)

An overwhelmingly high proportion of cases among the few selected cancers with reliable information on extent of disease are diagnosed, with a regional spread of disease ranging from 82% for larynx cancer to 44% for ovarian cancer. There is not much of a difference in the frequency of cases with a localized disease (14%) and a distant metastasis (12%) in breast cancer. Less than 4% of cases presented with localized disease among colorectal cancers. The extent of disease was unknown in 0–4%. The 5-year absolute survival by extent of disease followed the expected pattern: highest for localized cases followed by regional and distant metastasis cases among known categories of extent of disease.

Survival trend (Table 6)

The 5-year relative survival for cases registered in 1993–1997 compared to those in 1983–1992 [2] shows a marked decrease in cancers of the tongue, bone, skin melanoma, non-melanoma skin, vulva and penis. There has been an increase in survival in the corresponding period for cancers of the connective tissue, thyroid and Hodgkin lymphoma. For the rest, the absolute difference in survival is <10%. The level of complete follow-up in this volume has decreased in 25 out of 33 cancers compared to previous volume.

References

1. Parkin DM, Whelan SL, Ferlay J and Storm H. *Cancer Incidence in Five Continents, Vol I to VIII: IARC Cancerbase No. 7*. IARCPress, Lyon, 2005.

2. Martin N, Srisukho S, Kunpradist O and Suttajit M. Cancer survival in Chiang Mai, Thailand. In: *Cancer Survival in Developing Countries* (eds) R Sankaranarayanan, RJ Black and DM Parkin. IARC Scientific Publications No. 145. IARCPress, Lyon, 1998.

Figure 2. Absolute survival (%) from selected cancers by extent of disease, Chiang Mai, Thailand

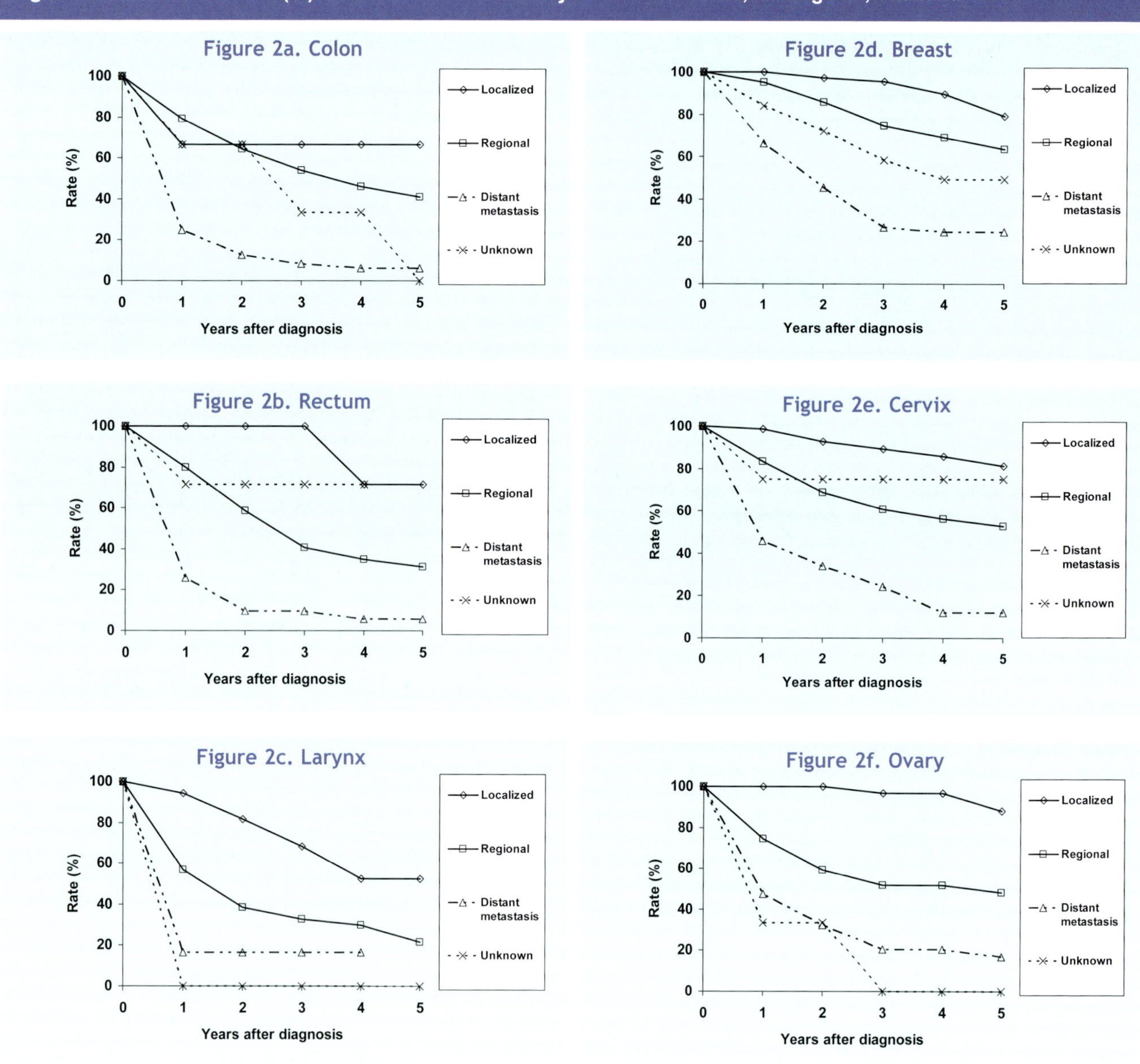

Table 1. Data quality indices - Proportion of histologically verified and death certificate only cases, number and proportion of included and excluded cases by site: Chiang Mai, Thailand, 1993–1997 cases followed-up until 2000

Site	ICD-10	Total registered	%		Excluded cases					Included cases	
			HV	DCO	DCO	Follow-up	Others	Total	%	No.	%
Tongue	C01-02	101	94.1	0.0	0	16	0	16	15.8	85	84.2
Oral cavity	C03-06	124	95.2	1.6	2	19	2	23	18.5	101	81.5
Tonsil	C09	59	98.3	0.0	0	7	1	8	13.6	51	86.4
Nasopharynx	C11	167	81.4	9.0	15	19	0	34	20.4	133	79.6
Hypopharynx	C12-13	78	94.9	0.0	0	9	0	9	11.5	69	88.5
Oesophagus	C15	109	75.2	0.9	1	20	0	21	19.3	88	80.7
Stomach	C16	408	77.7	2.2	9	82	1	92	22.5	316	77.5
Colon	C18	310	81.9	1.6	5	66	2	73	23.5	237	76.5
Rectum	C19-20	219	83.1	0.0	0	29	0	29	13.2	190	86.8
Liver	C22	993	42.5	12.0	119	168	1	288	29.0	705	71.0
Gall bladder	C23-24	182	62.1	1.6	3	44	0	47	25.8	135	74.2
Pancreas	C25	132	46.2	0.8	1	24	1	26	19.7	106	80.3
Gastrointestinal tract	C26	93	28.0	55.9	52	10	0	62	66.7	31	33.3
Nose/Sinuses	C30-31	39	76.9	0.0	0	6	0	6	15.4	33	84.6
Larynx	C32	184	83.2	1.6	3	28	0	31	16.8	153	83.2
Lung	C33-34	2 135	61.4	10.4	223	267	3	493	23.1	1 642	76.9
Bone	C40-41	45	64.4	15.6	7	3	0	10	22.2	35	77.8
Melanoma of skin	C43	31	100.0	0.0	0	4	0	4	12.9	27	87.1
Other skin	C44	268	98.1	1.9	5	92	2	99	36.9	169	63.1
Connective tissue	C47+C49	53	100.0	0.0	0	8	0	8	15.1	45	84.9
Breast	C50	621	93.6	1.4	9	65	3	77	12.4	544	87.6
Vulva	C51	31	100.0	0.0	0	3	0	3	9.7	28	90.3
Cervix	C53	973	96.8	0.4	4	81	3	88	9.0	885	91.0
Corpus uteri	C54	125	86.4	8.8	11	16	0	27	21.6	98	78.4
Ovary	C56	197	88.8	0.5	1	33	1	35	17.8	162	82.2
Penis	C60	92	94.6	0.0	0	20	0	20	21.7	72	78.3
Prostate	C61	148	92.6	0.0	0	39	2	41	27.7	107	72.3
Kidney	C64	58	70.7	5.2	3	16	1	20	34.5	38	65.5
Urinary bladder	C67	273	87.5	0.4	1	48	1	50	18.3	223	81.7
Brain & nervous system	C70-72	103	68.0	13.6	14	13	1	28	27.2	75	72.8
Thyroid	C73	164	93.9	0.0	0	34	0	34	20.7	130	79.3
Hodgkin lymphoma	C81	42	100.0	0.0	0	12	0	12	28.6	30	71.4
Non-Hodgkin lymphoma	C82-85+C96	369	99.7	0.3	1	67	3	71	19.2	298	80.8
Lymphoid leukaemia	C91	76	100.0	0.0	0	6	0	6	7.9	70	92.1
Myeloid leukaemia	C92-94	135	100.0	0.0	0	13	0	13	9.6	122	90.4
Leukaemia unspecified	C95	64	75.0	25.0	16	4	1	21	32.8	43	67.2

HV: histologically verified; DCO: death certificate only

Table 2. Number and proportion of cases with complete/incomplete follow-up (in years) and median follow-up (in months) by site: Chiang Mai, Thailand, 1993–1997 cases followed-up until 2000

Site	ICD-10	Cases included	Complete FU Alive/dead at end of FU		Incomplete FU: lost to FU						% with complete FU at 5 years	Median FU (in months)
							% lost to FU: years from diagnosis					
			No.	%	No.	%	< 1	1-3	3-5	> 5		
Tongue	C01-02	85	68	80.0	17	20.0	7.0	5.9	4.7	2.4	82.4	6.6
Oral cavity	C03-06	101	71	70.3	30	29.7	11.8	9.9	5.0	3.0	73.3	9.8
Tonsil	C09	51	33	64.7	18	35.3	17.6	11.8	5.9	0.0	64.7	7.4
Nasopharynx	C11	133	104	78.2	29	21.8	6.7	9.8	2.3	3.0	81.2	19.9
Hypopharynx	C12-13	69	54	78.3	15	21.7	8.7	4.3	2.9	5.8	84.1	8.6
Oesophagus	C15	88	77	87.5	11	12.5	8.0	2.3	1.1	1.1	88.6	2.7
Stomach	C16	316	261	82.6	55	17.4	8.5	3.2	4.4	1.3	83.9	5.7
Colon	C18	237	174	73.4	63	26.6	9.4	8.4	4.6	4.2	77.6	14.6
Rectum	C19-20	190	142	74.7	48	25.3	9.0	8.4	6.8	1.1	75.8	16.4
Liver	C22	705	638	90.5	67	9.5	7.1	1.1	0.4	0.9	91.4	2.1
Gall bladder	C23-24	135	107	79.3	28	20.7	11.9	7.4	0.0	1.5	80.8	3.8
Pancreas	C25	106	90	84.9	16	15.1	9.5	3.8	0.9	0.9	85.8	3.6
Gastrointestinal tract	C26	31	29	93.5	2	6.5	3.3	3.2	0.0	0.0	93.5	2.2
Nose/Sinuses	C30-31	33	24	72.7	9	27.3	9.1	12.1	0.0	6.1	78.8	20.5
Larynx	C32	153	112	73.2	41	26.8	8.5	8.5	5.9	3.9	77.1	12.1
Lung	C33-34	1 642	1 451	88.4	191	11.6	8.1	2.4	0.7	0.4	88.8	3.8
Bone	C40-41	35	27	77.1	8	22.9	8.6	2.9	5.7	5.7	82.8	12.1
Melanoma of skin	C43	27	20	74.1	7	25.9	7.4	3.7	11.1	3.7	77.8	16.6
Other skin	C44	169	87	51.5	82	48.5	15.3	17.8	7.7	7.7	59.2	23.2
Connective tissue	C47+C49	45	28	62.2	17	37.8	13.3	11.1	8.9	4.5	66.7	13.3
Breast	C50	544	354	65.1	190	34.9	7.1	12.5	8.5	6.8	71.9	39.0
Vulva	C51	28	22	78.6	6	21.4	7.1	10.7	0.0	3.6	82.2	22.8
Cervix	C53	885	621	70.2	264	29.8	6.7	8.4	10.1	4.8	75.0	38.0
Corpus uteri	C54	98	56	57.1	42	42.9	10.2	10.2	13.3	9.2	66.3	39.0
Ovary	C56	162	112	69.1	50	30.9	9.9	9.9	6.2	4.9	74.0	20.4
Penis	C60	72	44	61.1	28	38.9	16.7	13.9	8.3	0.0	61.1	12.0
Prostate	C61	107	82	76.6	25	23.4	5.6	5.6	7.5	4.7	81.3	27.2
Kidney	C64	38	31	81.6	7	18.4	10.5	5.3	0.0	2.6	84.2	6.6
Urinary bladder	C67	223	161	72.2	62	27.8	10.3	8.5	4.5	4.5	76.7	13.1
Brain & nervous system	C70-72	75	48	64.0	27	36.0	12.0	10.7	12.0	1.3	65.3	10.7
Thyroid	C73	130	82	63.1	48	36.9	7.7	11.5	10.8	6.9	70.0	37.5
Hodgkin lymphoma	C81	30	21	70.0	9	30.0	13.3	6.7	6.7	3.3	73.3	10.3
Non-Hodgkin lymphoma	C82-85+C96	298	232	77.9	66	22.1	10.4	8.1	2.3	1.3	79.2	8.2
Lymphoid leukaemia	C91	70	62	88.6	8	11.4	7.1	2.9	0.0	1.4	90.0	8.7
Myeloid leukaemia	C92-94	122	111	91.0	11	9.0	5.7	2.5	0.0	0.8	91.8	2.1
Leukaemia unspecified	C95	43	42	97.7	1	2.3	0.0	0.0	0.0	2.3	100.0	1.4

FU: follow-up

Table 3. Comparison of 1-, 3- and 5-year absolute and relative survival and 5-year age-standardized relative survival by site: Chiang Mai, Thailand, 1993–1997 cases followed-up until 2000

Site	ICD-10	Cases included	% Absolute survival			% Relative survival			% ASRS at 5-years	
			1-year	3-year	5-year	1-year	3-year	5-year	all ages	0-74 years
Tongue	C01-02	85	35.4	16.6	16.6	36.1	17.4	17.8	21.7	24.3
Oral cavity	C03-06	101	55.8	32.0	21.5	56.6	33.4	23.2	24.8	22.0
Tonsil	C09	51	48.4	26.7	20.0	49.1	27.6	21.0	26.9	30.6
Nasopharynx	C11	133	72.8	40.6	35.6	73.3	41.5	36.7	32.5	41.5
Hypopharynx	C12-13	69	45.5	23.1	20.9	46.3	24.3	22.6	27.0	30.0
Oesophagus	C15	88	21.9	8.9	8.9	22.2	9.4	9.8	11.0	6.4
Stomach	C16	316	38.4	19.5	12.1	38.8	20.2	12.8	12.9	12.1
Colon	C18	237	61.5	39.7	29.3	62.1	40.8	30.8	27.8	32.5
Rectum	C19-20	190	69.7	36.9	27.9	70.5	38.3	29.7	28.7	30.4
Liver	C22	705	17.0	4.5	3.0	17.1	4.7	3.2	3.2	3.3
Gall bladder	C23-24	135	32.3	11.9	6.0	32.7	12.4	6.3	4.8	6.4
Pancreas	C25	106	18.2	10.6	10.6	18.4	11.0	11.6	14.7	10.6
Gastrointestinal tract	C26	31	14.8			14.9				
Nose/Sinuses	C30-31	33	61.9	41.3	35.8	62.5	42.2	36.9	26.4	30.8
Larynx	C32	153	58.4	35.8	24.6	59.3	37.5	26.6	27.4	28.0
Lung	C33-34	1 642	24.1	6.8	4.5	24.3	7.0	4.8	5.8	4.8
Bone	C40-41	35	58.2	38.8	20.7	58.5	39.2	21.0	8.5	8.5
Melanoma of skin	C43	27	69.2	28.0	21.8	70.2	29.4	23.2	22.6	23.3
Other skin	C44	169	79.0	59.8	41.6	80.4	63.1	45.6	46.4	59.2
Connective tissue	C47+C49	45	64.3	45.1	45.1	64.7	45.9	46.6	44.6	44.6
Breast	C50	544	92.0	71.4	60.8	92.4	72.3	62.1	55.8	57.3
Vulva	C51	28	77.8	47.8	36.4	78.8	49.7	39.4	42.9	39.0
Cervix	C53	885	86.0	66.8	58.8	86.4	67.7	60.2	57.0	60.0
Corpus uteri	C54	98	90.3	71.1	66.2	90.7	72.2	67.9	48.8	64.4
Ovary	C56	162	71.4	52.0	47.1	71.7	52.6	47.9	35.2	44.7
Penis	C60	72	63.9	50.5	32.0	64.7	52.8	34.6	33.6	36.7
Prostate	C61	107	78.8	44.9	30.4	80.7	48.5	34.9	34.5	35.0
Kidney	C64	38	38.9	18.6	18.6	39.3	19.1	19.4	16.5	23.1
Urinary bladder	C67	223	60.3	39.5	28.8	61.1	41.1	30.7	26.5	33.2
Brain & nervous system	C70-72	75	56.0	30.2	20.4	56.2	30.5	20.6	15.3	16.4
Thyroid	C73	130	76.0	70.6	65.7	76.4	71.5	66.9	65.1	65.4
Hodgkin lymphoma	C81	30	60.7	56.7	51.5	61.1	57.7	53.0	69.7	73.1
Non-Hodgkin lymphoma	C82-85+C96	298	51.9	32.4	25.4	52.2	33.0	26.3	26.0	28.1
Lymphoid leukaemia	C91	70	52.6	24.2	20.3	52.7	24.3	20.4	15.4	15.4
Myeloid leukaemia	C92-94	122	28.3	16.1	10.5	28.4	16.3	10.7	8.7	10.9
Leukaemia unspecified	C95	43	18.6	9.3	9.3	18.8	9.6	9.7	8.9	11.0

ASRS: age-standardized relative survival

Table 4a. Site-wise number of cases, 5-year absolute and relative survival by sex: Chiang Mai, Thailand, 1993–1997 cases followed-up until 2000

Site	ICD-10	Cases included	Male			Female		
				% 5-year survival			% 5-year survival	
			No.	Abs	Rel	No.	Abs	Rel
Tongue	C01-02	85	61	14.7	16.0	24	21.5	22.5
Oral cavity	C03-06	101	60	16.7	18.1	41	28.9	31.3
Tonsil	C09	51	39	17.9	18.7	12		
Nasopharynx	C11	133	93	31.3	32.5	40	44.0	45.2
Hypopharynx	C12-13	69	56	23.2	25.1	13		
Oesophagus	C15	88	56	5.8	6.2	32	14.6	16.3
Stomach	C16	316	180	13.7	14.7	136	10.0	10.4
Colon	C18	237	126	31.6	33.4	111	26.8	28.1
Rectum	C19-20	190	102	29.2	31.4	88	26.2	27.6
Liver	C22	705	497	2.4	2.5	208	5.3	5.6
Gall bladder	C23-24	135	50	0.0	0.0	85	10.1	10.6
Pancreas	C25	106	49	12.2	13.9	57	9.3	9.6
Gastrointestinal tract	C26	31	18	0.0	0.0	13		
Nose/Sinuses	C30-31	33	21	33.1	34.2	12	40.4	41.3
Larynx	C32	153	116	30.9	33.7	37	3.7	3.9
Lung	C33-34	1 642	945	4.2	4.5	697	5.0	5.3
Bone	C40-41	35	27	15.3	15.6	8	44.6	45.1
Melanoma of skin	C43	27	14			13	35.9	38.2
Other skin	C44	169	87	35.3	38.8	82	47.4	51.8
Connective tissue	C47+C49	45	19	44.8	47.0	26	45.1	46.1
Breast	C50	544	2	100.0	101.7	542	60.6	61.9
Vulva	C51	28				28	36.4	39.4
Cervix	C53	885				885	58.8	60.2
Corpus uteri	C54	98				98	66.2	67.9
Ovary	C56	162				162	47.1	47.9
Penis	C60	72	72	32.0	34.6			
Prostate	C61	107	107	30.4	34.9			
Kidney	C64	38	22	16.7	17.7	16	21.2	21.6
Urinary bladder	C67	223	163	30.9	33.1	60	22.7	24.1
Brain & nervous system	C70-72	75	39	11.9	12.1	36	32.0	32.2
Thyroid	C73	130	31	47.2	49.0	99	71.8	72.8
Hodgkin lymphoma	C81	30	18	57.1	59.0	12	43.6	44.3
Non-Hodgkin lymphoma	C82-85+C96	298	179	20.2	21.0	119	33.3	34.4
Lymphoid leukaemia	C91	70	49	18.8	18.9	21	23.8	23.9
Myeloid leukaemia	C92-94	122	60	11.6	11.8	62	9.3	9.5
Leukaemia unspecified	C95	43	22	0.0	0.0	21	19.0	19.6

Abs: absolute survival; Rel: relative survival

Table 4b. Site-wise number of cases and relative survival by age group: Chiang Mai, Thailand, 1993–1997 cases followed-up until 2000

Site	ICD-10	Cases included	Number of cases by age group					Relative survival by age group % 5-year survival				
			< 45	45-54	55-64	65-74	> 75	< 45	45-54	55-64	65-74	> 75
Tongue	C01-02	85	12	9	14	25	25	19.7		28.0	18.3	0.0
Oral cavity	C03-06	101	8	13	31	24	25	31.4	32.5	20.9	9.9	35.5
Tonsil	C09	51	7	7	9	15	13	40.2		34.7		0.0
Nasopharynx	C11	133	30	32	38	24	9	41.1	63.4	36.7	6.1	0.0
Hypopharynx	C12-13	69	0	3	17	26	23		33.9	39.4	14.9	21.1
Oesophagus	C15	88	2	13	23	34	16	0.0	17.0	5.5	6.0	23.8
Stomach	C16	316	48	49	90	87	42	17.3	9.0	16.0	5.8	15.8
Colon	C18	237	45	38	56	68	30	26.2	33.4	46.5	24.0	19.8
Rectum	C19-20	190	40	22	41	57	30	29.6	37.7	30.4	28.5	23.3
Liver	C22	705	171	138	194	150	52	1.1	6.1	4.4	1.2	
Gall bladder	C23-24	135	12	15	29	61	18		0.0	8.2	7.5	0.0
Pancreas	C25	106	10	13	31	36	16		0.0	11.5		19.1
Gastrointestinal tract	C26	31	7	5	8	5	6	0.0	0.0	0.0		0.0
Nose/Sinuses	C30-31	33	10	3	12	5	3	60.0	0.0	32.5		
Larynx	C32	153	9	10	36	65	33	33.8	37.5	18.2	29.8	28.3
Lung	C33-34	1 642	102	248	632	516	144	10.3	4.3	3.8	4.4	7.6
Bone	C40-41	35	24	4	3	4	0	29.3	0.0	0.0		
Melanoma of skin	C43	27	6	3	4	9	5	33.6	0.0	68.7		
Other skin	C44	169	16	14	36	57	46	83.0	46.2	79.2	42.3	16.1
Connective tissue	C47+C49	45	23	8	6	5	3	46.2		43.7	40.6	38.5
Breast	C50	544	222	164	91	45	22	70.6	63.0	56.6	31.5	50.3
Vulva	C51	28	2	5	6	10	5	0.0	72.3	63.3	0.0	75.2
Cervix	C53	885	360	215	183	97	30	64.0	63.2	60.2	44.8	34.6
Corpus uteri	C54	98	25	24	35	12	2	86.3	78.0	62.8	41.5	0.0
Ovary	C56	162	69	42	30	16	5	61.1	50.7	31.9		0.0
Penis	C60	72	21	10	16	16	9			36.3	61.3	
Prostate	C61	107	0	5	18	43	41		40.8	25.8	39.4	34.2
Kidney	C64	38	8	8	7	9	6	38.6		14.7	21.8	0.0
Urinary bladder	C67	223	21	24	64	82	32	71.2	25.5	30.1	27.1	9.9
Brain & nervous system	C70-72	75	47	9	12	6	1	31.9		0.0		0.0
Thyroid	C73	130	68	17	17	26	2	91.3	63.6	48.0	19.1	0.0
Hodgkin lymphoma	C81	30	12	3	7	8	0	91.3	67.7	30.1	0.0	
Non-Hodgkin lymphoma	C82-85+C96	298	118	50	58	56	16	36.6	28.5	25.8	10.8	13.8
Lymphoid leukaemia	C91	70	55	5	5	5	0	25.2	0.0		0.0	0.0
Myeloid leukaemia	C92-94	122	66	14	20	18	4	14.2	8.1	15.3		0.0
Leukaemia unspecified	C95	43	23	0	6	8	6	8.8				0.0

Table 5. Proportion of cases and 5-year absolute survival by extent of disease and site: Chiang Mai, Thailand, 1993–1997

Site	ICD-10	Cases included	% of cases by extent of disease				% 5-year absolute survival			
			Localized	Regional	Dist. met.	Unknown	Localized	Regional	Dist. met.	Unknown
Colon	C18	237	1.3	65.8	31.6	1.3	66.7	40.8	6.0	0.0
Rectum	C19-20	190	3.7	74.2	20.0	2.1	71.4	31.2	5.9	
Larynx	C32	153	11.8	82.4	3.8	2.0	52.4	21.4	16.7	0.0
Breast	C50	544	14.3	70.0	11.9	3.8	79.3	63.7	24.8	49.4
Cervix	C53	885	26.1	69.7	3.7	0.5	81.2	52.7	12.2	75.0
Ovary	C56	162	24.1	43.8	30.2	1.9	88.2	48.3	16.9	0.0

Dis. met.: distant metastasis

Table 6. Comparison of 5-year absolute and relative survival of cases diagnosed between 1985–1992 and 1993–1997, Chiang Mai, Thailand

Site	ICD-10	% Complete FU at 5 years		% 5-year absolute survival		% 5-year relative survival	
		1985–1992	1993–1997	1985–1992	1993–1997	1985–1992	1993–1997
Tongue	C01-02	86.6	82.4	27.4	16.6	35.9	17.8
Oral cavity	C03-06	93.3	73.3	14.8	21.5	19.4	23.2
Tonsil	C09	86.4	64.7	16.9	20.0	23.3	21.0
Nasopharynx	C11	86.0	81.2	27.2	35.6	29.4	36.7
Hypopharynx	C12-13	87.2	84.1	15.5	20.9	21.4	22.6
Oesophagus	C15	96.8	88.6	2.9	8.9	3.8	9.8
Stomach	C16	95.0	83.9	7.5	12.1	8.6	12.8
Colon	C18	75.3	77.6	33.3	29.3	38.4	30.8
Rectum	C19-20	85.2	75.8	21.9	27.9	25.2	29.7
Liver	C22	97.9	91.4	0.4	3.0	0.5	3.2
Gall bladder	C23-24	94.8	80.8	3.5	6.0	4.1	6.3
Pancreas	C25	93.0	85.8	3.2	10.6	3.7	11.6
Larynx	C32	92.1	77.1	16.2	24.6	20.2	26.6
Lung	C33-34	95.8	88.8	2.7	4.5	3.1	4.8
Bone	C40-41	75.6	82.8	33.7	20.7	36.1	21.0
Melanoma of skin	C43	83.3	77.8	36.5	21.8	43.7	23.2
Other skin	C44	66.9	59.2	73.9	41.6	92.7	45.6
Connective tissue	C47+C49	88.0	66.7	35.3	45.1	37.9	46.6
Breast	C50	67.8	71.9	59.4	60.8	63.7	62.1
Vulva	C51	73.5	82.2	51.2	36.4	59.2	39.4
Cervix	C53	71.4	75.0	65.0	58.8	68.2	60.2
Corpus uteri	C54	51.3	66.3	64.1	66.2	69.5	67.9
Ovary	C56	82.7	74.0	42.6	47.1	44.9	47.9
Penis	C60	77.7	61.1	48.9	32.0	56.8	34.6
Prostate	C61	80.3	81.3	28.7	30.4	42.3	34.9
Kidney	C64	92.9	84.2	14.0	18.6	15.3	19.4
Urinary bladder	C67	82.7	76.7	31.0	28.8	38.3	30.7
Brain & nervous system	C70-72	90.9	65.3	17.9	20.4	18.7	20.6
Thyroid	C73	73.9	70.0	48.3	65.7	52.7	66.9
Hodgkin lymphoma	C81	82.4	73.3	27.2	51.5	29.6	53.0
Non-Hodgkin lymphoma	C82-85+C96	84.4	79.2	22.4	25.4	24.7	26.3
Lymphoid leukaemia	C91	97.7	90.0	13.2	20.3	13.7	20.4
Myeloid leukaemia	C92-94	93.2	91.8	10.1	10.5	10.9	10.7

FU: follow-up

Chapter 26

Cancer survival in Khon Kaen, Thailand, 1993–1997

Suwanrungruang K, Vatanasapt P, Kamsa-Ard S, Sriamporn S and Wiangnon S

Abstract

The Khon Kaen cancer registry was established in 1984 as a hospital-based cancer registry, and population-based cancer registration started in 1988 with retrospective data collection from 1985. Cancer registration is done by passive and active methods. Data on survival for 13 cancer sites or types registered during 1993–1997 were reported. Follow-up was done by active methods, with median follow-up ranging between 8–32 months for different cancers. The proportion with histologically verified diagnosis for various cancers ranged between 54–100%; death certificates only (DCOs) comprised 0–5%; 85–97% of total registered cases were included for survival analysis. Five-year follow-up ranged from 40–83%. Five-year age-standardized relative survival rates for common cancers were cervix (58%), breast (61%), colon (39%), ovary (43%), non-Hodgkin lymphoma (42%) and rectum (43%). Five-year relative survival by age group portrayed an inverse relationship or was fluctuating. Five-year survival was the highest for localized disease, followed by the regional and distant metastasis categories. Trends in 5-year relative survival in 1993–1997 compared to 1985–1992 showed a marked increase for cancers of the rectum, breast, ovary, Hodgkin and non-Hodgkin lymphomas and decrease for cancers of the lip and larynx.

Khon Kaen cancer registry

The Khon Kaen cancer registry was established in 1984 as a hospital-based cancer registry at the Faculty of Medicine, Srinagarind Hospital, Khon Kaen University. Population-based cancer registration started in 1988 with retrospective data collection from 1985, and the registry has been contributing data to the quinquennial IARC publication *Cancer Incidence in Five Continents* since volume VI [1]. Cancer registration is done by both passive and active methods. The principal sources of information on cancer cases are the hospital and pathology records. The registry covers an area of 10 866 km^2 and caters to a mixed urban and rural population of about 1.6 million with a sex ratio of 1008 females to 1000 males in 1995. The average annual age-standardized incidence rate is 179 per 100 000 among males and 128 per 100 000 among females, with a lifetime cumulative risk of one in 6 of developing cancer for both sexes in the period 1993–1997. The top-ranking cancers among males are liver, lung and colon, among females, the order is liver, cervix and breast.

The registry has contributed data on survival from 33 cancer sites or types for the first volume of the IARC publication on *Cancer Survival in Developing Countries* [2]. In the present volume, data on survival from 13 cancer sites or types registered during 1993–1997 are reported.

Data quality indices (Table 1)

The proportion of cases having a histologically verified cancer diagnosis in this series is 77%, varying between 100% for the lymphomas and 54% for colon cancer. The proportion of cases registered as death certificate only (DCO) is 2%, ranging between 0% for many cancers and 5% for cancer of the cervix. Cases excluded without any follow-up constitute 7%. The exclusion of cases from the survival analysis is the greatest among those with cancer of the cervix (15%) and the least among rectal cancer (3%). Thus, 85–97% of the total cases registered among selected cancers are included in the estimation of the survival probability.

Outcome of follow-up (Table 2)

Follow-up has been carried out predominantly by active methods. These include abstraction of cancer mortality from death certificates with a mention of cancer from the office of the Ministry of the Interior. Death certificates in remote villages are filled in by the headman of the village and are sent to the registry. The data collected are matched with the incident cancer database. The vital status information of the unmatched incident cases is obtained by repeated scrutiny of records in the hospitals, postal enquiry and house visits.

The closing date of follow-up was 31st December 2000. The median follow-up time ranged between 8 months for cancer of the urinary bladder to 32 months for lip cancer. Complete follow-up information at five years from the incidence date ranged from 83% for rectal cancer to 40% for cancer of the cervix. The proportion of cases lost to follow-up was generally the highest within one year from the incidence date.

Survival statistics

All ages and both sexes together (Table 3)

The 5-year relative survival is the highest in Hodgkin disease (70%) and the lowest in tongue cancer (30%). Among head and neck cancers, the survival figures are lip (64%), oral cavity with tongue excluded (39%), nasopharynx (33%) and larynx (35%). The survival is similar for colon and rectal cancers (43%). Non-Hodgkin lymphoma has a relative survival of 40% at 5 years from incidence date.

Figure 1a. Top ten cancers (ranked by survival), Khon Kaen, Thailand, 1993–1997

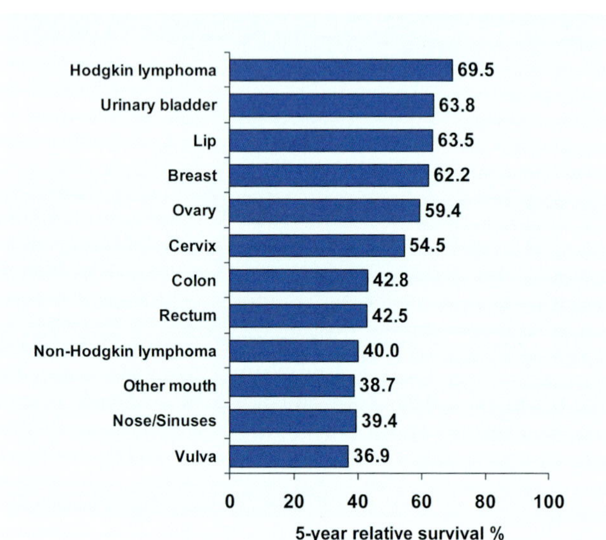

The 5-year age-standardized relative survival (ASRS) probability for all ages together is generally less than or similar to the corresponding unadjusted one for most cancers. Also, the 5-year ASRS (0–74 years of age) is generally higher than or similar to the corresponding ASRS (all ages) for a majority of cancers.

Sex

Male (Table 4a)

The top ranking cancers on the basis of 5-year relative survival are Hodgkin lymphoma (71%), cancers of the urinary bladder (65%), lip (64%) and rectum (42%), and non-Hodgkin lymphoma (38%).

Figure 1b. Top five cancers (ranked by survival), Male, Khon Kaen, Thailand, 1993–1997

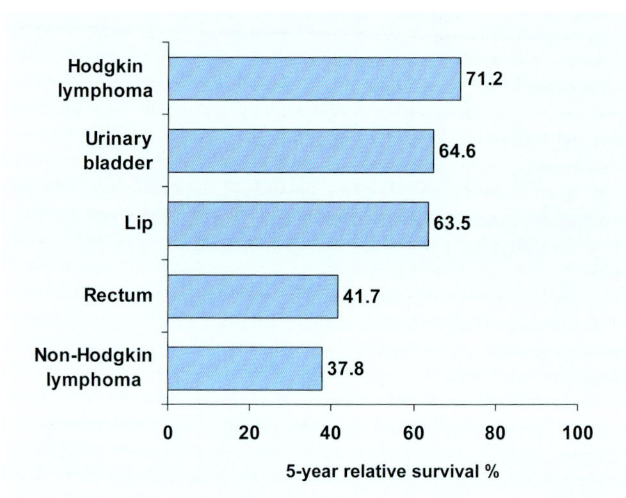

Female (Table 4a)

The top five cancers ranked on 5-year relative survival are Hodgkin lymphoma (69%), breast (62%), lip and bladder (60%), ovary (60%) and cervix (55%). Survival is distinctly higher among females than males for cancers of the tongue, oral cavity, nasopharynx and colon.

Figure 1c. Top five cancers (ranked by survival), Female, Khon Kaen, Thailand, 1993–1997

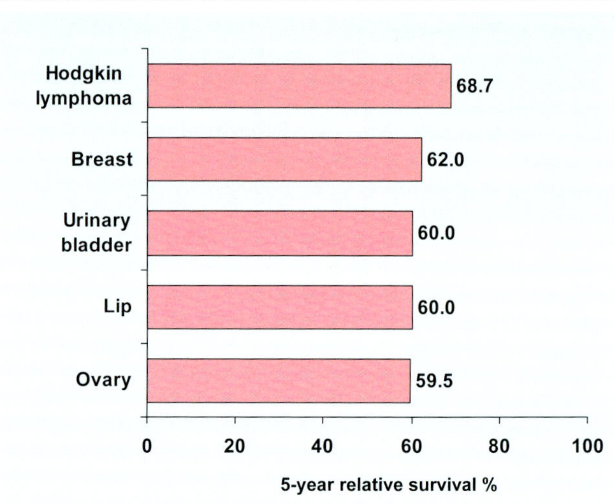

Age group (Table 4b)

The 5-year relative survival by age group reveals an inverse relationship, a decreasing survival with increasing age at diagnosis, for lip cancer. In the rest, it is observed to be fluctuating.

Extent of disease (Table 5; Figure 2)

The proportion of cases by extent of disease among breast cancer is 5% localized, 42% regional and 21% distant metastasis. The corresponding figures for cancer of the cervix are 17%, 54% and 6%, respectively. Ovarian cancer is represented equally by cases with localized and distant metastatic disease. The extent of disease is unknown in 19–32%. The 5-year absolute survival by extent of disease follows the expected pattern: highest for localized cases followed by regional and distant metastasis cases among known categories of extent of disease.

Survival trend (Table 6)

The 5-year relative survival for cases registered in 1993–1997 compared to those in 1985–1992 [2] shows a marked increase in cancers of the rectum, breast, ovary, Hodgkin and non-Hodgkin lymphomas. A decrease in survival in the corresponding period is observed for cancers of the lip and larynx. For the rest, the absolute difference in survival is <10% percent units.

References

1. Parkin DM, Whelan SL, Ferlay J and Storm H. *Cancer Incidence in Five Continents, Vol I to VIII: IARC Cancerbase No. 7*. IARCPress, Lyon, 2005.

2. Vatanasapt V, Sriamporn S, Kamsa-Ard S, Suwanrungruang K, Pengsaa P, Charoensiri DJ, Chaiyakum J and Pesee M. Cancer survival in Khon Kaen, Thailand. In: *Cancer Survival in Developing Countries* (eds) R Sankaranarayanan, RJ Black and DM Parkin. IARC Scientific Publications No. 145. IARCPress, Lyon, 1998, pp 123–134.

Figure 2. Absolute survival (%) from selected cancers by extent of disease, Khon Kaen, Thailand

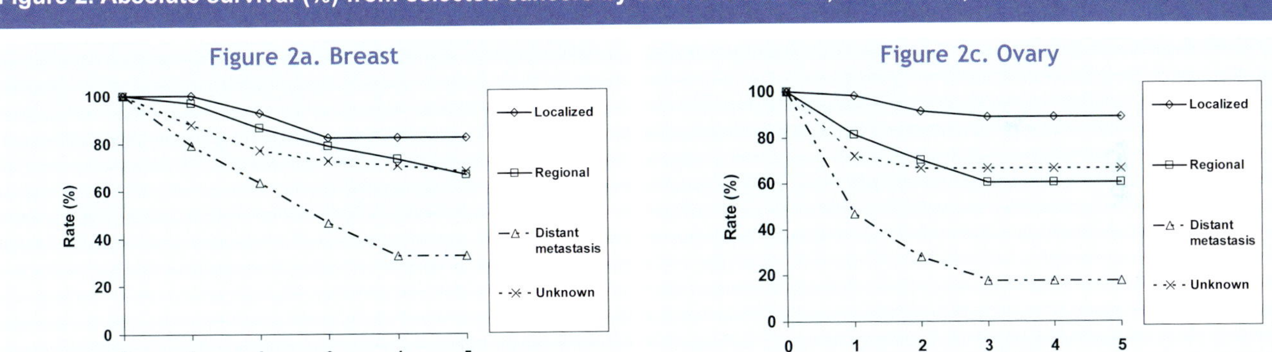

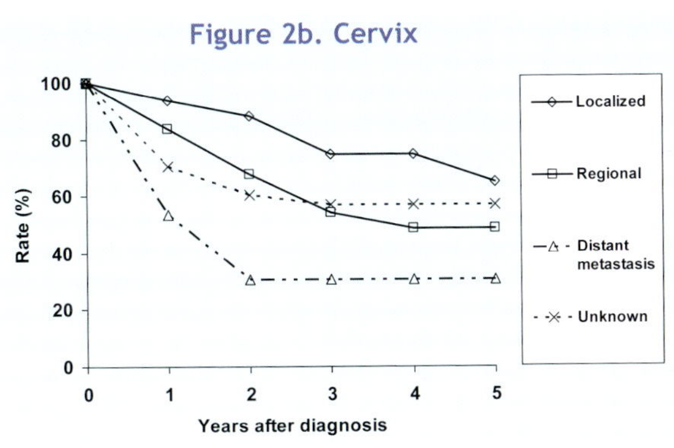

Table 1. Data quality indices - Proportion of histologically verified and death certificate only cases, number and proportion of included and excluded cases by site: Khon Kaen, Thailand, 1993–1997 cases followed-up until 2000

Site	ICD-10	Total registered	%		Excluded cases					Included cases	
			HV	DCO	DCO	Follow-up	Others	Total	%	No.	%
Lip	C00	88	85.2	1.1	1	8	0	9	10.2	79	89.8
Tongue	C01-02	57	77.2	0.0	0	3	0	3	5.3	54	94.7
Oral cavity	C03-06	120	80.8	3.3	4	9	0	13	10.8	107	89.2
Nasopharynx	C11	123	84.6	0.0	0	4	1	5	4.1	118	95.9
Colon	C18	258	54.3	1.6	4	11	1	16	6.2	242	93.8
Rectum	C19-20	143	67.1	0.0	0	3	1	4	2.8	139	97.2
Larynx	C32	38	68.4	0.0	0	2	0	2	5.3	36	94.7
Breast	C50	446	83.6	1.1	5	22	1	28	6.3	418	93.7
Cervix	C53	655	75.0	5.0	33	66	2	101	15.4	554	84.6
Ovary	C56	230	75.2	0.9	2	22	0	24	10.4	206	89.6
Urinary bladder	C67	114	77.2	0.0	0	10	1	11	9.6	103	90.4
Hodgkin lymphoma	C81	31	100.0	0.0	0	2	0	2	6.5	29	93.5
Non-Hodgkin lymphoma	C82-85+C96	191	100.0	0.0	0	23	0	23	12.0	168	88.0

HV: histologically verified; DCO: death certificate only

Table 2. Number and proportion of cases with complete/incomplete follow-up (in years) and median follow-up (in months) by site: Khon Kaen, Thailand, 1993–1997 cases followed-up until 2000

Site	ICD-10	No. of cases included	Complete FU Alive/dead at end of FU		Incomplete FU: loss to FU*		% lost to FU: years from diagnosis				% with complete FU at 5 years	Median FU (in months)
			No.	%	No.	%	< 1	1-3	3-5	> 5		
Lip	C00	79	53	67.1	26	32.9	19.0	5.1	6.3	2.5	69.6	32.0
Tongue	C01-02	54	42	77.8	12	22.2	20.4	1.9	0.0	0.0	77.8	8.4
Oral cavity	C03-06	107	79	73.8	28	26.2	19.6	2.8	1.9	1.9	75.7	12.3
Nasopharynx	C11	118	95	80.5	23	19.5	12.7	4.2	0.8	1.7	82.2	18.1
Colon	C18	242	193	79.8	49	20.2	6.6	6.2	5.4	2.0	81.8	18.2
Rectum	C19-20	139	112	80.6	27	19.4	10.1	6.5	0.7	2.1	82.7	18.6
Larynx	C32	36	29	80.6	7	19.4	19.4	0.0	0.0	0.0	80.6	13.8
Breast	C50	418	173	41.4	245	58.6	24.4	22.2	7.7	4.3	45.7	21.5
Cervix	C53	554	210	37.9	344	62.1	39.2	15.9	5.1	1.9	39.8	9.9
Ovary	C56	206	97	47.1	109	52.9	28.6	12.6	8.7	3.0	50.1	11.5
Urinary bladder	C67	103	43	41.7	60	58.3	35.9	10.7	8.7	3.0	44.7	7.8
Hodgkin lymphoma	C81	29	11	37.9	18	62.1	27.6	17.2	6.9	10.4	48.3	24.3
Non-Hodgkin lymphoma	C82-85+C96	168	89	53.0	79	47.0	28.0	10.1	6.0	2.9	55.9	9.1

*FU: follow-up; * non-random*

Table 3. Comparison of 1-, 3- and 5-year absolute and relative survival and 5-year age-standardized relative survival by site: Khon Kaen, Thailand, 1993–1997 cases followed-up until 2000

Site	ICD-10	Cases included	% Absolute survival			% Relative survival			% ASRS at 5-years	
			1-year	3-year	5-year	1-year	3-year	5-year	all ages	0-74 years
Lip	C00	79	93.0	65.3	59.4	94.1	67.8	63.5	70.2	72.9
Tongue	C01-02	54	58.8	37.6	28.5	59.3	38.9	29.9	30.0	32.4
Oral cavity	C03-06	107	67.0	46.4	36.7	67.7	47.8	38.7	41.1	41.9
Nasopharynx	C11	118	76.5	43.9	31.8	77.1	44.8	32.9	28.4	34.6
Colon	C18	242	64.5	50.5	40.8	65.1	51.8	42.8	38.7	44.3
Rectum	C19-20	139	70.5	44.4	40.2	71.1	45.7	42.5	42.5	42.8
Larynx	C32	36	75.4	32.3	32.3	76.5	33.7	34.5	26.2	26.5
Breast	C50	418	90.5	70.2	60.8	90.9	71.2	62.2	61.0	65.6
Cervix	C53	554	80.5	57.7	53.3	80.9	58.4	54.5	58.3	53.9
Ovary	C56	206	74.6	58.6	58.6	74.8	59.1	59.4	42.5	58.1
Urinary bladder	C67	103	76.3	59.6	59.6	77.3	61.9	63.8	67.3	59.7
Hodgkin lymphoma	C81	29	80.3	75.5	68.3	80.7	76.3	69.5	67.6	67.7
Non-Hodgkin lymphoma	C82-85+C96	168	63.3	46.6	38.2	63.8	47.7	40.0	42.0	39.3

ASRS: age-standardized relative survival

Table 4a. Site-wise number of cases, 5-year absolute and relative survival by sex: Khon Kaen, Thailand, 1993–1997 cases followed-up until 2000

Site	ICD-10	Cases included	Male % 5-year survival			Female % 5-year survival		
			No.	Abs	Rel	No.	Abs	Rel
Lip	C00	79	9	59.4	63.5	70	56.0	60.0
Tongue	C01-02	54	24	19.5	20.9	30	35.5	37.0
Oral cavity	C03-06	107	42	30.4	31.7	65	40.5	43.0
Nasopharynx	C11	118	82	24.5	25.5	36	50.6	51.8
Colon	C18	242	146	34.4	36.1	96	51.1	53.7
Rectum	C19-20	139	71	39.2	41.7	68	41.5	43.4
Larynx	C32	36	35	33.3	35.7	1	0.0	0.0
Breast	C50	418	5	60.0	71.6	413	60.7	62.0
Cervix	C53	554				554	53.3	54.5
Ovary	C56	206				206	58.6	59.5
Urinary bladder	C67	103	87	60.2	64.6	16	57.0	60.0
Hodgkin lymphoma	C81	29	18	69.9	71.2	11	67.7	68.7
Non-Hodgkin lymphoma	C82-85+C96	168	95	35.7	37.8	73	40.4	41.6

Abs: absolute survival; Rel: relative survival

Table 4b. Site-wise number of cases and relative survival by age group: Khon Kaen, Thailand, 1993–1997 cases followed-up until 2000

Site	ICD-10	Cases included	Number of cases by age group					Relative survival by age group % 5-year survival				
			< 45	45-54	55-64	65-74	> 75	< 45	45-54	55-64	65-74	> 75
Lip	C00	79	5	9	21	33	11	101.5	88.2	62.8	59.2	45.6
Tongue	C01-02	54	13	4	17	16	4	36.2	33.7	46.5	11.6	30.0
Oral cavity	C03-06	107	5	15	42	28	17	60.7	36.0	39.3	38.0	36.9
Nasopharynx	C11	118	36	17	38	17	10	55.2	26.8	20.7	26.1	21.3
Colon	C18	242	60	49	64	50	19	44.7	47.6	38.4	47.4	33.0
Rectum	C19-20	139	19	22	49	38	11	28.3	66.9	40.4	39.9	42.9
Larynx	C32	36	3	1	11	13	8	0.0	0.0	57.1	27.0	
Breast	C50	418	161	140	73	31	13	64.0	52.4	77.8	70.8	31.4
Cervix	C53	554	169	183	132	57	13	59.7	56.2	40.7	59.9	120.9
Ovary	C56	206	81	60	45	19	1	76.6	48.4	43.4	61.0	0.0
Urinary bladder	C67	103	14	14	22	37	16	82.9	62.7	49.2	60.5	81.4
Hodgkin lymphoma	C81	29	17	7	2	2	1	61.9	86.0			
Non-Hodgkin lymphoma	C82-85+C96	168	75	34	15	31	13	41.2	20.7	44.3	32.6	84.2

Table 5. Proportion of cases and 5-year absolute survival by extent of disease and site: Khon Kaen, Thailand, 1993–1997

Site	ICD-10	Cases included	% of cases by extent of disease				% 5-year absolute survival			
			Localized	Regional	Dist. met.	Unknown	Localized	Regional	Dist. met.	Unknown
Breast	C50	418	5.3	41.6	21.1	32.0	82.3	66.9	32.8	67.9
Cervix	C53	554	17.3	53.8	6.3	22.6	65.1	48.7	30.6	57.0
Ovary	C56	206	29.6	21.4	29.6	19.4	88.8	60.6	17.5	66.6

Dis. met.: distant metastasis

Table 6. Comparison of 5-year absolute and relative survival of cases diagnosed between 1985–1992 and 1993–1997, Khon Kaen, Thailand

Site	ICD-10	% 5-year absolute survival		% 5-year relative survival	
		1985–1992	1993–1997	1985–1992	1993–1997
Lip	C00	63.1	59.4	74.4	63.5
Tongue	C01-02	20.1	28.5	23.2	29.9
Oral cavity	C03-06	31.7	36.7	39.3	38.7
Nasopharynx	C11	26.8	31.8	29.1	32.9
Colon	C18	31.9	40.8	36.6	42.8
Rectum	C19-20	29.1	40.2	32.7	42.5
Larynx	C32	36.4	32.3	44.5	34.5
Breast	C50	44.9	60.8	47.1	62.2
Cervix	C53	54.5	53.3	57.5	54.5
Ovary	C56	34.0	58.6	35.6	59.4
Urinary bladder	C67	49.7	59.6	57.2	63.8
Hodgkin lymphoma	C81	29.4	68.3	31.1	69.5
Non-Hodgkin lymphoma	C82-85+C96	26.2	38.2	28.0	40.0

Chapter 27

Cancer survival in Lampang, Thailand, 1990–2000

Martin N, Pongnikorn S, Patel N and Daoprasert K

Abstract

The Lampang cancer registry was established in 1995, with retrospective data collection since 1988. Cancer registration is currently done by passive methods. The registry is contributing data on survival for 40 cancer sites or types registered during 1990–2000. Follow-up has been carried out by passive and active methods with median follow-up ranging from 1–74 months for different cancers. The proportion having a histologically verified diagnosis for various cancers ranged between 30–100%; death certificate only (DCO) cases comprised 0–33%; 67–100% of total registered cases were included for survival analysis. Complete follow-up at five years ranged from 96–100% for different cancers. The 5-year age-standardized relative survival rate was the highest for skin non-melanoma (85%) followed by lip (81%), thyroid (74%), corpus uteri (71%) and penis (71%). The 5-year relative survival by age group showed a fluctuating trend. An overwhelmingly high proportion of cases were diagnosed with a regional spread of disease, ranging from 35–68% for different cancers, and survival was decreasing with increasing extent of disease for most cancers studied.

Chiang Mai tumour registry

The Lampang cancer registry was established in 1995 in the Lampang Cancer Centre, Lampang, under the supervision of the National Cancer Institute for cancer prevention and control in the northern part of Thailand. The population-based cancer registration started with retrospective data collection on cancer incidence and mortality from 1988. The registry contributed data to the quinquennial IARC publication *Cancer Incidence in Five Continents* for the first time in volume VIII [1]. Data collection for the years 1988–1993 was done by active methods. Cancer registration is currently done by the passive method of notification from 21 sources comprising cancer centres, hospitals in the government and private sectors, provincial public health services and pathological laboratories [2]. The registry covers an area of 12 534 km^2 and caters to a mixed urban and rural population of about 0.8 million with a sex ratio of 1004 females to 1000 males in 2000. The average annual age-standardized incidence rate is 180 per 100 000 among males and 155 per 100 000 among females, with a lifetime cumulative risk of one in 6 of developing cancer for both sexes in the period 1993–1997. The top-ranking cancers among males are lung, liver and colon, and among females, the order is lung, cervix and breast.

The registry is contributing data on survival from 40 cancer sites or types for the first time in this volume of the IARC publication on *Cancer Survival in Africa, Asia, the Caribbean and Central America*.

Data quality indices (Table 1)

The proportion of cases with histologically verified cancer diagnosis in our series is 71%, varying from 30% in liver cancer to 100% in skin melanoma, lymphomas and leukaemias. The proportion of cases registered as death certificates only (DCOs) was 6%, ranging between nil for many cancers and 33%, for bone cancer. Cases excluded without any follow-up are negligible. The exclusion of cases from the survival analysis is the greatest among bone cancer (33%) while none were excluded from many cancers. Thus, 67–100% of the total cases registered are included in the estimation of the survival probability.

Outcome of follow-up (Table 2)

Follow-up has been carried out by passive and active methods. These included notification of cancer mortality information from the Lampang provincial public health service records. The mortality data are matched with the incident cancer database. Unmatched incident cases are then subjected to one or more of the following to obtain vital status information: repeated scrutiny of records in the respective sources of registration, postal enquiry and house visits.

The closing date of follow-up was 31st December 2003. The median follow-up time ranged from less than one month in unspecified leukaemia to 74 months for non melanoma skin cancer. Complete follow-up information at five years from the incidence date ranged from 96–100%.

Survival statistics

All ages and both sexes together (Table 3)

The top-ranking cancers in terms of 5-year relative survival are non-melanoma skin (85%), corpus uteri (73%), lip (73%), thyroid (67%) and penis (65%). The lowest survival rate is encountered in ill-defined digestive organs (1%) followed by unspecified leukaemia (11%). Major salivary gland (62%) and tonsil (44%), among other head and neck cancers, and colon (39%) and rectum (38%), among gastrointestinal cancers, have higher survival than others. Survival from cancers of the urinary system is 47% for urinary bladder, 34% for kidney and 27% for renal pelvis. Hodgkin and non-Hodgkin lymphoma have similar survival (42%). The survival figures for leukaemias are 41% for lymphoid, 34% for myeloid and 11% for unspecified.

Figure 1a. Top ten cancers (ranked by survival), Lampang, Thailand, 1990–2000

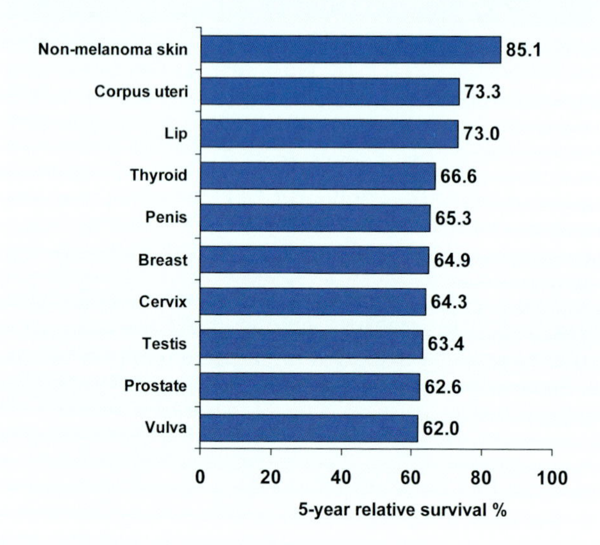

The 5-year age-standardized relative survival (ASRS) probability for all ages together is generally less than or similar to the corresponding unadjusted one for most cancers. Also, the 5-year ASRS (0–74 years of age) is generally higher than or similar to the corresponding ASRS (all ages) for a majority of cancers.

Sex

Male (Table 4a)

The top five cancers ranked on the 5-year relative survival are non-melanoma skin (86%), lip (73%), penis (65%), testis and prostate (63%). Survival from tongue and kidney is markedly higher among males than females.

Figure 1b. Top five cancers (ranked by survival), Male, Lampang, Thailand, 1990–2000

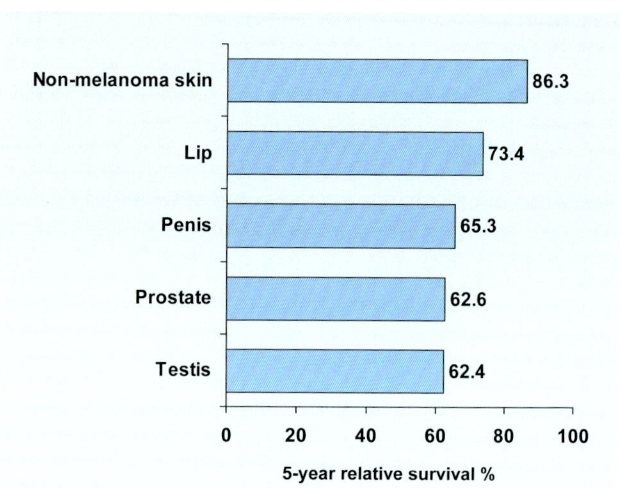

Female (Table 4a)

The highest 5-year relative survival is observed in non-melanoma skin (84%), followed by corpus uteri (73%), lip (73%), thyroid (72%) and major salivary gland (67%). Survival probabilities for cancers of the breast, cervix and ovary are 65%, 64% and 50%, respectively. The survival is noticeably higher among females than males in cancers of the salivary gland, tonsil, hypopharynx, bone, connective tissue, renal pelvis and thyroid.

Figure 1c. Top five cancers (ranked by survival), Female, Lampang, Thailand, 1990–2000

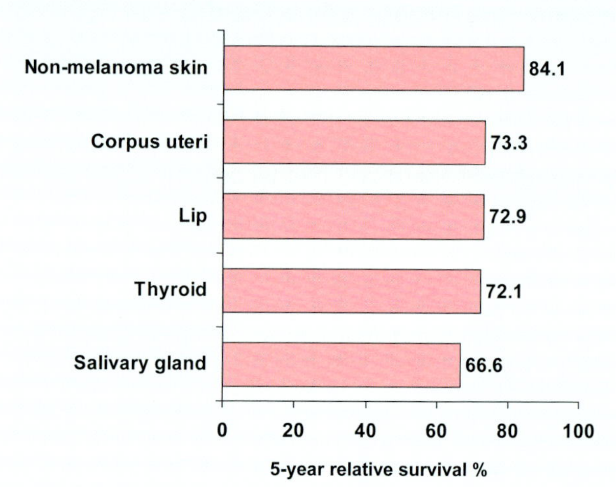

Age group (Table 4b)

The 5-year relative survival by age group reveals an inverse relationship: a decreasing survival with increasing age at diagnosis for cancer of the vulva only. In the rest, it is observed to be fluctuating.

Extent of disease (Table 5; Figure 2)

An overwhelmingly high proportion of cases among the few selected cancers with reliable information on extent of disease are diagnosed with a regional spread of disease, ranging from 68% for tongue cancer to 35% for ovarian cancer.

In colon cancer, 44% are classified under regional and one third under distant metastasis. The extent of disease was unknown in 4–14%. The 5-year absolute survival by extent of disease generally follows a trend: highest survival for localized disease followed by regional and distant metastasis for cancers of larynx, breast, cervix and ovary.

References

1. Parkin DM, Whelan SL, Ferlay J and Storm H. *Cancer Incidence in Five Continents, Vol I to VIII: IARC Cancerbase No. 7*. IARCPress, Lyon, 2005.

2. Pongnikorn S, Martin N, Pornruangwong W, Daoprasert K. *Cancer Incidence and Mortality in Lampang, Thailand, 1990–2000, Vol. III*. Lampang Cancer Centre, Lampang, 2004.

Figure 2. Absolute survival (%) from selected cancers by extent of disease, Lampang, Thailand

Figure 2a. Tongue

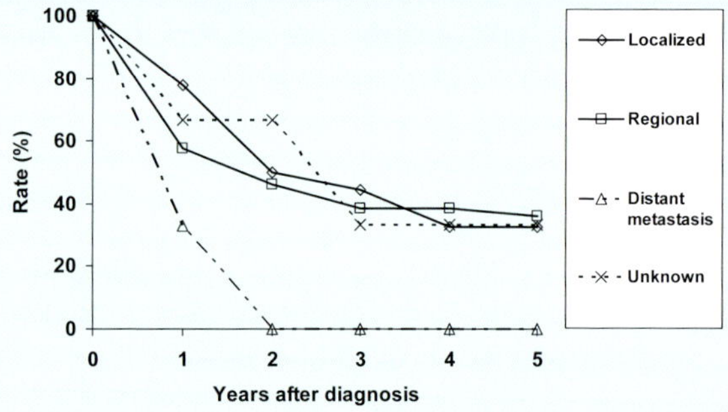

Figure 2e. Larynx

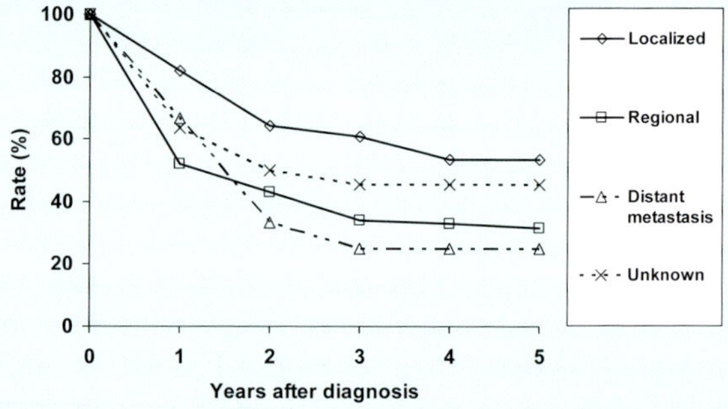

Figure 2b. Oral cavity

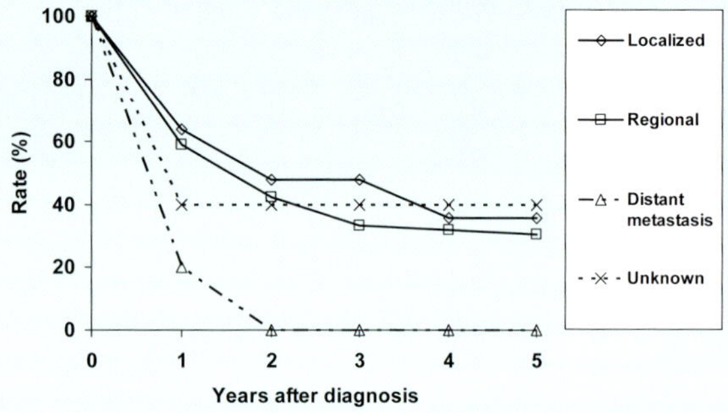

Figure. 2f. Breast

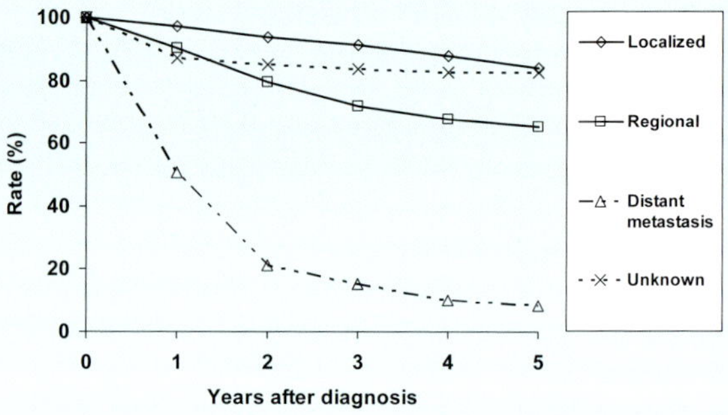

Figure 2c. Colon

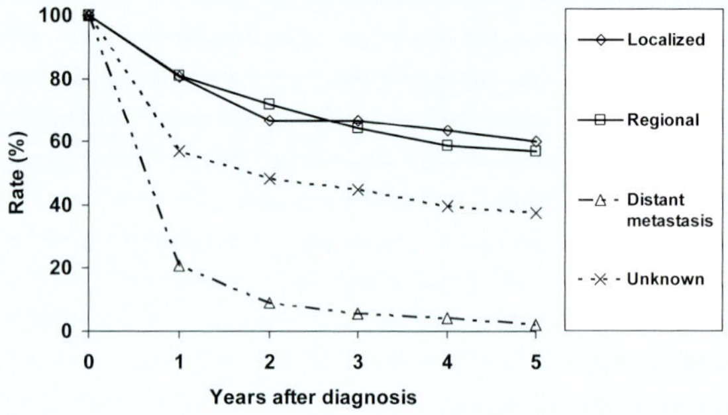

Figure 2g. Cervix

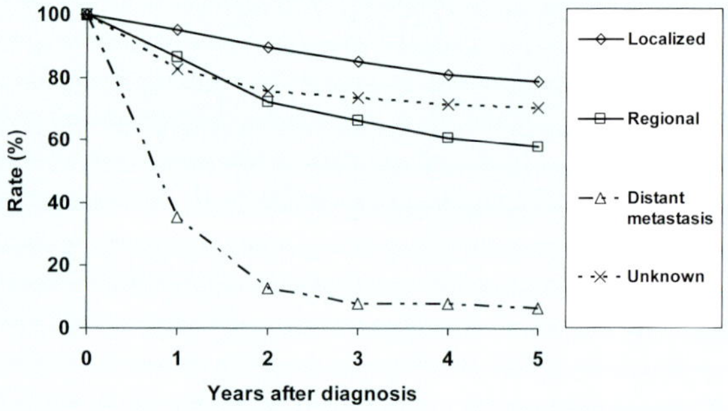

Figure 2d. Rectum

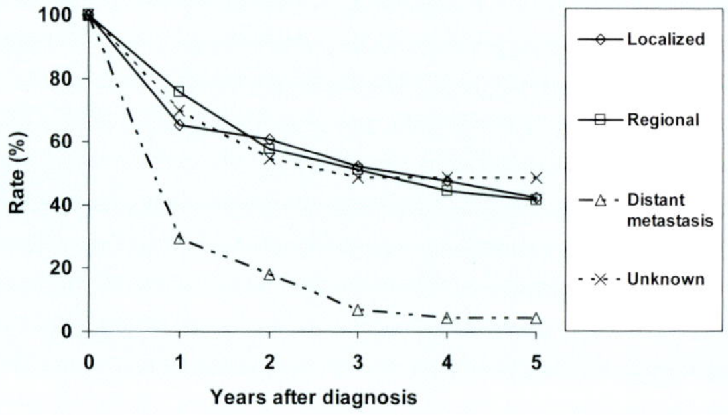

Figure 2h. Ovary

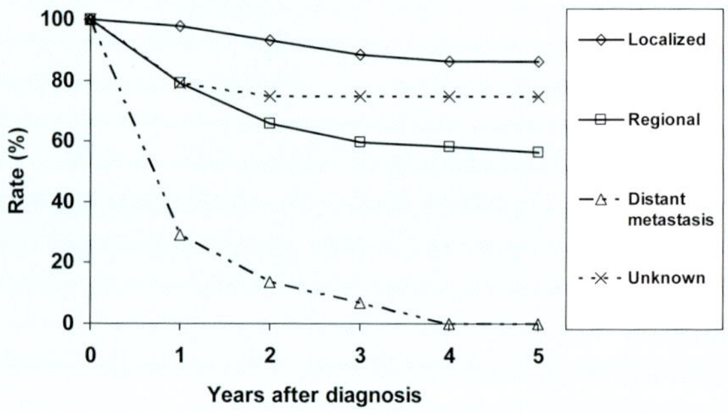

Table 1. Data quality indices - Proportion of histologically verified and death certificate only cases, number and proportion of included and excluded cases by site: Lampang, Thailand, 1990–2000 cases followed-up until 2003

Site	ICD-10	Total registered	%		Excluded cases					Included cases	
			HV	DCO	DCO	Follow-up	Others	Total	%	No.	%
Lip	C00	33	97.0	0.0	0	0	0	0	0.0	33	100.0
Tongue	C01-02	76	93.4	0.0	0	0	0	0	0.0	76	100.0
Oral cavity	C03-06	124	83.9	4.8	6	0	0	6	4.8	118	95.2
Salivary gland	C07-08	33	75.8	3.0	1	0	0	1	3.0	32	97.0
Tonsil	C09	47	91.5	0.0	0	0	0	0	0.0	47	100.0
Nasopharynx	C11	169	85.2	0.0	0	0	0	0	0.0	169	100.0
Hypopharynx	C12-13	43	95.3	0.0	0	0	0	0	0.0	43	100.0
Oesophagus	C15	118	61.0	4.2	5	0	0	5	4.2	113	95.8
Stomach	C16	424	70.0	6.4	27	1	0	28	6.6	396	93.4
Colon	C18	522	59.0	18.4	96	0	1	97	18.6	425	81.4
Rectum	C19-20	250	83.6	0.4	1	0	0	1	0.4	249	99.6
Liver	C22	1 707	29.7	14.7	251	1	0	252	14.8	1 455	85.2
Gall bladder	C23-24	277	58.8	3.6	10	1	0	11	4.0	266	96.0
Pancreas	C25	162	45.7	2.5	4	0	0	4	2.5	158	97.5
Gastrointestinal tract	C26	151	51.7	7.3	11	0	0	11	7.3	140	92.7
Nose/Sinuses	C30-31	42	85.7	0.0	0	0	0	0	0.0	42	100.0
Larynx	C32	168	86.3	2.4	4	2	0	6	3.6	162	96.4
Lung	C33-34	3 278	65.9	7.8	257	6	1	264	8.1	3 014	91.9
Bone	C40-41	39	56.4	33.3	13	0	0	13	33.3	26	66.7
Melanoma of skin	C43	50	100.0	0.0	0	0	0	0	0.0	50	100.0
Other skin	C44	296	95.9	1.4	4	0	0	4	1.4	292	98.6
Connective tissue	C47+C49	71	94.4	0.0	0	1	0	1	1.4	70	98.6
Breast	C50	842	89.9	1.4	12	0	0	12	1.4	830	98.6
Vulva	C51	30	96.7	0.0	0	0	0	0	0.0	30	100.0
Cervix	C53	1 088	92.2	0.8	9	0	0	9	0.8	1 079	99.2
Corpus uteri	C54	112	77.7	9.8	11	0	0	11	9.8	101	90.2
Ovary	C56	193	80.3	0.0	0	0	0	0	0.0	193	100.0
Penis	C60	71	88.7	1.4	1	0	0	1	1.4	70	98.6
Prostate	C61	176	88.1	2.8	5	0	0	5	2.8	171	97.2
Testis	C62	31	74.2	0.0	0	0	0	0	0.0	31	100.0
Kidney	C64	53	47.2	13.2	7	0	0	7	13.2	46	86.8
Renal pelvis	C65	39	97.4	0.0	0	0	0	0	0.0	39	100.0
Urinary bladder	C67	269	84.4	0.7	2	2	0	4	1.5	265	98.5
Brain & nervous system	C70-72	84	65.5	13.1	11	0	0	11	13.1	73	86.9
Thyroid	C73	140	76.4	5.0	7	0	0	7	5.0	133	95.0
Hodgkin lymphoma	C81	55	100.0	0.0	0	0	1	1	1.8	54	98.2
Non-Hodgkin lymphoma	C82-85+C96	368	100.0	0.0	0	0	0	0	0.0	368	100.0
Lymphoid leukaemia	C91	109	100.0	0.0	0	0	0	0	0.0	109	100.0
Myeloid leukaemia	C92-94	137	100.0	0.0	0	0	0	0	0.0	137	100.0
Leukaemia unspecified	C95	90	100.0	0.0	0	0	0	0	0.0	90	100.0

HV: histologically verified; DCO: death certificate only

Table 2. Number and proportion of cases with complete/incomplete follow-up (in years) and median follow-up (in months) by site: Lampang, Thailand, 1990–2000 cases followed-up until 2003

Site	ICD-10	Cases included	Complete FU Alive/dead at end of FU		Incomplete FU: lost to FU		% lost to FU: years from diagnosis				% with complete FU at 5 years	Median FU (in months)
			No.	%	No.	%	< 1	1-3	3-5	> 5		
Lip	C00	33	32	97.0	1	3.0	0.0	0.0	0.0	3.0	100.0	72.8
Tongue	C01-02	76	76	100.0	0	0.0	0.0	0.0	0.0	0.0	100.0	22.1
Oral cavity	C03-06	118	117	99.2	1	0.8	0.0	0.0	0.8	0.0	99.2	15.7
Salivary gland	C07-08	32	31	96.9	1	3.1	0.0	0.0	3.1	0.0	96.9	56.5
Tonsil	C09	47	47	100.0	0	0.0	0.0	0.0	0.0	0.0	100.0	37.4
Nasopharynx	C11	169	169	100.0	0	0.0	0.0	0.0	0.0	0.0	100.0	28.4
Hypopharynx	C12-13	43	43	100.0	0	0.0	0.0	0.0	0.0	0.0	100.0	15.7
Oesophagus	C15	113	113	100.0	0	0.0	0.0	0.0	0.0	0.0	100.0	9.6
Stomach	C16	396	395	99.7	1	0.3	0.0	0.0	0.3	0.0	99.7	7.3
Colon	C18	425	424	99.8	1	0.2	0.0	0.0	0.0	0.2	100.0	19.4
Rectum	C19-20	249	247	99.2	2	0.8	0.0	0.0	0.4	0.4	99.6	24.0
Liver	C22	1 455	1 452	99.8	3	0.2	0.0	0.0	0.2	0.0	99.8	2.2
Gall bladder	C23-24	266	266	100.0	0	0.0	0.0	0.0	0.0	0.0	100.0	4.5
Pancreas	C25	158	158	100.0	0	0.0	0.0	0.0	0.0	0.0	100.0	3.4
Gastrointestinal tract	C26	140	140	100.0	0	0.0	0.0	0.0	0.0	0.0	100.0	1.4
Nose/Sinuses	C30-31	42	42	100.0	0	0.0	0.0	0.0	0.0	0.0	100.0	43.5
Larynx	C32	162	160	98.8	2	1.2	0.0	0.0	1.2	0.0	98.8	20.6
Lung	C33-34	3 014	3 009	99.8	5	0.2	0.0	0.0	0.1	0.1	99.9	4.9
Bone	C40-41	26	26	100.0	0	0.0	0.0	0.0	0.0	0.0	100.0	17.0
Melanoma of skin	C43	50	50	100.0	0	0.0	0.0	0.0	0.0	0.0	100.0	42.2
Other skin	C44	292	289	99.0	3	1.0	0.0	0.0	0.3	0.7	99.7	74.4
Connective tissue	C47+C49	70	69	98.6	1	1.4	0.0	0.0	0.0	1.4	100.0	47.5
Breast	C50	830	821	98.9	9	1.1	0.0	0.0	1.0	0.1	99.0	59.0
Vulva	C51	30	30	100.0	0	0.0	0.0	0.0	0.0	0.0	100.0	61.2
Cervix	C53	1 079	1 064	98.6	15	1.4	0.0	0.0	0.6	0.7	99.4	63.6
Corpus uteri	C54	101	101	100.0	0	0.0	0.0	0.0	0.0	0.0	100.0	67.3
Ovary	C56	193	192	99.5	1	0.5	0.0	0.0	0.5	0.0	99.5	46.2
Penis	C60	70	69	98.6	1	1.4	0.0	0.0	1.4	0.0	98.6	60.7
Prostate	C61	171	170	99.4	1	0.6	0.0	0.0	0.0	0.6	100.0	49.6
Testis	C62	31	31	100.0	0	0.0	0.0	0.0	0.0	0.0	100.0	55.8
Kidney	C64	46	46	100.0	0	0.0	0.0	0.0	0.0	0.0	100.0	6.1
Renal pelvis	C65	39	38	97.4	1	2.6	0.0	0.0	0.0	2.6	100.0	5.5
Urinary bladder	C67	265	260	98.1	5	1.9	0.0	0.0	1.5	0.4	98.5	28.1
Brain & nervous system	C70-72	73	70	95.9	3	4.1	0.0	0.0	4.1	0.0	95.9	28.9
Thyroid	C73	133	133	100.0	0	0.0	0.0	0.0	0.0	0.0	100.0	59.3
Hodgkin lymphoma	C81	54	52	96.3	2	3.7	0.0	0.0	1.9	1.9	98.1	24.1
Non-Hodgkin lymphoma	C82-85+C96	368	366	99.5	2	0.5	0.0	0.0	0.3	0.3	99.7	25.5
Lymphoid leukaemia	C91	109	107	98.2	2	1.8	0.0	0.0	0.0	1.8	100.0	25.1
Myeloid leukaemia	C92-94	137	136	99.3	1	0.7	0.0	0.0	0.7	0.0	99.3	8.9
Leukaemia unspecified	C95	90	90	100.0	0	0.0	0.0	0.0	0.0	0.0	100.0	0.7

FU: follow-up

Table 3. Comparison of 1-, 3- and 5-year absolute and relative survival and 5-year age-standardized relative survival by site: Lampang, Thailand, 1990–2000 cases followed-up until 2003

Site	ICD-10	Cases included	% Absolute survival			% Relative survival			% ASRS at 5-years	
			1-year	3-year	5-year	1-year	3-year	5-year	all ages	0-74 years
Lip	C00	33	93.9	69.7	66.6	95.5	73.6	73.0	80.6	87.4
Tongue	C01-02	76	61.8	38.2	33.8	62.6	39.8	36.4	32.8	33.2
Oral cavity	C03-06	118	56.8	33.9	31.2	57.8	35.8	34.5	37.2	37.2
Salivary gland	C07-08	32	84.4	59.4	59.4	85.2	61.0	62.0	48.8	50.9
Tonsil	C09	47	63.8	51.1	40.1	64.8	53.4	43.5	43.6	43.4
Nasopharynx	C11	169	68.6	45.6	39.3	69.1	46.5	40.6	35.4	39.9
Hypopharynx	C12-13	43	53.5	37.2	22.2	54.3	38.8	23.9	29.1	32.8
Oesophagus	C15	113	44.2	32.7	28.7	44.8	34.2	31.1	30.4	26.8
Stomach	C16	396	42.2	25.0	19.7	42.7	26.0	21.2	21.5	20.4
Colon	C18	425	57.4	42.1	35.9	58.1	43.5	38.0	35.0	39.4
Rectum	C19-20	249	65.9	43.0	36.2	66.7	44.7	38.9	42.3	36.8
Liver	C22	1 455	19.4	13.2	12.2	19.6	13.7	13.0	14.0	11.9
Gall bladder	C23-24	266	29.7	17.7	15.2	30.1	18.4	16.4	19.5	18.5
Pancreas	C25	158	22.8	14.6	13.9	23.1	15.1	15.0	15.1	15.0
Gastrointestinal tract	C26	140	5.7	2.1	0.7	5.8	2.2	0.7	0.5	0.6
Nose/Sinuses	C30-31	42	78.6	57.1	52.1	79.5	59.2	55.0	55.5	50.7
Larynx	C32	162	59.9	39.5	36.8	60.8	41.4	39.9	44.4	49.1
Lung	C33-34	3 014	26.4	14.0	12.0	26.7	14.5	12.9	14.5	12.1
Bone	C40-41	26	57.7	38.5	34.4	57.9	38.8	34.8	14.6	19.9
Melanoma of skin	C43	50	82.0	52.0	43.3	82.9	54.0	46.2	43.6	46.2
Other skin	C44	292	89.7	82.9	77.6	91.2	87.3	85.1	84.7	85.4
Connective tissue	C47+C49	70	80.0	57.1	50.9	80.6	58.6	53.1	49.2	52.6
Breast	C50	830	85.9	69.4	63.1	86.4	70.5	64.9	63.6	63.3
Vulva	C51	30	76.7	66.7	58.8	77.4	68.7	62.0	59.8	63.4
Cervix	C53	1 079	85.9	69.4	62.6	86.3	70.5	64.3	61.9	63.3
Corpus uteri	C54	101	86.1	75.2	70.7	86.7	76.8	73.3	70.9	74.4
Ovary	C56	193	68.4	52.3	48.5	68.7	53.0	49.6	44.1	46.3
Penis	C60	70	81.4	65.7	60.9	82.5	68.4	65.3	70.6	73.1
Prostate	C61	171	80.7	64.9	53.1	82.9	70.9	62.6	66.5	58.3
Testis	C62	31	80.6	67.7	60.4	81.3	69.5	63.4	61.4	61.1
Kidney	C64	46	43.5	37.0	32.5	43.8	38.0	34.1	36.8	29.0
Renal pelvis	C65	39	33.3	25.6	25.6	33.6	26.2	26.6	28.0	28.0
Urinary bladder	C67	265	67.2	48.7	42.8	68.2	51.1	46.6	46.9	49.5
Brain & nervous system	C70-72	73	67.1	47.9	43.5	67.4	48.6	44.6	45.8	43.4
Thyroid	C73	133	75.2	67.7	63.5	75.9	69.5	66.6	73.9	73.1
Hodgkin lymphoma	C81	54	66.7	44.4	40.6	67.3	45.5	42.1	53.9	56.4
Non-Hodgkin lymphoma	C82-85+C96	368	58.2	45.4	40.1	58.8	46.8	42.3	43.6	44.3
Lymphoid leukaemia	C91	109	63.3	44.0	39.8	63.7	44.5	40.5	35.8	44.1
Myeloid leukaemia	C92-94	137	47.4	35.0	32.6	47.8	35.7	33.5	31.7	35.0
Leukaemia unspecified	C95	90	21.1	12.2	11.1	21.2	12.4	11.4	10.5	12.9

ASRS: age-standardized relative survival

Table 4a. Site-wise number of cases, 5-year absolute and relative survival by sex: Lampang, Thailand, 1990–2000 cases followed-up until 2003

Site	ICD-10	Cases included	Male % 5-year survival			Female % 5-year survival		
			No.	Abs	Rel	No.	Abs	Rel
Lip	C00	33	10	70.0	73.4	23	65.1	72.9
Tongue	C01-02	76	45	37.8	41.0	31	26.8	28.6
Oral cavity	C03-06	118	49	34.5	38.7	69	29.0	31.6
Salivary gland	C07-08	32	15	53.3	56.7	17	64.7	66.6
Tonsil	C09	47	37	37.4	39.4	10	50.0	60.1
Nasopharynx	C11	169	109	38.3	39.5	60	41.5	43.2
Hypopharynx	C12-13	43	32	18.3	20.0	11	33.0	34.6
Oesophagus	C15	113	65	28.6	31.5	48	28.9	30.5
Stomach	C16	396	235	20.9	22.9	161	18.1	18.8
Colon	C18	425	236	37.4	39.8	189	34.0	35.8
Rectum	C19-20	249	148	33.5	36.5	101	40.2	42.4
Liver	C22	1 455	976	11.3	12.1	479	13.9	14.9
Gall bladder	C23-24	266	126	15.1	16.0	140	15.3	16.7
Pancreas	C25	158	74	13.5	14.6	84	14.3	15.3
Gastrointestinal tract	C26	140	80	0.0	0.0	60	1.7	1.7
Nose/Sinuses	C30-31	42	19	52.1	55.6	23	52.0	54.5
Larynx	C32	162	115	38.2	41.7	47	33.1	35.2
Lung	C33-34	3 014	1 936	12.1	13.1	1 078	11.7	12.4
Bone	C40-41	26	7	14.3	14.6	19	41.8	42.2
Melanoma of skin	C43	50	30	46.7	49.6	20	40.0	42.9
Other skin	C44	292	132	78.4	86.3	160	76.9	84.1
Connective tissue	C47+C49	70	40	40.7	42.3	30	63.3	66.4
Breast	C50	830	16	43.8	47.0	814	63.5	65.3
Vulva	C51	30				30	58.8	62.0
Cervix	C53	1 079				1 079	62.6	64.3
Corpus uteri	C54	101				101	70.7	73.3
Ovary	C56	193				193	48.5	49.6
Penis	C60	70	70	60.9	65.3			
Prostate	C61	171	171	53.1	62.6			
Testis	C62	31	31	60.4	63.4			
Kidney	C64	46	26	42.3	44.5	20	19.4	20.3
Renal pelvis	C65	39	30	16.7	17.4	9	55.6	57.3
Urinary bladder	C67	265	192	42.5	46.5	73	43.5	46.9
Brain & nervous system	C70-72	73	40	42.4	43.6	33	44.4	45.4
Thyroid	C73	133	25	40.0	43.3	108	69.2	72.1
Hodgkin lymphoma	C81	54	38	41.9	43.7	16	37.5	38.5
Non-Hodgkin lymphoma	C82-85+C96	368	216	36.6	38.7	152	44.9	47.5
Lymphoid leukaemia	C91	109	68	37.5	38.4	41	43.6	44.1
Myeloid leukaemia	C92-94	137	81	29.4	30.2	56	37.3	38.4
Leukaemia unspecified	C95	90	51	11.8	12.1	39	10.3	10.5

Abs: absolute survival; Rel: relative survival

Table 4b. Site-wise number of cases and relative survival by age group: Lampang, Thailand, 1990–2000 cases followed-up until 2003

Site	ICD-10	Cases included	Number of cases by age group					Relative survival by age group % 5-year survival				
			< 45	45-54	55-64	65-74	> 75	< 45	45-54	55-64	65-74	> 75
Lip	C00	33	3	2	8	12	8	101.2	101.6	65.1	91.0	32.3
Tongue	C01-02	76	12	7	24	18	15	25.3	14.5	43.4	43.7	32.6
Oral cavity	C03-06	118	10	8	32	24	44	20.3	63.5	22.7	40.4	38.8
Salivary gland	C07-08	32	12	3	6	7	4	92.6	33.8	34.5	62.5	29.3
Tonsil	C09	47	7	6	12	13	9	43.5	50.9	32.6	50.3	43.1
Nasopharynx	C11	169	54	41	34	32	8	61.1	32.0	27.2	30.2	45.2
Hypopharynx	C12-13	43	2	3	16	11	11	0.0	67.9	21.4	29.4	10.7
Oesophagus	C15	113	6	13	32	42	20	16.9	15.7	38.3	28.2	39.5
Stomach	C16	396	72	60	96	106	62	17.0	12.5	26.9	21.4	24.3
Colon	C18	425	84	60	101	122	58	40.6	43.2	36.9	38.9	28.9
Rectum	C19-20	249	39	36	53	78	43	38.9	50.2	38.4	27.8	51.1
Liver	C22	1 455	211	279	426	374	165	12.4	11.5	11.9	11.8	23.4
Gall bladder	C23-24	266	18	37	85	92	34	33.7	13.8	14.4	13.7	22.8
Pancreas	C25	158	18	24	45	46	25	16.9	12.7	13.8	16.4	15.8
Gastrointestinal tract	C26	140	22	27	46	33	12	0.0	0.0	2.2	0.0	0.0
Nose/Sinuses	C30-31	42	10	11	8	6	7	40.4	63.6	64.7	35.8	71.3
Larynx	C32	162	8	17	37	63	37	88.8	53.9	36.4	38.7	27.9
Lung	C33-34	3 014	178	487	1 007	970	372	14.7	10.3	10.8	13.4	20.3
Bone	C40-41	26	18	3	3	1	1	44.4	0.0	34.3	0.0	0.0
Melanoma of skin	C43	50	8	7	12	16	7	37.7	58.1	33.6	60.5	33.8
Other skin	C44	292	30	31	77	73	81	80.4	88.5	87.0	85.7	83.1
Connective tissue	C47+C49	70	30	17	8	9	6	53.2	59.8	38.7	61.0	32.5
Breast	C50	830	299	245	150	87	49	70.6	64.5	58.0	58.4	65.7
Vulva	C51	30	8	4	5	8	5	75.5	67.6	62.0	50.8	47.9
Cervix	C53	1 079	413	286	210	123	47	74.5	60.8	59.4	50.4	51.4
Corpus uteri	C54	101	22	25	27	21	6	72.5	73.1	76.2	75.7	57.1
Ovary	C56	193	77	36	52	21	7	59.9	39.4	53.2	25.3	33.9
Penis	C60	70	14	16	20	8	12	58.0	61.7	56.6	109.6	64.0
Prostate	C61	171	2	1	27	58	83	101.4	102.1	33.8	63.0	71.0
Testis	C62	31	20	5	2	2	2	60.9	54.4	52.2	110.2	80.9
Kidney	C64	46	13	7	11	11	4	62.0	29.1	9.4	19.8	60.4
Renal pelvis	C65	39	6	6	18	9	0	33.8	33.8	23.0	23.9	
Urinary bladder	C67	265	20	23	72	88	62	50.2	70.8	37.3	49.6	43.5
Brain & nervous system	C70-72	73	48	7	10	7	1	43.9	43.5	31.3	59.8	119.8
Thyroid	C73	133	40	18	31	32	12	90.7	74.2	59.8	40.4	56.9
Hodgkin lymphoma	C81	54	18	5	14	13	4	67.3	40.7	37.3	24.8	0.0
Non-Hodgkin lymphoma	C82-85+C96	368	103	41	91	83	50	47.8	46.1	35.5	43.9	37.1
Lymphoid leukaemia	C91	109	78	6	7	11	7	42.1	50.6	44.1	47.5	0.0
Myeloid leukaemia	C92-94	137	64	18	23	19	13	37.7	32.9	40.7	23.0	18.0
Leukaemia unspecified	C95	90	54	13	12	8	3	7.3	15.6	17.1	26.7	0.0

Table 5. Proportion of cases and 5-year absolute survival by extent of disease and site: Lampang, Thailand, 1990–2000

Site	ICD-10	Cases included	% of cases by extent of disease				% 5-year absolute survival			
			Localized	Regional	Dist. met.	Unknown	Localized	Regional	Dist. met.	Unknown
Tongue	C01-02	76	23.6	68.4	4.0	4.0	32.6	36.2	0.0	33.3
Oral cavity	C03-06	118	21.2	66.1	4.2	8.5	35.6	30.7	0.0	40.0
Colon	C18	425	8.4	44.2	33.7	13.7	60.0	56.8	2.1	37.5
Rectum	C19-20	249	9.2	59.8	17.7	13.3	42.3	41.8	4.5	48.5
Larynx	C32	162	17.3	61.7	7.4	13.6	53.4	31.6	25.0	45.5
Breast	C50	830	22.5	52.9	14.2	10.4	84.1	65.2	8.2	82.5
Cervix	C53	1 079	31.2	53.9	5.8	9.2	78.7	57.9	6.5	70.6
Ovary	C56	193	22.8	34.7	30.1	12.4	86.2	56.6	0.0	75.0

Dis. met.: distant metastasis

Chapter 28

Cancer survival in Songkhla, Thailand, 1990–1999

Sriplung H and Prechavittayakul P

Abstract

The Songkhla registry, besides being hospital-based, has population-based cancer registration data available since 1990. Cancer registration is done by active methods. The registry is contributing data on survival for 36 cancer sites or types registered during 1990–1999. Follow-up has been carried out by passive and active methods with median follow-up ranging from 3–71 months for different cancers. The proportion with histologically verified diagnosis for various cancers ranged between 52–100%; death certificate only (DCO) cases comprised 0–34%; 54–93% of total registered cases were included for survival analysis. Complete follow-up at five years ranged from 50–85% for different cancers. Five-year age-standardized relative survival rates of common cancers were cervix (59%), lung (7%), breast (59%), thyroid (86%), oesophagus (11%), liver (2%), non-melanoma skin (75%), colon (45%) and oral cavity (33%). Five-year relative survival by age group did not reveal any pattern or trend and was fluctuating. A majority were diagnosed with regional spread of disease, and survival decreased with increasing clinical extent of disease.

Khon Kaen cancer registry

The Songkhla registry is located within the Faculty of Medicine, Prince of Songkhla University. Besides a hospital cancer registry at the University hospital, the data on incident cancer cases based on population-based cancer registration have been available since 1990. The registry contributed data to the quinquennial IARC publication *Cancer Incidence in Five Continents* for the first time in volume VIII [1]. The cancer registration is done by active methods. Case-finding is carried out from 23 sources of registration, comprising government and private sector hospitals, provincial health and population registration offices. The network of cancer registries in Thailand also provides data to the registry. The principal sources of information on cancer cases are hospital and pathology records. The registry caters to a mixed urban and rural population of about 1.1 million with a sex ratio of 1027 females to 1000 males in 1995. The average annual age-standardized incidence rate is 100 per 100 000 among males and 83 per 100 000 among females, with a lifetime cumulative risk of one in 10 of developing cancer in the period 1993–1996. The top-ranking cancers among males are lung followed by oesophagus and oral cavity. Among females, the order is cervix, breast and thyroid.

The registry is contributing data on survival from 36 cancer sites or types for the first time in this volume of the IARC publication on *Cancer Survival in Africa, Asia, the Caribbean and Central America*.

Data quality indices (Table 1)

The proportion of cases with histologically verified cancer diagnosis in this series is 88%, varying between 52% for liver cancer and 100% for many cancers. The proportion of cases registered as death certificate only (DCO) is 2%, ranging from nil for many cancers to 34% for unspecified leukaemia. Cases excluded for having no follow-up information constitute 15%. The exclusion of cases from the survival analysis is the greatest in unspecified leukaemia (46%) and the least in cancer of the tonsil (7%). Thus, 54–93% of the total cases registered are included in the estimation of the survival probability.

Outcome of follow-up (Table 2)

Follow-up has been carried out predominantly by passive methods. These include abstraction of cancer mortality information from the vital statistics division records. The abstracted data are matched with the incident cancer database. Unmatched incident cases are then subjected to one or more of the following to obtain the vital status information: repeated scrutiny of records in the hospitals and linkage with referral system, government free health service and insurance system.

The closing date of follow-up was 31st December 2003. The median follow-up ranged from 3 months for liver cancer to 71 months for thyroid cancer. Complete follow-up information at five years from the incidence date ranged from 85% for myeloid leukaemia to 50% for non-melanoma skin cancer. The losses to follow-up occurred evenly in all the time periods of <1 year, 1–3 years, 3-5 years and >5 years and are ascertained to be random.

Survival statistics

All ages and both sexes together (Table 3)

The 5-year relative survival is the highest in thyroid cancer (88%) followed by non-melanoma skin (74%). The lowest survival rate was encountered with liver cancer 2%. Lip (69%) and nasopharynx (46%), among other head and neck cancers, and colon (48%) and rectum (35%), among gastrointestinal cancers, have a higher survival than others. Survival from cancers of the urinary system is 46% for urinary bladder and 36% for kidney. Hodgkin lymphoma had a better survival (56%) than non-Hodgkin (44%). The survival figures for leukaemias are 49% for lymphoid, 15% for myeloid and 25% for unspecified.

Figure 1a. Top ten cancers (ranked by survival), Songkhla, Thailand, 1990–1999

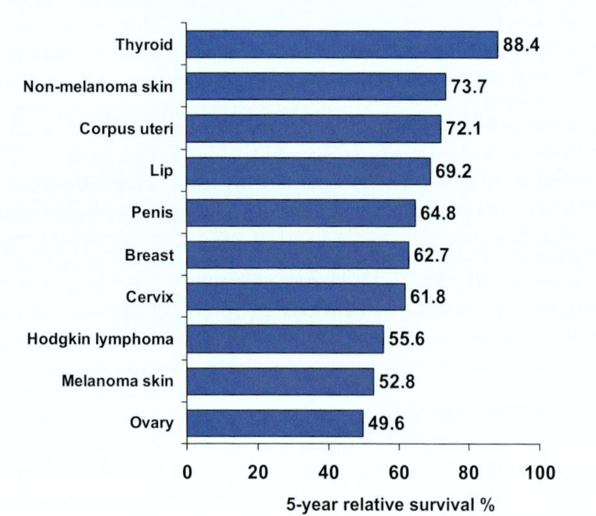

The 5-year age-standardized relative survival (ASRS) probability for all ages together is generally less than or similar to the corresponding unadjusted one for most cancers. Also, the 5-year ASRS (0–74 years of age) is generally higher than or similar to the corresponding ASRS (all ages) for a majority of cancers.

Sex

Male (Table 4a)

The top-ranking cancers in terms of 5-year relative survival are thyroid (82%), Hodgkin lymphoma (71%), lip (69%), non-melanoma skin (65%) and penis (65%). Survival probabilities from cancers of the gall bladder, pancreas, bone, Hodgkin lymphoma and multiple myeloma are noticeably higher among males than females.

Figure 1b. Top five cancers (ranked by survival), Male, Songkhla, Thailand, 1990–1999

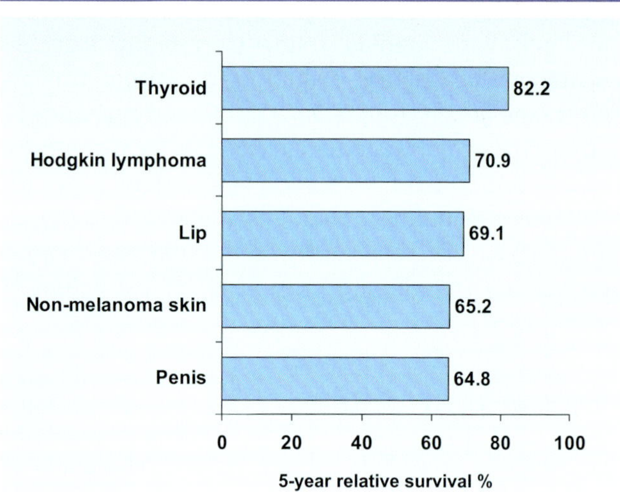

Female (Table 4a)

The highest 5-year relative survival was observed in thyroid cancer (90%) followed by non-melanoma skin (82%) and corpus uteri (72%). The figures for breast,

Figure 1c. Top five cancers (ranked by survival), Female, Songkhla, Thailand, 1990–1999

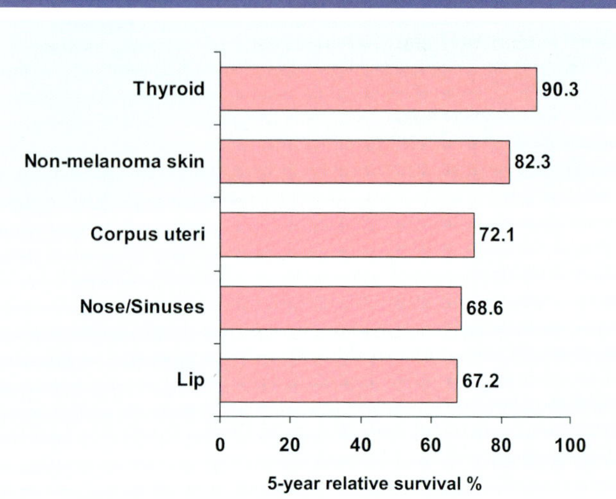

cervix and ovary are 63%, 62% and 50%, respectively. Survival was distinctly higher among females than males in most cancers of the head and neck, rectum, nose and sinuses, skin, connective tissue, kidney and brain.

Age group (Table 4b)

The 5-year relative survival by age group does not reveal any pattern or trend and is observed to be fluctuating.

Extent of disease (Table 5; Figure 2)

Among the known categories of extent of disease for selected cancers, most cases were diagnosed with regional spread of disease at the time of diagnosis: tongue (31%), larynx (40%), breast (35%), cervix (55%) and ovary (29%). The extent of disease is unknown in a substantial proportion ranging from 17–42%. The 5-year absolute survival by extent of disease followed the expected pattern: highest for localized cases followed by regional and distant metastasis cases among known categories of extent of disease with the exception of laryngeal cancer.

References

1. Parkin DM, Whelan SL, Ferlay J and Storm H. *Cancer Incidence in Five Continents, Vol I to VIII: IARC Cancerbase No. 7*. IARCPress, Lyon, 2005.

Figure 2. Absolute survival (%) from selected cancers by extent of disease, Songkhla, Thailand

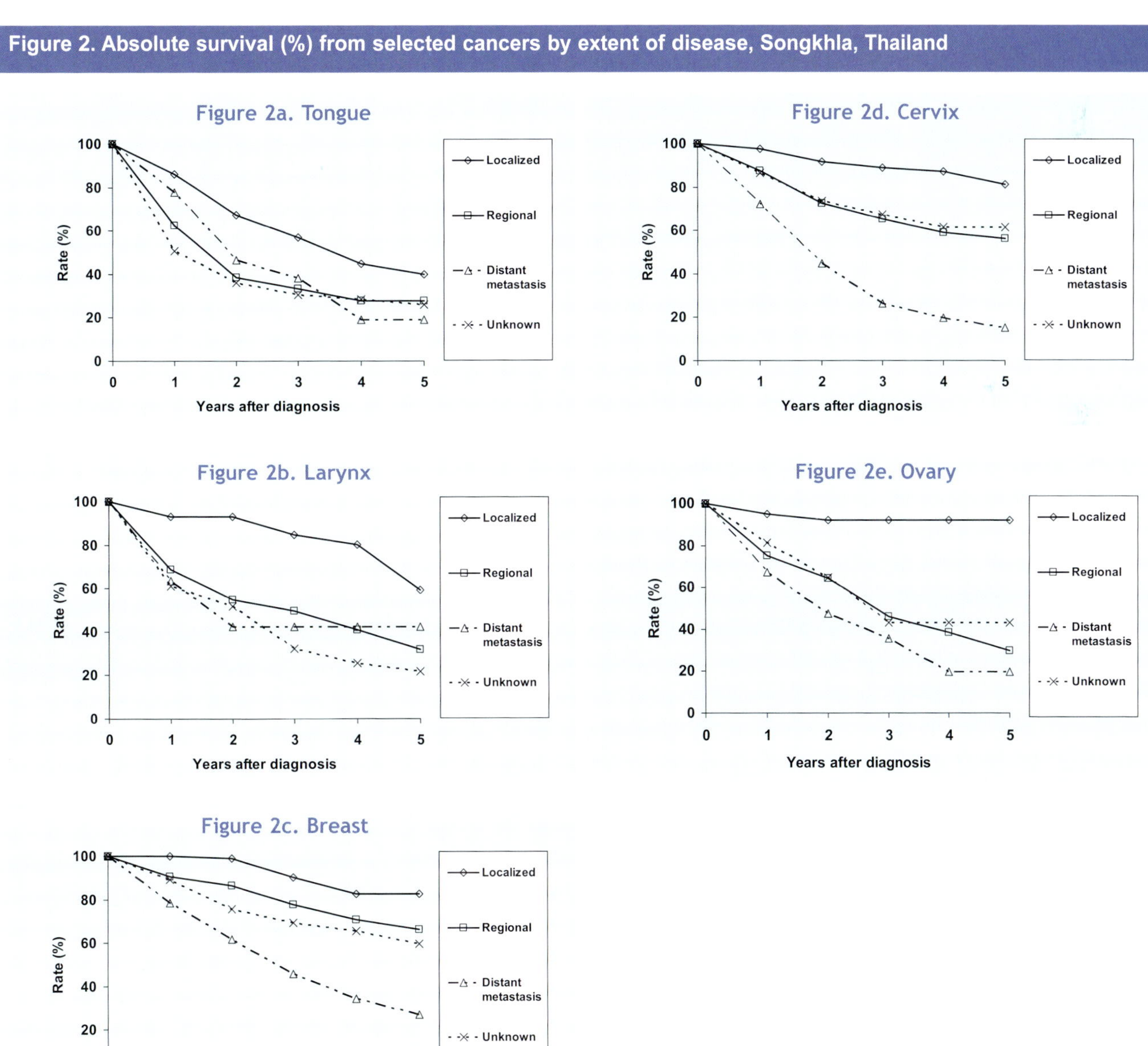

Table 1. Data quality indices - Proportion of histologically verified and death certificate only cases, number and proportion of included and excluded cases by site: Songkhla, Thailand, 1990–1999 cases followed-up until 2003

Site	ICD-10	Total registered	%		Excluded cases					Included cases	
			HV	DCO	DCO	Follow-up	Others	Total	%	No.	%
Lip	C00	38	92.1	0.0	0	7	0	7	18.4	31	81.6
Tongue	C01-02	230	93.5	0.0	0	34	0	34	14.8	196	85.2
Oral cavity	C03-06	275	94.5	1.5	4	37	0	41	14.9	234	85.1
Tonsil	C09	86	93.0	1.2	1	5	0	6	7.0	80	93.0
Nasopharynx	C11	193	95.9	0.5	1	24	0	25	13.0	168	87.0
Hypopharynx	C12-13	148	91.2	0.0	0	19	0	19	12.8	129	87.2
Oesophagus	C15	399	83.7	1.5	6	72	0	78	19.5	321	80.5
Stomach	C16	176	88.6	2.8	5	28	0	33	18.8	143	81.3
Colon	C18	314	83.1	3.2	10	57	0	67	21.3	247	78.7
Rectum	C19-20	232	91.4	0.0	0	29	0	29	12.5	203	87.5
Liver	C22	383	52.0	9.1	35	77	0	112	29.2	271	70.8
Gall bladder	C23-24	78	75.6	1.3	1	16	0	17	21.8	61	78.2
Pancreas	C25	109	55.0	3.7	4	21	0	25	22.9	84	77.1
Nose/Sinuses	C30-31	47	95.7	0.0	0	5	0	5	10.6	42	89.4
Larynx	C32	167	88.6	1.8	3	26	0	29	17.4	138	82.6
Lung	C33-34	850	78.0	5.1	43	136	1	180	21.2	670	78.8
Bone	C40-41	44	88.6	9.1	4	7	0	11	25.0	33	75.0
Melanoma of skin	C43	37	100.0	0.0	0	8	0	8	21.6	29	78.4
Other skin	C44	352	99.1	0.6	2	91	1	94	26.7	258	73.3
Connective tissue	C47+C49	80	100.0	0.0	0	13	0	13	16.3	67	83.8
Breast	C50	665	91.6	1.2	8	95	0	103	15.5	562	84.5
Cervix	C53	904	95.2	0.9	8	116	0	124	13.7	780	86.3
Corpus uteri	C54	110	90.0	4.5	5	11	0	16	14.5	94	85.5
Ovary	C56	218	95.9	0.5	1	43	1	45	20.6	173	79.4
Penis	C60	100	91.0	0.0	0	30	0	30	30.0	70	70.0
Prostate	C61	174	90.8	0.6	1	29	0	30	17.2	144	82.8
Kidney	C64	53	84.9	3.8	2	5	0	7	13.2	46	86.8
Urinary bladder	C67	199	89.4	0.0	0	44	0	44	22.1	155	77.9
Brain & nervous system	C70-72	158	55.7	13.9	22	30	0	52	32.9	106	67.1
Thyroid	C73	376	97.1	0.3	1	42	0	43	11.4	333	88.6
Hodgkin lymphoma	C81	41	100.0	0.0	0	5	0	5	12.2	36	87.8
Non-Hodgkin lymphoma	C82-85+C96	353	99.2	0.6	2	32	0	34	9.6	319	90.4
Multiple myeloma	C90	59	100.0	0.0	0	5	0	5	8.5	54	91.5
Lymphoid leukaemia	C91	107	100.0	0.0	0	8	0	8	7.5	99	92.5
Myeloid leukaemia	C92-94	191	100.0	0.0	0	18	0	18	9.4	173	90.6
Leukaemia unspecified	C95	74	66.2	33.8	25	9	0	34	45.9	40	54.1

HV: histologically verified; DCO: death certificate only

Table 2. Number and proportion of cases with complete/incomplete follow-up (in years) and median follow-up (in months) by site: Songkhla, Thailand, 1990–1999 cases followed-up until 2003

Site	ICD-10	No. of cases included	Complete FU Alive/dead at end of FU		Incomplete FU: loss to FU*						% with complete FU at 5 years	Median FU (in months)
							% lost to FU: years from diagnosis					
			No.	%	No.	%	< 1	1-3	3-5	> 5		
Lip	C00	31	17	54.8	14	45.2	12.9	6.5	16.1	9.7	64.5	39.6
Tongue	C01-02	196	130	66.3	66	33.7	13.8	8.2	4.6	7.1	73.5	12.2
Oral cavity	C03-06	234	160	68.4	74	31.6	13.2	6.8	4.7	6.8	75.2	12.6
Tonsil	C09	80	58	72.5	22	27.5	13.8	10.0	1.3	2.5	75.0	9.7
Nasopharynx	C11	168	104	61.9	64	38.1	8.9	15.5	6.0	7.7	69.6	26.7
Hypopharynx	C12-13	129	87	67.4	42	32.6	13.2	7.0	6.2	6.2	73.6	13.2
Oesophagus	C15	321	259	80.7	62	19.3	12.8	4.0	1.6	0.9	81.6	7.1
Stomach	C16	143	108	75.5	35	24.5	13.3	5.6	4.9	0.7	76.2	7.1
Colon	C18	247	130	52.6	117	47.4	17.8	12.1	7.7	9.7	62.3	17.3
Rectum	C19-20	203	133	65.5	70	34.5	10.3	9.9	7.9	6.4	71.9	20.3
Liver	C22	271	216	79.7	55	20.3	16.6	2.6	0.4	0.7	80.4	3.0
Gall bladder	C23-24	61	37	60.7	24	39.3	21.3	13.1	4.9	0.0	60.7	9.1
Pancreas	C25	84	65	77.4	19	22.6	15.5	3.6	3.6	0.0	77.4	6.3
Nose/Sinuses	C30-31	42	30	71.4	12	28.6	7.1	14.3	2.4	4.8	76.2	11.3
Larynx	C32	138	92	66.7	46	33.3	13.0	8.0	4.3	8.0	74.6	20.3
Lung	C33-34	670	539	80.4	131	19.6	13.6	3.4	0.9	1.6	82.1	5.0
Bone	C40-41	33	22	66.7	11	33.3	18.2	6.1	6.1	3.0	69.7	15.2
Melanoma of skin	C43	29	16	55.2	13	44.8	13.8	10.3	6.9	13.8	69.0	18.3
Other skin	C44	258	95	36.8	163	63.2	22.9	14.3	12.8	13.2	50.0	29.4
Connective tissue	C47+C49	67	46	68.7	21	31.3	10.4	9.0	6.0	6.0	74.6	10.2
Breast	C50	562	288	51.2	274	48.8	12.1	9.8	11.0	15.8	67.1	40.4
Cervix	C53	780	422	54.1	358	45.9	13.2	12.1	8.6	12.1	66.2	33.5
Corpus uteri	C54	94	44	46.8	50	53.2	16.0	14.9	11.7	10.6	57.4	36.4
Ovary	C56	173	84	48.6	89	51.4	16.2	19.7	8.1	7.5	56.1	23.3
Penis	C60	70	25	35.7	45	64.3	21.4	17.1	10.0	15.7	51.4	22.5
Prostate	C61	144	91	63.2	53	36.8	11.8	10.4	5.6	9.0	72.2	24.9
Kidney	C64	46	24	52.2	22	47.8	19.6	13.0	6.5	8.7	60.9	11.1
Urinary bladder	C67	155	89	57.4	66	42.6	11.0	11.6	9.7	10.3	67.7	28.8
Brain & nervous system	C70-72	106	65	61.3	41	38.7	11.3	16.0	6.6	4.7	66.0	11.2
Thyroid	C73	333	213	64.0	120	36.0	7.5	9.3	7.8	11.4	75.4	71.0
Hodgkin lymphoma	C81	36	14	38.9	22	61.1	16.7	13.9	16.7	13.9	52.8	32.6
Non-Hodgkin lymphoma	C82-85+C96	319	190	59.6	129	40.4	17.9	8.5	6.3	7.8	67.4	11.1
Multiple myeloma	C90	54	38	70.4	16	29.6	13.0	9.3	5.6	1.9	72.2	15.2
Lymphoid leukaemia	C91	99	69	69.7	30	30.3	10.1	8.1	4.0	8.1	77.8	24.3
Myeloid leukaemia	C92-94	173	140	80.9	33	19.1	6.4	5.8	2.3	4.6	85.5	6.6
Leukaemia unspecified	C95	40	31	77.5	9	22.5	15.0	2.5	5.0	0.0	77.5	5.0

*FU: follow-up; * non-random*

Table 3. Comparison of 1-, 3- and 5-year absolute and relative survival and 5-year age-standardized relative survival by site: Songkhla, Thailand, 1990–1999 cases followed-up until 2003

Site	ICD-10	Cases included	% Absolute survival			% Relative survival			% ASRS at 5-years	
			1-year	3-year	5-year	1-year	3-year	5-year	all ages	0-74 years
Lip	C00	31	89.7	74.0	58.3	92.3	81.3	69.2	74.9	77.1
Tongue	C01-02	196	63.3	37.2	28.7	64.3	38.9	30.9	31.3	31.4
Oral cavity	C03-06	234	62.9	34.6	26.7	64.1	36.6	29.4	33.4	35.3
Tonsil	C09	80	55.7	23.5	10.7	56.5	24.5	11.4	12.1	13.5
Nasopharynx	C11	168	83.2	57.0	44.3	83.7	58.0	45.6	40.8	47.4
Hypopharynx	C12-13	129	65.1	36.8	28.0	66.2	38.7	30.5	24.0	24.0
Oesophagus	C15	321	40.4	10.4	7.6	41.1	11.0	8.4	10.5	9.9
Stomach	C16	143	44.6	20.6	8.7	45.2	21.5	9.3	10.1	8.8
Colon	C18	247	77.8	51.4	45.0	78.9	53.6	48.3	45.4	52.8
Rectum	C19-20	203	74.0	44.8	33.2	74.9	46.4	35.4	36.2	31.9
Liver	C22	271	29.2	8.1	2.2	29.4	8.3	2.3	2.2	2.5
Gall bladder	C23-24	61	59.6	25.1	10.0	60.5	26.1	10.7	11.0	14.4
Pancreas	C25	84	41.9	15.0	12.2	42.5	15.5	13.0	8.7	15.9
Nose/Sinuses	C30-31	42	50.6	33.5	33.5	51.2	34.5	35.2	26.0	25.9
Larynx	C32	138	71.3	51.6	35.9	72.5	54.1	38.9	36.3	44.6
Lung	C33-34	670	36.3	11.0	7.2	36.7	11.4	7.6	6.9	8.6
Bone	C40-41	33	73.3	45.6	31.9	73.5	45.9	32.3	27.5	27.5
Melanoma of skin	C43	29	74.1	55.1	49.8	74.9	56.9	52.8	56.1	53.8
Other skin	C44	258	88.2	75.6	65.2	90.0	80.8	73.7	74.8	76.6
Connective tissue	C47+C49	67	57.5	42.4	32.7	57.9	43.4	34.2	29.9	32.0
Breast	C50	562	90.0	72.5	61.2	90.4	73.6	62.7	59.3	62.4
Cervix	C53	780	88.7	68.7	60.4	89.1	69.6	61.8	58.9	61.3
Corpus uteri	C54	94	85.0	77.5	69.7	85.4	79.0	72.1	69.2	72.5
Ovary	C56	173	81.1	56.2	48.6	81.5	57.0	49.6	41.5	48.7
Penis	C60	70	85.6	68.3	58.7	86.8	72.0	64.8	65.3	64.6
Prostate	C61	144	80.8	51.9	32.1	83.2	57.0	38.1	39.0	32.7
Kidney	C64	46	65.9	40.1	35.1	66.5	41.1	36.4	35.3	37.0
Urinary bladder	C67	155	80.9	58.8	41.4	82.3	62.0	45.5	45.6	45.9
Brain & nervous system	C70-72	106	58.0	37.9	37.9	58.2	38.3	38.4	32.0	31.1
Thyroid	C73	333	93.8	89.0	86.6	94.2	90.1	88.4	85.5	86.9
Hodgkin lymphoma	C81	36	84.8	70.5	54.4	85.3	71.6	55.6	53.1	55.9
Non-Hodgkin lymphoma	C82-85+C96	319	63.9	46.5	41.8	64.5	47.8	43.8	45.6	47.7
Multiple myeloma	C90	54	68.3	33.4	27.6	68.9	34.4	29.0	28.9	32.3
Lymphoid leukaemia	C91	99	70.2	54.3	48.1	70.5	54.7	48.6	34.5	36.5
Myeloid leukaemia	C92-94	173	47.5	25.1	14.4	47.8	25.6	14.7	13.4	15.4
Leukaemia unspecified	C95	40	48.6	29.0	24.6	48.8	29.3	24.8	17.0	17.0

ASRS: age-standardized relative survival

Table 4a. Site-wise number of cases, 5-year absolute and relative survival by sex: Songkhla, Thailand, 1990–1999 cases followed-up until 2003

Site	ICD-10	Cases included	Male % 5-year survival			Female % 5-year survival		
			No.	Abs	Rel	No.	Abs	Rel
Lip	C00	31	8	57.1	69.1	23	56.9	67.2
Tongue	C01-02	196	161	23.6	25.5	35	54.6	58.6
Oral cavity	C03-06	234	164	23.8	25.9	70	33.8	38.1
Tonsil	C09	80	71	5.8	6.2	9	46.9	48.7
Nasopharynx	C11	168	117	40.3	41.6	51	53.8	54.8
Hypopharynx	C12-13	129	114	25.1	27.4	15	48.2	50.9
Oesophagus	C15	321	234	6.8	7.6	87	9.2	9.9
Stomach	C16	143	96	8.9	9.5	47	8.7	9.4
Colon	C18	247	136	42.8	45.9	111	48.3	51.8
Rectum	C19-20	203	119	29.0	31.0	84	38.7	41.2
Liver	C22	271	225	2.2	2.4	46	0.0	0.0
Gall bladder	C23-24	61	23	36.8	39.9	38	4.5	4.7
Pancreas	C25	84	51	16.7	17.5	33	4.0	4.4
Nose/Sinuses	C30-31	42	29	20.3	21.7	13	66.7	68.6
Larynx	C32	138	129	36.0	39.1	9	33.0	34.7
Lung	C33-34	670	482	6.4	6.8	188	9.3	9.8
Bone	C40-41	33	22	39.6	40.0	11	14.8	15.1
Melanoma of skin	C43	29	14	38.0	40.7	15	57.2	60.1
Other skin	C44	258	134	58.7	65.2	124	71.8	82.3
Connective tissue	C47+C49	67	40	29.3	30.8	27	39.8	41.3
Breast	C50	562	6	30.0	32.1	556	61.6	63.1
Cervix	C53	780				780	60.4	61.8
Corpus uteri	C54	94				94	69.7	72.1
Ovary	C56	173				173	48.6	49.6
Penis	C60	70	70	58.7	64.8			
Prostate	C61	144	144	32.1	38.1			
Kidney	C64	46	30	24.5	25.6	16	58.6	60.6
Urinary bladder	C67	155	122	40.9	44.8	33	44.0	49.0
Brain & nervous system	C70-72	106	57	31.4	31.9	49	47.9	48.2
Thyroid	C73	333	78	79.8	82.2	255	88.6	90.3
Hodgkin lymphoma	C81	36	27	69.0	70.9	9	35.9	36.3
Non-Hodgkin lymphoma	C82-85+C96	319	193	39.4	41.3	126	45.9	47.9
Multiple myeloma	C90	54	30	33.9	35.9	24	16.8	17.2
Lymphoid leukaemia	C91	99	51	44.0	44.3	48	52.7	53.4
Myeloid leukaemia	C92-94	173	90	15.5	15.9	83	12.8	13.1
Leukaemia unspecified	C95	40	19	23.5	23.7	21	25.6	25.9

Abs: absolute survival; Rel: relative survival

Table 4b. Site-wise number of cases and relative survival by age group: Songkhla, Thailand, 1990–1999 cases followed-up until 2003

Site	ICD-10	Cases included	Number of cases by age group					Relative survival by age group % 5-year survival				
			< 45	45-54	55-64	65-74	> 75	< 45	45-54	55-64	65-74	> 75
Lip	C00	31	0	1	6	5	19			77.9	76.8	65.2
Tongue	C01-02	196	10	25	62	62	37		39.7	29.0	30.4	32.6
Oral cavity	C03-06	234	16	21	48	88	61	58.1	28.7	33.8	28.3	19.6
Tonsil	C09	80	9	11	19	29	12	43.4	0.0	14.3	10.3	
Nasopharynx	C11	168	64	36	37	24	7	52.2	56.6	34.0	30.1	0.0
Hypopharynx	C12-13	129	4	19	26	51	29	0.0	31.0	16.1	49.3	11.8
Oesophagus	C15	321	7	30	105	114	65	27.6	8.8	9.5	4.4	12.0
Stomach	C16	143	18	24	38	35	28	0.0	0.0	5.1	10.9	12.0
Colon	C18	247	41	31	54	58	63	54.9	61.8	44.9	54.1	32.9
Rectum	C19-20	203	29	26	67	48	33	32.6	34.4	43.7	20.7	43.8
Liver	C22	271	59	54	69	64	25	7.0	0.0	3.5	0.0	0.0
Gall bladder	C23-24	61	7	6	22	11	15	0.0		10.7	40.7	0.0
Pancreas	C25	84	11	12	25	21	15	15.2	25.6	23.4	0.0	0.0
Nose/Sinuses	C30-31	42	13	3	13	6	7	39.9	0.0	58.4		26.1
Larynx	C32	138	7	21	35	50	25	52.7	36.6	38.3	55.3	0.0
Lung	C33-34	670	57	91	217	212	93	14.2	11.3	6.3	7.4	2.4
Bone	C40-41	33	30	1	1	1	0	32.6	102.2	0.0	0.0	
Melanoma of skin	C43	29	6	3	5	12	3	84.1		51.3	41.7	71.0
Other skin	C44	258	28	31	53	62	84	88.5	80.4	71.5	69.3	71.2
Connective tissue	C47+C49	67	30	12	12	8	5	46.9	24.9	13.8	40.3	26.0
Breast	C50	562	200	174	106	56	26	64.5	65.0	63.7	55.2	46.0
Cervix	C53	780	304	200	160	84	32	69.6	59.7	60.2	49.6	36.8
Corpus uteri	C54	94	14	33	26	19	2	67.2	69.0	82.9	69.9	59.0
Ovary	C56	173	61	45	42	18	7	72.8	46.5	34.8	38.3	0.0
Penis	C60	70	12	10	19	14	15	71.9	65.9	56.5	65.4	66.6
Prostate	C61	144	0	4	17	45	78		0.0	32.4	38.3	42.4
Kidney	C64	46	13	6	14	8	5	51.3	79.1	17.8	29.5	
Urinary bladder	C67	155	13	17	38	46	41	57.4	47.0	40.6	46.1	45.6
Brain & nervous system	C70-72	106	74	9	17	4	2	44.1		32.6	0.0	
Thyroid	C73	333	181	51	53	30	18	100.8	88.4	74.7	66.4	37.3
Hodgkin lymphoma	C81	36	17	11	5	2	1	56.7	64.6	55.2		0.0
Non-Hodgkin lymphoma	C82-85+C96	319	103	51	62	54	49	57.4	52.4	38.0	32.9	28.6
Multiple myeloma	C90	54	8	14	13	15	4	31.6	24.2	49.2	15.2	0.0
Lymphoid leukaemia	C91	99	86	4	2	4	3	51.8	72.6	0.0	0.0	
Myeloid leukaemia	C92-94	173	80	28	29	26	10	18.9	14.1	21.1	0.0	0.0
Leukaemia unspecified	C95	40	33	3	1	3	0	28.5		0.0	0.0	

Table 5. Proportion of cases and 5-year absolute survival by extent of disease and site: Songkhla, Thailand, 1990–1999

Site	ICD-10	Cases included	% of cases by extent of disease				% 5-year absolute survival			
			Localized	Regional	Dist. met.	Unknown	Localized	Regional	Dist. met.	Unknown
Tongue	C01-02	196	19.9	30.6	7.1	42.3	40.0	27.9	19.1	26.0
Larynx	C32	138	21.0	39.9	8.7	30.4	59.5	31.9	42.4	21.9
Breast	C50	562	17.1	34.7	14.4	33.8	82.8	66.2	27.0	59.6
Cervix	C53	780	22.3	54.6	5.8	17.3	81.2	56.3	15.4	61.3
Ovary	C56	173	24.3	28.9	12.7	34.1	92.1	30.0	19.8	43.0

Dis. met.: distant metastasis

Chapter 29

Cancer survival in Izmir, Turkey, 1995–1997

Eser S

Abstract

The Izmir cancer registry, the first population-based cancer registry in Turkey, was established in 1992. Cancer registration is now done by active methods. The registry contributed data on survival for 12 cancer sites or types registered in 1995–1997. Follow-up was predominantly done by active methods with median follow-up ranging between 17–72 months for different cancers. The proportion with histologically verified diagnosis for various cancers ranged between 84–100%; there were no death certificate only (DCO) cases; 98–100% of total registered cases were included for the survival analysis. Complete follow-up at five years ranged from 79–98% for different cancers. Five-year age-standardized relative survival rates of common cancers were breast (77%), urinary bladder (70%), larynx (69%), colon (53%), rectum (52%), non-Hodgkin lymphoma (50%) and cervix (58%). Five-year relative survival by age group portrayed decreasing survival with increasing age at diagnosis for cancer of the cervix, and was fluctuating for other cancers. Decreasing survival with increasing clinical extent of disease was also noted.

Izmir cancer registry

The Izmir cancer registry was the first population-based cancer registry in Turkey, established in 1992 by the Ministry of Health and Ege University, in collaboration with the Turkish-American Collaboration for Health Research and Programming, University of Massachusetts at the Izmir provincial health directorate. The Ministry of Health had earlier established a passive cancer registration system for the entire country in 1983, which ended registering one fourth of expected cancers. Cancer registration is now done by active methods. Over 40 sources of registration, comprising government and private sector hospitals, clinics, pathology laboratories and hospices, are visited for data collection from the hospital cancer registries and other medical records. The registry covers an area of 11 530 km^2, of the entire Izmir province and caters to a population of about 3.3 million in 1998 with a sex ratio of 985 females to 1000 males. The average annual age-standardized incidence rate is 157 per 100 000 among males and 94 per 100 000 among females in 1993–1994. The top-ranking cancers among males are lung followed by non-melanoma skin, larynx and bladder. Among females, the order is breast, non-melanoma skin, corpus uteri and ovary [1].

The registry contributed data on survival for 12 cancer sites or types for the first time in this volume of the IARC publication on *Cancer Survival in Africa, Asia, the Caribbean and Central America.*

Data quality indices (Table 1)

The proportion of cases having a histologically verified cancer diagnosis in our series is 95%, varying between 100% for haematopoietic malignancies and 84% for colon cancer. None are registered based on a death certificate only (DCO) in the series. The exclusion of cases from the survival analysis due to the non-availability of any follow-up information or other reasons was negligible. Thus, 98–100% of the total cases in the series are included in the estimation of the survival probability.

Outcome of follow-up (Table 2)

The registry collects copies of death certificates mentioning cancer from the provincial health directorate, but because of poor quality and lack of information regarding socio-demographic data and addresses, these data could not be matched with the records of incident cases. Thus, follow-up information on the vital status of all incident cases are collected by one or more of the following ways: repeated scrutiny of records in the respective sources of registration, postal/telephone enquiries and house visits.

The closing date of follow-up was 31st December 2003. The median follow-up ranged between 17 months for myeloid leukaemia and 72 months for breast cancer. The availability of complete follow-up information at five years from the incidence date varied from 79% in rectal cancer to 98% in lymphoid leukaemia. The proportion of losses to follow-up was generally the highest in the extremities of the classified follow-up intervals (within the first year and five or more years of follow-up) for all cancers. This minimizes the bias of estimation of 5-year survival probability, as a sizeable proportion of cases lost to follow-up after five years would have had a complete follow-up until 5 years from the incidence date.

Survival statistics

All ages and both sexes together (Table 3)

The top-ranking cancers in terms of 5-year relative survival are breast (77%), larynx (71%), urinary bladder (70%), Hodgkin lymphoma (69%) and cervix (62%). Survival estimates for colon and rectum cancers were 53% and 50%, respectively. The survival figures for haematopoietic malignancies were 51% for lymphoid leukaemia, 32% for myeloid leukaemia and multiple myeloma.

Figure 1a. Top five cancers (ranked by survival), Izmir, Turkey, 1995–1997

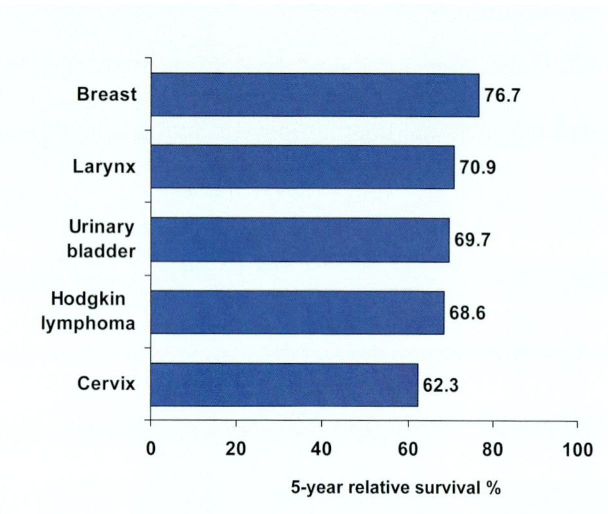

The 5-year age-standardized relative survival (ASRS) estimate for all ages together is generally less than or similar to the corresponding unadjusted one with a few exceptions. Also, the 5-year ASRS (0–74 years of age) is generally higher than or similar to the corresponding ASRS (all ages) for most cancers.

Sex

Male (Table 4a)

The rank order on the 5-year relative survival reveals breast (76%) at the top, followed by larynx (71%), urinary bladder (69%), Hodgkin lymphoma (68%) and rectum (56%). Survival from rectal cancer is noticeably higher among males than females.

Figure 1b. Top five cancers (ranked by survival), Male, Izmir, Turkey, 1995–1997

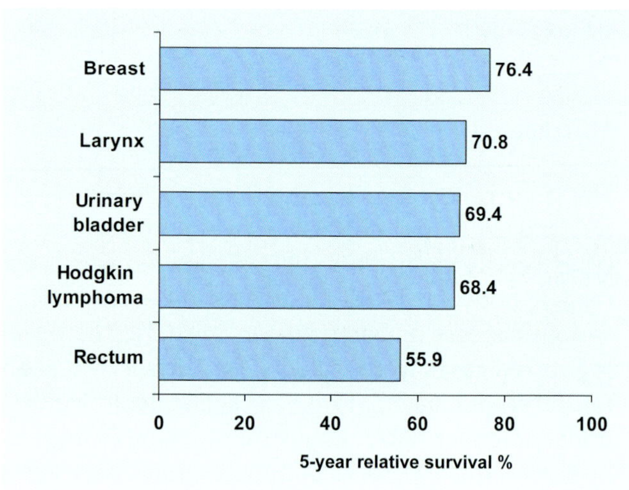

Female (Table 4a)

The highest 5-year relative survival was observed in cancer of the breast (77%) followed by larynx (73%), urinary bladder (72%), Hodgkin lymphoma (69%) and cervix (62%). Survival from ovarian cancer is 59%. The survival is markedly higher among females than males in non-Hodgkin lymphoma and myeloid leukaemia.

Figure 1c. Top five cancers (ranked by survival), Female, Izmir, Turkey, 1995–1997

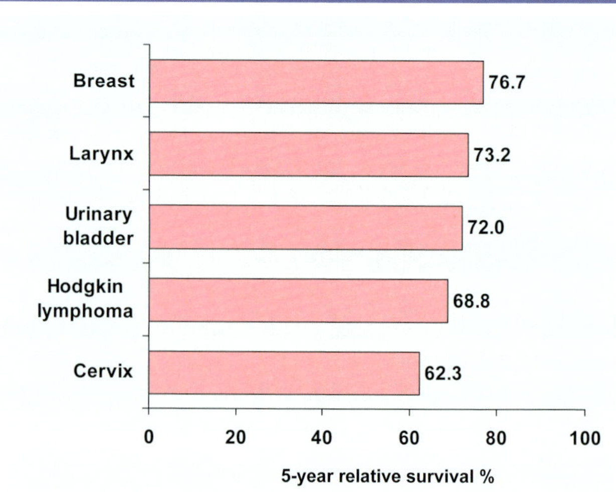

Age group (Table 4b)

The 5-year relative survival by age group portrays an inverse relationship: decreasing survival with increasing age at diagnosis for cancer of the cervix. In the rest, it is observed to be fluctuating.

Extent of disease (Table 5; Figure 2)

A majority of cases among cancer of the larynx (32%) have been diagnosed with localized disease. In ovarian cancer, the proportion of cases with distant metastasis (47%) is higher than other categories. Regional spread of disease is the most common among cancers of the colon (44%), rectum (41%), breast (34%) and cervix (42%). The extent of disease was unknown in 23–40%. The 5-year absolute survival by extent of disease reveals no differences in localized, regional and unknown categories for cancer of the rectum; distant metastasis cases among cancer of the larynx fare as well as cases with regional spread of disease. Cases with localized cervix cancer have survival similar to those classified as unknown.

References

1. Fidaner C, Eser SY, Parkin DM. Incidence in Izmir in 1993–1994: first results from Izmir Cancer Registry. *Eur J Cancer* 2001; 37: 83–92.

Figure 2. Absolute survival (%) from selected cancers by extent of disease, Izmir, Turkey

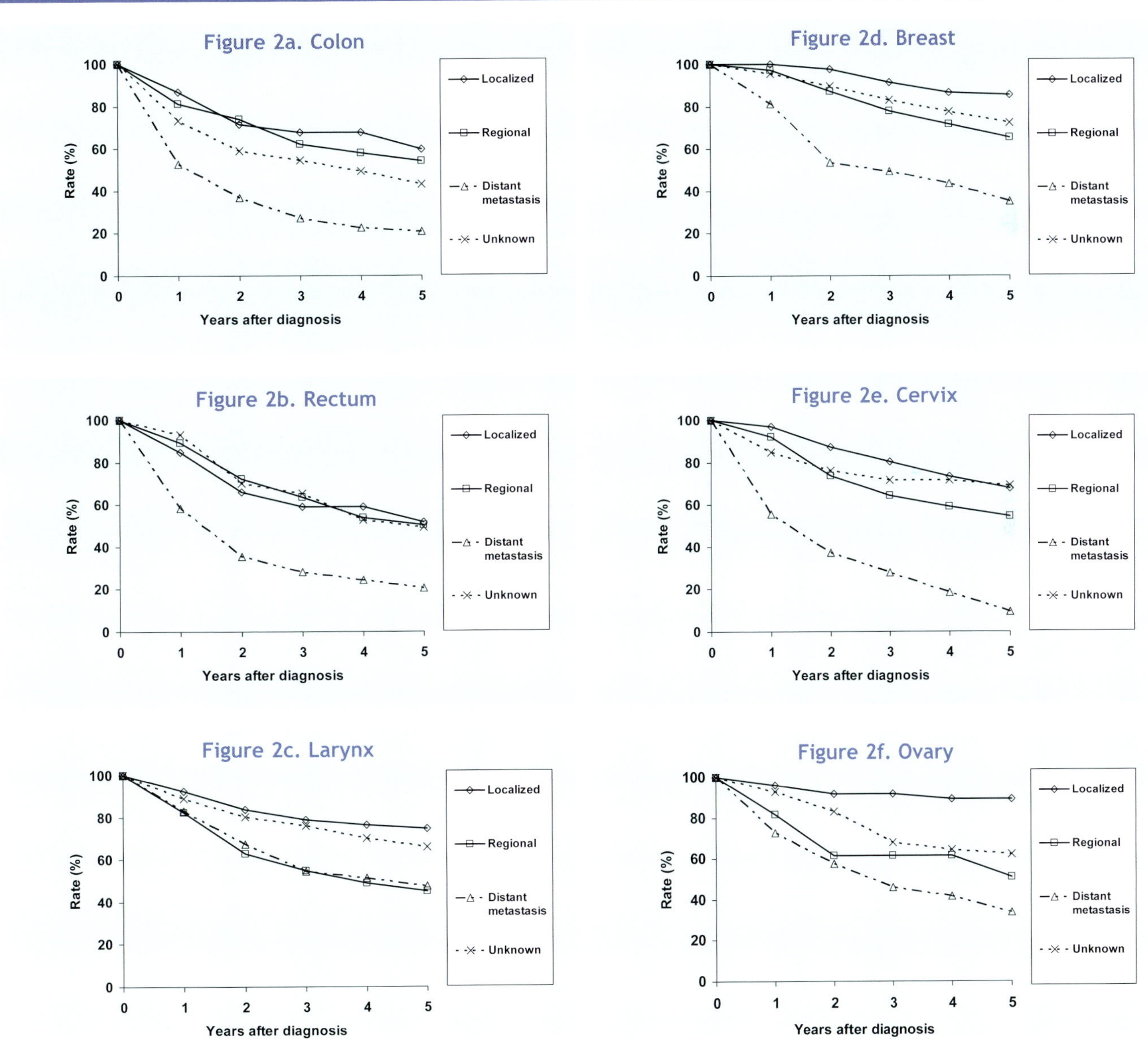

Table 1. Data quality indices - Proportion of histologically verified and death certificate only cases, number and proportion of included and excluded cases by site: Izmir, Turkey, 1995–1997 cases followed-up until 2003

Site	ICD-10	Total registered	%		Excluded cases					Included cases	
			HV	DCO	DCO	Follow-up	Others	Total	%	No.	%
Colon	C18	380	84.2	0.0	0	3	6	9	2.4	371	97.6
Rectum	C19-20	349	92.8	0.0	0	3	2	5	1.4	344	98.6
Larynx	C32	481	95.6	0.0	0	1	2	3	0.6	478	99.4
Breast	C50	1 346	95.6	0.0	0	6	11	17	1.3	1 329	98.7
Cervix	C53	248	98.0	0.0	0	0	2	2	0.8	246	99.2
Ovary	C56	232	98.3	0.0	0	0	2	2	0.9	230	99.1
Urinary bladder	C67	571	91.2	0.0	0	3	2	5	0.9	566	99.1
Hodgkin lymphoma	C81	85	100.0	0.0	0	0	0	0	0.0	85	100.0
Non-Hodgkin lymphoma	C82-85+C96	350	100.0	0.0	0	1	5	6	1.7	344	98.3
Multiple myeloma	C90	79	100.0	0.0	0	0	0	0	0.0	79	100.0
Lymphoid leukaemia	C91	161	100.0	0.0	0	0	0	0	0.0	161	100.0
Myeloid leukaemia	C92-94	149	100.0	0.0	0	1	0	1	0.7	148	99.3

HV: histologically verified; DCO: death certificate only

Table 2. Number and proportion of cases with complete/incomplete follow-up (in years) and median follow-up (in months) by site: Izmir, Turkey, 1995–1997 cases followed-up until 2003

Site	ICD-10	Cases included	Complete FU Alive/dead at end of FU		Incomplete FU: lost to FU		% lost to FU: years from diagnosis				% with complete FU at 5 years	Median FU (in months)
			No.	%	No.	%	< 1	1-3	3-5	> 5		
Colon	C18	371	266	71.7	105	28.3	11.1	3.0	1.3	12.9	84.6	28.2
Rectum	C19-20	344	232	67.5	112	32.5	16.0	2.9	2.0	11.6	79.1	24.6
Larynx	C32	478	308	64.4	170	35.6	9.8	1.7	1.5	22.6	87.0	64.0
Breast	C50	1 329	806	60.7	523	39.3	10.9	2.3	1.8	24.3	85.0	72.0
Cervix	C53	246	127	51.6	119	48.4	10.6	3.7	2.4	31.7	83.3	51.9
Ovary	C56	230	141	61.3	89	38.7	10.9	1.3	2.6	23.9	85.2	49.6
Urinary bladder	C67	566	350	61.8	216	38.2	13.3	2.7	1.2	21.0	82.9	49.3
Hodgkin lymphoma	C81	85	56	65.8	29	34.2	11.8	5.9	1.2	15.3	81.1	65.0
Non-Hodgkin lymphoma	C82-85+C96	344	256	74.5	88	25.5	11.6	3.2	2.0	8.7	83.2	22.4
Multiple myeloma	C90	79	68	86.0	11	14.0	7.6	1.3	1.3	3.8	89.8	19.4
Lymphoid leukaemia	C91	161	99	61.4	62	38.6	7.5	2.5	1.9	26.7	97.8	31.9
Myeloid leukaemia	C92-94	148	119	80.3	29	19.7	6.8	4.1	2.0	6.8	87.1	16.9

FU: follow-up

Table 3. Comparison of 1-, 3- and 5-year absolute and relative survival and 5-year age-standardized relative survival by site: Izmir, Turkey, 1995–1997 cases followed-up until 2003

Site	ICD-10	Cases included	% Absolute survival			% Relative survival			% ASRS at 5-years	
			1-year	3-year	5-year	1-year	3-year	5-year	all ages	0-74 years
Colon	C18	371	73.8	53.6	44.9	76.0	58.7	52.5	53.2	52.2
Rectum	C19-20	344	82.9	55.9	44.1	85.0	60.1	50.4	51.6	52.0
Larynx	C32	478	87.9	70.2	62.2	90.0	75.6	70.9	68.9	71.4
Breast	C50	1 329	96.3	81.3	71.1	97.6	84.9	76.7	76.6	77.2
Cervix	C53	246	89.7	68.2	58.8	90.7	70.5	62.3	57.6	63.5
Ovary	C56	230	83.4	62.9	54.7	84.7	65.7	59.0	60.2	59.7
Urinary bladder	C67	566	84.7	67.3	57.7	87.7	75.1	69.7	69.9	70.7
Hodgkin lymphoma	C81	85	92.5	77.4	65.6	93.3	79.3	68.6	67.9	65.8
Non-Hodgkin lymphoma	C82-85+C96	344	72.6	51.0	45.1	73.9	53.8	49.5	49.8	50.6
Multiple myeloma	C90	79	65.8	43.0	28.5	67.3	46.2	32.3	31.6	31.1
Lymphoid leukaemia	C91	161	78.1	55.5	48.2	79.2	57.6	51.4	52.6	50.1
Myeloid leukaemia	C92-94	148	65.7	41.2	29.5	67.0	43.4	32.2	33.0	34.2

ASRS: age-standardized relative survival

Table 4a. Site-wise number of cases, 5-year absolute and relative survival by sex: Izmir, Turkey, 1995–1997 cases followed-up until 2003

Site	ICD-10	Cases included	Male % 5-year survival			Female % 5-year survival		
			No.	Abs	Rel	No.	Abs	Rel
Colon	C18	371	217	42.8	50.1	154	48.0	56.1
Rectum	C19-20	344	192	47.8	55.9	152	39.6	43.8
Larynx	C32	478	450	61.9	70.8	28	66.2	73.2
Breast	C50	1 329	36	66.5	76.4	1 293	71.2	76.7
Cervix	C53	246				246	58.8	62.3
Ovary	C56	230				230	54.7	59.0
Urinary bladder	C67	566	508	57.5	69.4	58	59.2	72.0
Hodgkin lymphoma	C81	85	56	65.1	68.4	29	66.4	68.8
Non-Hodgkin lymphoma	C82-85+C96	344	194	40.3	43.9	150	51.4	56.7
Multiple myeloma	C90	79	41	26.0	30.4	38	31.5	34.6
Lymphoid leukaemia	C91	161	93	45.8	49.6	68	51.3	53.8
Myeloid leukaemia	C92-94	148	78	23.4	26.2	70	38.0	40.4

Abs: absolute survival; Rel: relative survival

Table 4b. Site-wise number of cases and relative survival by age group: Izmir, Turkey, 1995–1997 cases followed-up until 2003

Site	ICD-10	Cases included	Number of cases by age group					Relative survival by age group % 5-year survival				
			< 45	45-54	55-64	65-74	> 75	< 45	45-54	55-64	65-74	> 75
Colon	C18	371	49	60	97	120	45	48.0	57.8	51.8	51.4	55.6
Rectum	C19-20	344	64	66	85	99	30	39.4	48.3	47.7	64.5	53.0
Larynx	C32	478	55	118	164	121	20	72.7	68.9	72.9	71.3	58.4
Breast	C50	1 329	387	360	310	211	61	73.1	75.2	80.4	82.5	72.2
Cervix	C53	246	66	71	66	39	4	70.9	63.3	60.0	54.4	0.0
Ovary	C56	230	58	47	66	48	11	66.9	64.2	49.5	57.1	64.6
Urinary bladder	C67	566	35	85	168	197	81	84.7	73.3	66.6	68.1	67.0
Hodgkin lymphoma	C81	85	58	11	9	5	2	72.5	53.7	62.8	32.7	138.2
Non-Hodgkin lymphoma	C82-85+C96	344	117	55	82	72	18	54.1	50.5	49.4	41.0	42.2
Multiple myeloma	C90	79	9	22	25	20	3	14.0	39.7	34.4	27.3	54.3
Lymphoid leukaemia	C91	161	96	20	16	19	10	53.4	47.1	49.8	37.7	73.7
Myeloid leukaemia	C92-94	148	60	20	22	32	14	38.7	37.4	22.3	23.2	25.3

Table 5. Proportion of cases and 5-year absolute survival by extent of disease and site: Izmir, Turkey, 1995–1997

Site	ICD-10	Cases included	% of cases by extent of disease				% 5-year absolute survival			
			Localized	Regional	Dist. met.	Unknown	Localized	Regional	Dist. met.	Unknown
Colon	C18	371	8.9	43.7	19.9	27.5	59.8	54.1	20.8	43.0
Rectum	C19-20	344	14.2	40.8	21.2	23.8	51.8	50.3	20.4	49.2
Larynx	C32	478	32.1	23.0	7.5	37.4	74.8	45.1	47.6	65.8
Breast	C50	1 329	20.5	34.3	4.7	40.5	85.5	65.4	35.1	72.3
Cervix	C53	246	28.9	41.8	6.1	23.2	67.7	54.6	9.3	69.1
Ovary	C56	230	22.6	5.2	47.4	24.8	89.4	51.1	33.6	62.3

Dis. met.: distant metastasis

Chapter 30

Cancer survival in Kampala, Uganda, 1993–1997

Wabinga H, Parkin DM, Nambooze S and Amero J

Abstract

The Kampala cancer registry was established in 1954 as a population-based cancer registry, and registration of cases is done by active methods. The registry contributed data on survival for 15 cancer sites or types registered in 1993–1997. For Kaposi sarcoma, only a random sample of the total incident cases was provided for survival study. Follow-up has been carried out predominantly by active methods, with median follow-up ranging from 4–26 months. The proportion with histologically verified diagnosis for various cancers ranged between 36–83%; death certificate only (DCO) cases were negligible; 58–92% of total registered cases were included for survival analysis. Complete follow-up at five years ranged between 47–87% for different cancers. Five-year age-standardized relative survival rates for selected cancers were Kaposi sarcoma (22%), cervix (19%), oesophagus (5%), non-Hodgkin lymphoma (26%), breast (36%) and prostate (46%). None survived beyond 5 years for cancers of the stomach and lung. Five-year relative survival by age group was fluctuating with no definite pattern or trend emerging and no survivors in many age intervals.

Kampala cancer registry

The Kampala cancer registry was established in 1954 as a population-based cancer registry at the department of pathology, Makerere University Medical School, to obtain information on cancer occurrence in Kyadondo county [1]. It contributed data to the quinquennial IARC publication *Cancer Incidence in Five Continents* in volumes I, VII and VIII [2] and cancer survival data for Kampala have been published [3]. Cancer is not a notifiable disease, and registration of cases is done by active methods. The principal sources of data are medical records in the hospitals in the government and non-government sectors, pathology laboratories and hospice. The registry caters to a population of about 1.1 million in 1995 with a sex ratio of 1029 females to 1000 males. The average annual age-standardized incidence rate is 162 per 100 000 among males and 171 per 100 000 among females in 1993–1997. The top-ranking cancers among males are Kaposi sarcoma, cancer of the prostate and non-Hodgkin lymphoma. Among females, the order is Kaposi sarcoma, cervix and breast.

The registry contributed data on survival from 15 cancer sites or types for the first time in this volume of the IARC publication on *Cancer Survival in Africa, Asia, the Caribbean and Central America*. For Kaposi sarcoma, only a random sample of the total incident cases (431 out of 1376 cases; 31%) was available for this survival study.

Data quality indices (Table 1)

The proportion of cases with histological confirmation of cancer diagnosis in this series is 66%, varying between 83% for cancer of the thyroid and 36% for liver. The proportion of cases registered based on a death certificate only was negligible. The exclusion of cases without any follow-up information is 21%, ranging from 5% in lung cancer to 39% in cancer of the eye. Thus, 58–92% of the total cases in different cancers registered are included in the estimation of the survival probability.

Outcome of follow-up (Table 2)

Follow-up has been carried out predominantly by active methods. Cancer mortality information obtained from accessible death certificates in health units of the county are matched with the registry database. The vital status of the unmatched incident cases are then ascertained by repeated scrutiny of hospital records, postal enquiries and house visits.

The closing date of follow-up was 31st December 1999. The median follow-up varied from 4 months in stomach cancer to 26 months for prostate cancer. Complete follow-up at five years from the incidence date ranged from 47% in cancer of the eye to 87% for liver and lung cancers. The bulk of the losses to follow-up have generally occurred in the first year of follow-up.

Survival statistics

All ages and both sexes together (Table 3)

The 5-year relative survival is the highest in cancer of the prostate (48%) followed by breast (44%) and non-Hodgkin lymphoma (34%) in the series. None survived for 5 years from incidence date among cancers of the stomach and lung.

Figure 1a. Top ten cancers (ranked by survival), Kampala, Uganda, 1993–1997

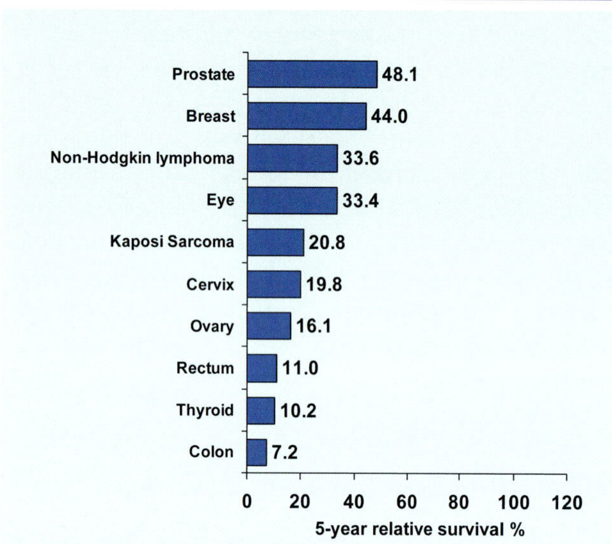

The 5-year age-standardized relative survival (ASRS) probability for all ages together is either less than or similar to the corresponding unadjusted one for a majority of cancers. The 5-year ASRS (0–74 years of age) is observed to be either higher than or similar to the corresponding ASRS (all ages) for all cancers.

Sex

Male (Table 4a)

The 5-year relative survival was the highest for cancer of the breast (n=5, 111%) followed in order by prostate (48%), eye (42%), thyroid and non-Hodgkin lymphoma (39%). None survived for 5 years from incidence date in cancers of the nasopharynx, stomach and lung. The 5-year relative survival was notably higher among males than females in cancers of the eye, thyroid and non-Hodgkin lymphoma.

Female (Table 4a)

The top-ranking cancers in terms of 5-year relative survival were breast (42%), non-Hodgkin lymphoma (26%) and Kaposi sarcoma (21%). Survival from cervix and ovarian cancers were 20% and 16%, respectively. None survived until 5 years from incidence date in cancers of the nasopharynx, stomach and thyroid.

Figure 1b. Top five cancers (ranked by survival), Male, Kampala, Uganda, 1993–1997

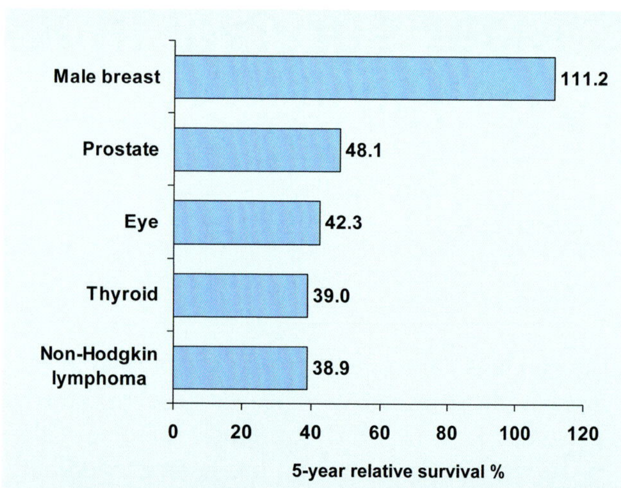

Figure 1c. Top five cancers (ranked by survival), Female, Kampala, Uganda, 1993–1997

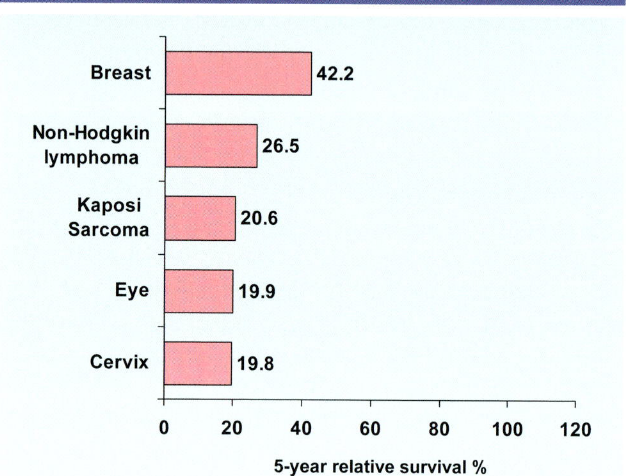

Age group (Table 4b)

The 5-year relative survival by age group is seen to fluctuate, with no definite pattern or trend emerging and no survivors in many age intervals.

References

1. Wabinga HR, Parkin DM, Wabwire-Mangen F, Nambooze S. Trends in cancer incidence in Kyadondo County, Uganda, 1960–1997. *Br J Cancer*. 2000; 82(9): 1585–1592.

2. Parkin DM, Whelan SL, Ferlay J and Storm H. *Cancer Incidence in Five Continents, Vol I to VIII: IARC Cancerbase No. 7*. IARCPress, Lyon, 2005.

3. Gondos A, Brenner H, Wabinga H, Parkin DM. Cancer survival in Kampala, Uganda. *Br J Cancer*. 2005; 92(9):1808–1812.

Table 1. Data quality indices - Proportion of histologically verified and death certificate only cases, number and proportion of included and excluded cases by site: Kampala, Uganda, 1993–1997 cases followed-up until 1999

Site	ICD-10	Total registered	%		Excluded cases					Included cases	
			HV	DCO	DCO	Follow-up	Others	Total	%	No.	%
Nasopharynx	C11	63	77.8	0.0	0	14	0	14	22.2	49	77.8
Oesophagus	C15	196	40.3	0.0	0	14	2	16	8.2	180	91.8
Stomach	C16	104	48.1	0.0	0	11	3	14	13.5	90	86.5
Colon	C18	56	57.1	0.0	0	4	1	5	8.9	51	91.1
Rectum	C19-20	59	67.8	0.0	0	8	1	9	15.3	50	84.7
Liver	C22	133	36.1	0.8	1	8	8	17	12.8	116	87.2
Lung	C33-34	55	61.8	1.8	1	3	4	8	14.5	47	85.5
Kaposi sarcoma	C46*	431	80.5	0.0	0	60	1	61	14.2	370	85.8
Breast	C50	233	63.9	0.0	0	66	5	71	30.5	162	69.5
Cervix	C53	461	63.8	0.2	1	166	11	178	38.6	283	61.4
Ovary	C56	75	54.7	0.0	0	9	0	9	12.0	66	88.0
Prostate	C61	213	76.5	0.0	0	40	19	59	27.7	154	72.3
Eye	C69	140	66.4	0.0	0	55	4	59	42.1	81	57.9
Thyroid	C73	53	83.0	0.0	0	11	3	14	26.4	39	73.6
Non-Hodgkin lymphoma	C82-85+C96	251	79.7	0.8	2	69	2	73	29.1	178	70.9

*HV: histologically verified; DCO: death certificate only; * random sample of total incident cases*

Table 2. Number and proportion of cases with complete/incomplete follow-up (in years) and median follow-up (in months) by site: Kampala, Uganda, 1993–1997 cases followed-up until 1999

Site	ICD-10	No. of cases included	Complete FU Alive/dead at end of FU		Incomplete FU: loss to FU*		% lost to FU: years from diagnosis				% with complete FU at 5 years	Median FU (in months)
			No.	%	No.	%	< 1	1-3	3-5	> 5		
Nasopharynx	C11	49	31	63.3	18	36.7	32.7	4.1	0.0	0.0	63.3	6.3
Oesophagus	C15	180	152	84.4	28	15.6	12.8	2.8	0.0	0.0	84.4	7.2
Stomach	C16	90	67	74.4	23	25.6	21.1	4.4	0.0	0.0	74.4	4.2
Colon	C18	51	41	80.4	10	19.6	19.6	0.0	0.0	0.0	80.4	6.6
Rectum	C19-20	50	40	80.0	10	20.0	18.0	2.0	0.0	0.0	80.0	9.4
Liver	C22	116	101	87.1	15	12.9	12.1	0.0	0.9	0.0	87.1	5.9
Lung	C33-34	47	41	87.2	6	12.8	12.8	0.0	0.0	0.0	87.2	4.8
Kaposi sarcoma	C46°	370	248	67.0	122	33.0	21.6	9.2	1.9	0.3	67.3	8.1
Breast	C50	162	96	59.3	66	40.7	27.8	9.3	1.9	1.9	61.1	10.9
Cervix	C53	283	149	52.7	134	47.3	35.0	11.3	0.7	0.4	53.0	8.3
Ovary	C56	66	48	72.7	18	27.3	15.2	7.6	3.0	1.5	74.2	5.0
Prostate	C61	154	119	77.3	35	22.7	16.2	3.9	2.6	0.0	77.3	26.2
Eye	C69	81	38	46.9	43	53.1	37.0	14.8	1.2	0.0	46.9	14.9
Thyroid	C73	39	22	56.4	17	43.6	25.6	15.4	0.0	2.6	59.0	7.5
Non-Hodgkin lymphoma	C82-85+C96	178	118	66.3	60	33.7	23.0	7.9	1.7	1.1	67.4	9.4

*FU: follow-up; ° from a random sample of total cases; * non-random*

Table 3. Comparison of 1-, 3- and 5-year absolute and relative survival and 5-year age-standardized relative survival by site: Kampala, Uganda, 1993–1997 cases followed-up until 1999

Site	ICD-10	Cases included	% Absolute survival			% Relative survival			% ASRS at 5-years	
			1-year	3-year	5-year	1-year	3-year	5-year	all ages	0-74 years
Nasopharynx	C11	49	58.5	27.2	0.0	59.8	29.0	0.0	0.0	0.0
Oesophagus	C15	180	36.5	10.3	2.5	38.3	12.3	3.4	4.6	3.0
Stomach	C16	90	39.1	7.5	0.0	40.9	8.5	0.0	0.0	0.0
Colon	C18	51	54.3	19.0	5.4	57.2	22.7	7.4	6.2	8.2
Rectum	C19-20	50	56.0	13.7	9.1	58.4	15.4	11.0	7.2	10.1
Liver	C22	116	33.0	8.0	2.7	34.0	8.7	3.1	1.1	1.4
Lung	C33-34	47	15.9	0.0	0.0	16.4	0.0	0.0	0.0	0.0
Kaposi sarcoma	C46*	370	58.5	33.8	18.6	59.7	36.1	20.8	21.9	35.6
Breast	C50	162	72.0	54.3	37.8	74.5	59.3	44.0	36.1	45.8
Cervix	C53	283	73.0	34.9	17.1	75.0	37.8	19.8	18.7	13.1
Ovary	C56	66	44.3	28.5	13.7	45.5	31.4	16.1	10.2	8.6
Prostate	C61	154	86.6	56.2	29.4	95.0	75.3	48.1	45.6	47.2
Eye	C69	81	92.4	55.1	30.4	94.3	58.4	33.4	35.7	35.7
Thyroid	C73	39	62.3	26.7	8.9	63.8	28.7	10.2	10.8	10.8
Non-Hodgkin lymphoma	C82-85+C96	178	61.4	40.7	31.9	62.3	42.2	33.6	26.1	25.1

*ASRS: age-standardized relative survival; * random sample of total incident cases*

Table 4a. Site-wise number of cases, 5-year absolute and relative survival by sex: Kampala, Uganda, 1993–1997 cases followed-up until 1999

Site	ICD-10	Cases included	Male % 5-year survival			Female % 5-year survival		
			No.	Abs	Rel	No.	Abs	Rel
Nasopharynx	C11	49	26	0.0	0.0	23	0.0	0.0
Oesophagus	C15	180	95	3.4	4.4	85	1.9	3.1
Stomach	C16	90	50	0.0	0.0	40	0.0	0.0
Colon	C18	51	25	5.6	8.8	26	5.3	6.2
Rectum	C19-20	50	27	9.7	12.3	23	9.2	10.5
Liver	C22	116	63	2.3	2.7	53	3.1	3.6
Lung	C33-34	47	28	0.0	0.0	19		
Kaposi sarcoma	C46*	370	219	18.5	20.9	151	18.7	20.6
Breast	C50	162	5	100.0	111.2	157	36.2	42.2
Cervix	C53	283				283	17.1	19.8
Ovary	C56	66				66	13.7	16.1
Prostate	C61	154	154	29.4	48.1			
Eye	C69	81	43	38.8	42.3	38	17.8	19.9
Thyroid	C73	39	3	33.3	39.0	36	0.0	0.0
Non-Hodgkin lymphoma	C82-85+C96	178	103	37.0	38.9	75	25.0	26.5

*Abs: absolute survival; Rel: relative survival; * random sample of total cases; * random sample of total incident cases*

Table 4b. Site-wise number of cases and relative survival by age group: Kampala, Uganda, 1993–1997 cases followed-up until 1999

Site	ICD-10	Cases included	Number of cases by age group					Relative survival by age group % 5-year survival				
			< 45	45-54	55-64	65-74	> 75	< 45	45-54	55-64	65-74	> 75
Nasopharynx	C11	49	39	5	5	0	0	0.0	0.0			
Oesophagus	C15	180	30	48	36	43	23	0.0	3.9		8.7	10.5
Stomach	C16	90	25	20	22	12	11	0.0	0.0	0.0		0.0
Colon	C18	51	10	14	8	11	8	0.0	13.1	0.0	18.7	0.0
Rectum	C19-20	50	21	8	8	9	4		40.5	0.0	0.0	0.0
Liver	C22	116	60	20	21	13	2	6.7	0.0	0.0	0.0	0.0
Lung	C33-34	47	21	8	11	6	1	0.0	0.0	0.0	0.0	0.0
Kaposi sarcoma	C46*	370	303	40	26	0	1	17.2	20.2	58.8	0.0	0.0
Breast	C50	162	77	36	22	14	13	50.8	46.9	57.4	26.8	0.0
Cervix	C53	283	151	71	31	23	7	32.3	16.6	0.0		56.2
Ovary	C56	66	39	9	9	6	3	26.2	18.6		0.0	
Prostate	C61	154	1	12	30	54	57	0.0	89.7	33.5	56.2	43.9
Eye	C69	81	74	6	1	0	0	32.1	64.1		0.0	0.0
Thyroid	C73	39	17	12	8	2	0	26.0	0.0	0.0		
Non-Hodgkin lymphoma	C82-85+C96	178	167	4	2	4	1	34.5				

** random sample of total incident cases*

Chapter 31

Cancer survival in Harare, Zimbabwe, 1993–1997

Chokunonga E, Borok MZ, Chirenje ZM, Nyabakau AM and Parkin DM

Abstract

The Zimbabwe national cancer registry was established in 1985 as a population-based cancer registry covering Harare city. Cancer is not a notifiable disease, and registration of cases is done by active methods. The registry contributed data on randomly drawn sub-samples of Harare resident cases among 17 common cancer sites or types registered during 1993–1997 from black and white populations. Follow-up was carried out predominantly by active methods with median follow-up ranging from 1–54 months for different cancers. The proportion with histologically verified diagnosis for various cancers ranged from 20–100%; death certificate only (DCO) cases comprised 0–34%; 58–97% of total registered cases were included for survival analysis. Complete follow-up at five years ranged from 94–100%. Five-year age-standardized relative survival rates of selected cancers among both races combined were cervix (42%), breast (68%), Kaposi sarcoma (4%), liver (3%), oesophagus (12%), stomach (20%) and lung (14%). Survival was markedly higher among white than black populations for most cancers with adequate cases. Five-year relative survival by age group was fluctuating, with no definite pattern or trend.

Zimbabwe cancer registry

The Zimbabwe national cancer registry was established in 1985 as a population-based cancer registry at the Parirenyatwa Hospital, Medical School of the University of Zimbabwe, Harare, under the support of the Ministry of Health and Child Welfare, IARC and other organizations. It contributed data to the quinquennial IARC publication Cancer Incidence in Five Continents in volumes VII (for African (black) and European (white) populations) and VIII (for black population only) [1]. Cancer is not a notifiable disease, and registration of cases is done by active methods. The principal sources of data are the medical records in the cancer departments, hospitals, pathology laboratories in the public and private sectors and specific clinical research studies. The registry covers the Harare city and caters to a population of about 1.5 million in 1997 with a sex ratio of 943 females to 1000 males. The average annual age-standardized incidence rate (ASR) of all cancers except non-melanoma skin among the black population was 223 per 100 000 among males and 219 per 100 000 among females in 1993–1997; the corresponding figures for the white population in 1990–1992 are 291 per 100 000 males and 298 per 100 000 females [1,2,3].

The registry has contributed data on survival from 17 cancer sites or types in this volume of the IARC publication on *Cancer Survival in Africa, Asia, the Caribbean and Central America*. For this study, only sub-samples of Harare resident cases among the 17 common cancers are included. For most cancers, it was intended that a minimum of 150 cases be randomly selected. For cervix and breast cancers and Kaposi sarcoma, the number intended is 300. For breast cancer, it is equally distributed among minority (white) and (black) races. For the rest of cancers, the inclusion of the minority races (other than white) is only by chance [4].

Data quality indices (Table 1)

The proportion of cases with histological confirmation of cancer diagnosis in this series is 65%, varying between 20% for liver cancer and 100% for Hodgkin lymphoma. The proportion of cases registered based on a death certificate only is 10%, ranging from nil to 34%. The exclusion of cases without any follow-up information or other inconsistencies ranged from 1–8%. Thus, 58–97% in the series among different cancers are included in the estimation of the survival probability.

Outcome of follow-up (Table 2)

Follow-up has been carried out predominantly by active methods. Cancer mortality information obtained from accessible death certificates in greater Harare is matched with the registry database. The vital status of the unmatched incident cases is then ascertained by repeated scrutiny of hospital records, postal enquiries and house visits.

The closing date of follow-up was 31st December 1999. The median follow-up varied from 1 month in liver cancer to 54 months for melanoma skin cancer. Complete follow-up at five years from the incidence date ranged from 95% in cancer of the larynx to 100% for many cancers.

Survival statistics (Tables 3a-3c)

All ages and both sexes together

The survival estimates for different cancers were tabulated separately for the black, white and all races together.

Black population (Table 3a)

The 5-year relative survival estimate was the highest in cancer of the eye (66%). The corresponding figures for melanoma skin and Hodgkin lymphoma are 58% and 51%, respectively. The lowest survival rate was encountered with liver cancer (4%).

Figure 1a. Top ten cancers (ranked by survival), Black, Harare, Zimbabwe, 1993–1997

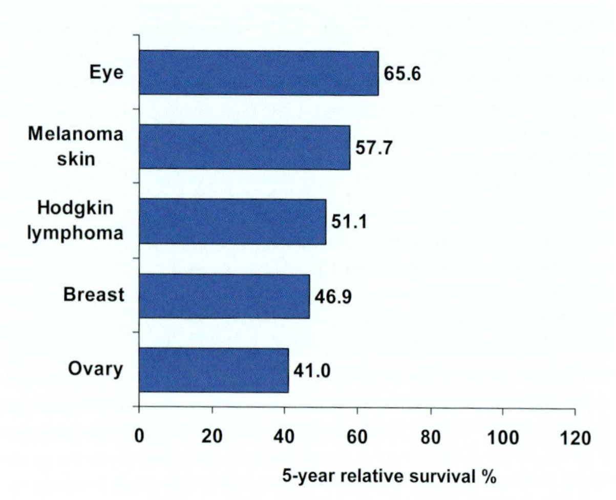

White population (Table 3b)

The top ranking cancers on 5-year relative survival estimate are melanoma skin (101%), urinary bladder (83%) and breast (79%). There are very few cases in half the number of cancers under study.

Figure 1b. Top five cancers (ranked by survival),White, Harare, Zimbabwe, 1993–1997

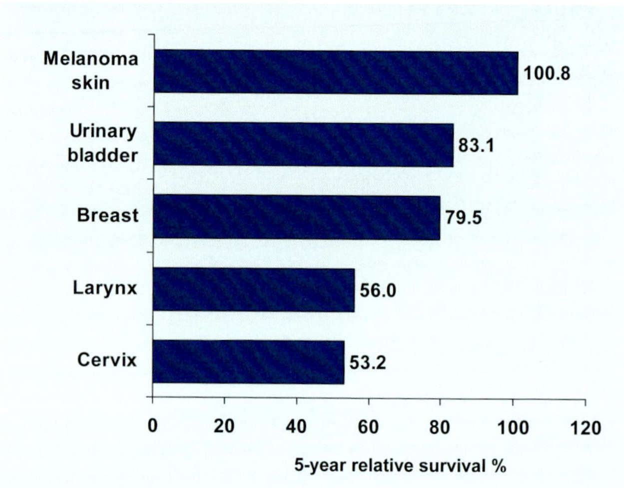

All races together (Table 3c)

For both races together, the 5-year age-standardized relative survival (ASRS) probability for all ages together is either greater than or similar to the corresponding unadjusted one for a majority of cancers. The 5-year ASRS (0–74 years of age) was observed to be either less than or similar to the corresponding ASRS (all ages) for all cancers.

Figure 1c. Top five cancers (ranked by survival), all races, Harare, Zimbabwe, 1993–1997

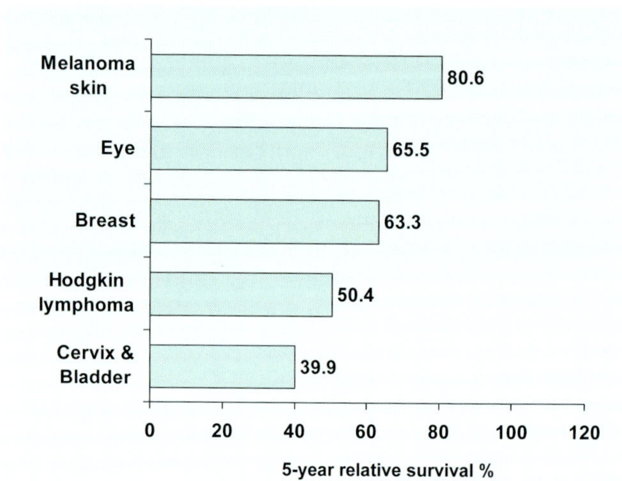

Black vs white populations

In most cancers where there was an adequate number of cases, the 5-year relative survival was markedly higher among the white than the black population. However, for colon cancer, a higher survival among black than white population was found. There is not much of a difference in survival from cancers of the rectum and lung between the two populations.

Figure 1d. Comparison of 5-year relative survival (%), Harare, Zimbabwe, 1993–1997

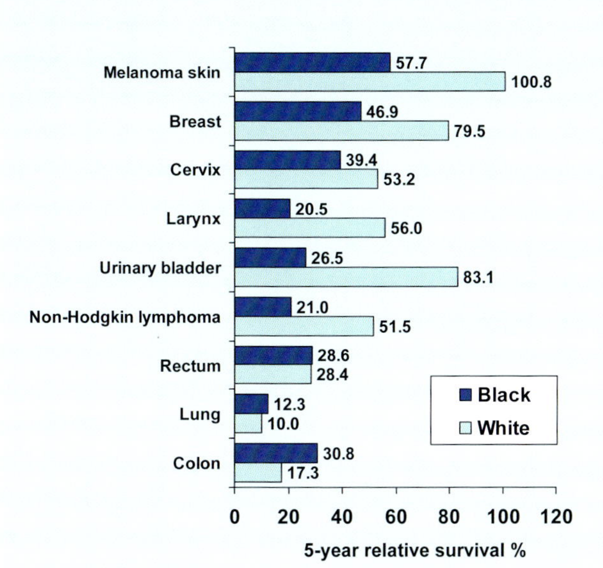

Sex

Male (Table 4a)

The 5-year relative survival was distinctly higher among males than females in cancers of the colon, rectum, larynx, breast and urinary bladder.

Female (Table 4a)

The highest 5-year relative survival is observed in melanoma skin (83%) followed by cancers of the eye (74%) and breast (62%). Survival rates from cervix and ovarian cancers were 40% and 37%, respectively. Survival is markedly higher among females than males in cancers of the oesophagus, eye and Hodgkin lymphoma.

Age group (Table 4b)

The 5-year relative survival by age group is seen to fluctuate, with no definite pattern or trend.

References

1. Parkin DM, Whelan SL, Ferlay J and Storm H. *Cancer Incidence in Five Continents, Vol I to VIII: IARC Cancerbase No. 7*. IARCPress, Lyon, 2005.

2. Chokunonga E, Levy LM, Bassett MT, Mauchaza BG, Thomas DB, Parkin DM. Cancer incidence in the African population of Harare, Zimbabwe: Second results from the cancer registry 1993–1995. *Int J Cancer*. 2000; 85: 54–59.

3. Bassett MT, Levy L, Chokunonga E, Mauchaza B, Ferlay J, Parkin DM. Cancer in the European population of Harare, Zimbabwe, 1990–1992. *Int J Cancer*. 1995; 63: 24–28.

4. Gondos A, Chokunonga E, Brenner H, Parkin DM, Sankila R, Borok MZ, Chirenje ZM, Nyakabau AM, Bassett MT. Cancer survival in a southern African urban population. *Int J Cancer*. 2004; 112(5):860–864.

Table 1. Data quality indices - Proportion of histologically verified and death certificate only cases, number and proportion of included and excluded cases by site: Harare, Zimbabwe, 1993–1997 cases* followed-up until 1999, all races together

Site	ICD-10	Total registered	%		Excluded cases					Included cases	
			HV	DCO	DCO	Follow-up	Others	Total	%	No.	%
Oesophagus	C15	146	51.4	8.9	13	0	2	15	10.3	131	89.7
Stomach	C16	144	67.4	9.0	13	2	0	15	10.4	129	89.6
Colon	C18	68	64.7	11.8	8	1	2	11	16.2	57	83.8
Rectum	C19-20	76	76.3	10.5	8	1	0	9	11.8	67	88.2
Liver	C22	149	20.1	10.7	16	1	0	17	11.4	132	88.6
Larynx	C32	80	73.8	7.5	6	1	0	7	8.8	73	91.3
Lung	C33-34	148	40.5	20.9	31	0	1	32	21.6	116	78.4
Melanoma of skin	C43	106	91.5	0.0	0	1	4	5	4.7	101	95.3
Kaposi sarcoma	C46	258	47.3	33.7	87	0	20	107	41.5	151	58.5
Breast	C50	287	77.7	7.7	22	5	2	29	10.1	258	89.9
Cervix	C53	284	72.5	2.1	6	9	5	20	7.0	264	93.0
Ovary	C56	66	62.1	4.5	3	0	0	3	4.5	63	95.5
Prostate	C61	73	57.5	9.6	7	2	0	9	12.3	64	87.7
Urinary bladder	C67	142	59.2	7.0	10	1	1	12	8.5	130	91.5
Eye	C69	130	90.8	0.0	0	6	8	14	10.8	116	89.2
Hodgkin lymphoma	C81	40	100.0	0.0	0	1	0	1	2.5	39	97.5
Non-Hodgkin lymphoma	C82-85+C96	103	91.3	1.0	1	3	0	4	3.9	99	96.1

*HV: histologically verified; DCO: death certificate only; * random sample of total incident cases*

Table 2. Number and proportion of cases with complete/incomplete follow-up (in years) and median follow-up (in months) by site: Harare, Zimbabwe, 1993–1997 cases* followed-up until 1999, all races together

Site	ICD-10	Cases included	Complete FU		Incomplete FU: lost to FU						% with complete FU at 5 years	Median FU (in months)
			Alive/dead at end of FU				% lost to FU: years from diagnosis					
			No.	%	No.	%	< 1	1-3	3-5	> 5		
Oesophagus	C15	131	131	100.0	0	0.0	0.0	0.0	0.0	0.0	100.0	2.3
Stomach	C16	129	127	98.4	2	1.6	1.6	0.0	0.0	0.0	98.4	4.8
Colon	C18	57	57	100.0	0	0.0	0.0	0.0	0.0	0.0	100.0	14.6
Rectum	C19-20	67	65	97.0	2	3.0	1.5	1.5	0.0	0.0	97.0	16.1
Liver	C22	132	131	99.2	1	0.8	0.8	0.0	0.0	0.0	99.2	1.0
Larynx	C32	73	69	94.5	4	5.5	5.5	0.0	0.0	0.0	94.5	14.1
Lung	C33-34	116	116	100.0	0	0.0	0.0	0.0	0.0	0.0	100.0	2.0
Melanoma of skin	C43	101	100	99.0	1	1.0	1.0	0.0	0.0	0.0	99.0	54.2
Kaposi sarcoma	C46	151	151	100.0	0	0.0	0.0	0.0	0.0	0.0	100.0	3.4
Breast	C50	258	250	96.9	8	3.1	2.7	0.4	0.0	0.0	96.9	39.3
Cervix	C53	264	260	98.5	4	1.5	1.1	0.4	0.0	0.0	98.5	26.2
Ovary	C56	63	63	100.0	0	0.0	0.0	0.0	0.0	0.0	100.0	18.7
Prostate	C61	64	61	95.3	3	4.7	4.7	0.0	0.0	0.0	95.3	16.6
Urinary bladder	C67	130	127	97.7	3	2.3	1.5	0.8	0.0	0.0	97.7	11.8
Eye	C69	116	114	98.3	2	1.7	0.9	0.9	0.0	0.0	98.3	42.1
Hodgkin lymphoma	C81	39	39	100.0	0	0.0	0.0	0.0	0.0	0.0	100.0	30.6
Non-Hodgkin lymphoma	C82-85+C96	99	97	98.0	2	2.0	2.0	0.0	0.0	0.0	98.0	7.8

*FU: follow-up; * from a random sample of total cases*

Table 3a. Comparison of 1-, 3- and 5-year absolute and relative survival and 5-year age-standardized relative survival by site: Harare, Zimbabwe, Black, 1993–1997 cases* followed-up until 1999

Site	ICD-10	Cases included	% Absolute survival			% Relative survival			% ASRS at 5-years	
			1-year	3-year	5-year	1-year	3-year	5-year	all ages	0-74 years
Oesophagus	C15	124	24.2	13.7	9.0	25.4	15.5	11.1	9.2	12.1
Stomach	C16	110	34.9	16.8	15.7	36.4	19.4	19.8	18.6	19.1
Colon	C18	30	53.3	29.7	25.7	55.4	33.1	30.8	24.9	40.6
Rectum	C19-20	43	55.3	22.6	22.6	57.3	25.3	28.6	66.3	40.3
Liver	C22	131	8.0	3.9	3.0	8.4	4.5	3.7	3.0	3.7
Larynx	C32	48	55.3	35.0	16.2	57.8	39.9	20.5	17.7	22.5
Lung	C33-34	91	14.3	9.8	9.8	14.9	11.2	12.3	16.0	10.8
Melanoma of skin	C43	45	68.9	50.8	47.1	71.4	57.1	57.7	55.6	54.1
Kaposi sarcoma	C46	150	20.7	8.3	5.0	21.0	8.7	5.4	4.4	4.4
Breast	C50	128	71.5	50.6	40.2	73.6	55.4	46.9	54.8	42.9
Cervix	C53	254	67.5	45.2	33.9	69.5	49.3	39.4	44.1	38.7
Ovary	C56	51	56.9	42.8	36.4	58.2	46.0	41.0	39.1	39.1
Prostate	C61	35	42.9	24.8		46.4	30.4			
Urinary bladder	C67	99	41.1	26.3	20.7	42.8	30.1	26.5	35.0	27.4
Eye	C69	115	83.4	71.5	58.3	85.5	76.9	65.6	69.9	69.9
Hodgkin lymphoma	C81	37	67.6	56.6	46.6	68.8	59.5	51.1	46.1	46.1
Non-Hodgkin lymphoma	C82-85+C96	89	39.8	22.8	18.3	40.9	25.0	21.0	31.4	18.0

*ASRS: age-standardized relative survival; * random sample of total incident cases*

Table 3b. Comparison of 1-, 3- and 5-year absolute and relative survival and 5-year age-standardized relative survival by site: Harare, Zimbabwe, White, 1993–1997 cases* followed-up until 1999

Site	ICD-10	Cases included	% Absolute survival			% Relative survival			% ASRS at 5-years	
			1-year	3-year	5-year	1-year	3-year	5-year	all ages	0-74 years
Oesophagus	C15	6	33.3	33.3	33.3	34.9	39.5	45.8	67.8	24.2
Stomach	C16	19	52.6	31.6	31.6	55.4	35.9	38.3	33.7	47.0
Colon	C18	25	56.0	20.0	12.0	60.6	25.2	17.3	13.1	20.1
Rectum	C19-20	24	83.3	37.5	21.9	87.9	44.3	28.4	40.5	34.0
Liver	C22	1	0.0	0.0	0.0	0.0	0.0	0.0	0.0	0.0
Larynx	C32	23	64.4	41.4	36.6	69.4	52.0	56.0	59.3	65.8
Lung	C33-34	24	25.0	7.5	7.5	26.3	8.6	10.0	6.7	10.4
Melanoma of skin	C43	54	92.5	86.9	81.4	96.2	98.0	100.8	105.3	96.2
Kaposi sarcoma	C46	1	0.0	0.0	0.0	0.0	0.0	0.0	0.0	0.0
Breast	C50	116	91.4	75.7	61.9	95.6	87.1	79.5	81.1	74.2
Cervix	C53	9	66.7	44.4	44.4	69.4	50.6	53.2	60.9	65.8
Ovary	C56	11	63.6	36.4	18.2	66.8	43.0	25.0	17.2	9.8
Prostate	C61	28	77.8	64.0		85.3	83.8			
Urinary bladder	C67	29	79.3	72.4	53.0	86.0	93.1	83.1	82.7	67.1
Eye	C69	1	100.0	0.0	0.0	131.5	0.0	0.0	0.0	0.0
Hodgkin lymphoma	C81	2	100.0	33.3		101.1	34.3			
Non-Hodgkin lymphoma	C82-85+C96	8	62.5	37.5	37.5	65.2	43.0	51.5	31.3	17.9

*ASRS: age-standardized relative survival; * random sample of total incident cases*

Table 3c. Comparison of 1-, 3- and 5-year absolute and relative survival and 5-year age-standardized relative survival by site: Harare, Zimbabwe, all races, 1993–1997 cases* followed-up until 1999

Site	ICD-10	Cases included	% Absolute survival			% Relative survival			% ASRS at 5-years	
			1-year	3-year	5-year	1-year	3-year	5-year	all ages	0-74 years
Oesophagus	C15	131	24.4	14.5	10.1	25.6	16.4	12.7	12.3	12.3
Stomach	C16	129	37.5	19.0	18.1	39.2	21.9	22.6	20.5	22.8
Colon	C18	57	54.4	26.1	18.3	57.5	30.7	23.8	18.8	28.6
Rectum	C19-20	67	65.4	28.0	21.5	68.2	32.2	27.4	45.3	30.3
Liver	C22	132	8.0	3.9	2.9	8.4	4.5	3.7	3.0	3.7
Larynx	C32	73	57.7	36.8	22.8	60.9	43.3	31.1	28.1	29.7
Lung	C33-34	116	17.2	9.3	9.3	18.0	10.7	11.8	13.6	11.4
Melanoma of skin	C43	101	82.1	70.0	65.5	85.2	78.8	80.6	82.7	77.4
Kaposi sarcoma	C46	151	20.5	8.3	5.0	20.9	8.7	5.4	4.4	4.4
Breast	C50	258	81.1	62.7	51.2	84.2	70.5	63.3	67.7	57.8
Cervix	C53	264	67.2	44.9	34.3	69.2	49.1	39.9	42.2	39.1
Ovary	C56	63	57.1	40.9	31.4	58.8	44.7	36.8	38.6	34.0
Prostate	C61	64	58.4	41.9		63.6	53.4			
Urinary bladder	C67	130	50.4	37.5	28.9	53.0	44.6	39.9	55.5	37.2
Eye	C69	116	83.6	70.8	57.7	85.8	76.7	65.5	64.5	69.9
Hodgkin lymphoma	C81	39	69.2	55.9	46.1	70.5	58.7	50.4	46.5	46.5
Non-Hodgkin lymphoma	C82-85+C96	99	41.8	23.6	19.8	43.1	26.0	23.6	41.1	26.0

*ASRS: age-standardized relative survival; * random sample of total incident cases*

Table 4a. Site-wise number of cases, 5-year absolute and relative survival by sex: Harare, Zimbabwe, 1993–1997 cases* followed-up until 1999, all races together

Site	ICD-10	Cases included	Male			Female		
			% 5-year survival			% 5-year survival		
			No.	Abs	Rel	No.	Abs	Rel
Oesophagus	C15	131	121	9.4	11.6	10	20.0	25.7
Stomach	C16	129	79	17.6	22.4	50	19.0	22.9
Colon	C18	57	47	20.2	26.5	10	10.0	12.6
Rectum	C19-20	67	25	29.4	37.8	42	16.3	20.5
Liver	C22	132	132	2.9	3.7	0		
Larynx	C32	73	64	24.6	33.9	9	12.7	15.8
Lung	C33-34	116	94	9.6	12.2	22		
Melanoma of skin	C43	101	51	61.6	78.1	50	69.9	83.4
Kaposi sarcoma	C46	151	110	5.0	5.3	41	6.5	7.3
Breast	C50	258	5	100.0	149.9	253	50.3	61.9
Cervix	C53	264				264	34.3	39.9
Ovary	C56	63				63	31.4	36.8
Prostate	C61	64	64					
Urinary bladder	C67	130	96	31.2	43.7	34	24.8	31.6
Eye	C69	116	57	48.7	55.4	59	65.2	73.6
Hodgkin lymphoma	C81	39	23	43.8	46.9	16	50.0	56.2
Non-Hodgkin lymphoma	C82-85+C96	99	73	19.0	22.9	26	21.6	24.9

*Abs: absolute survival; Rel: relative survival; * random sample of total cases; * random sample of total incident cases*

Table 4b. Site-wise number of cases and relative survival by age group: Harare, Zimbabwe, 1993–1997 cases* followed-up until 1999, all races together

Site	ICD-10	Cases included	Number of cases by age group					Relative survival by age group				
								% 5-year survival				
			< 45	45-54	55-64	65-74	> 75	< 45	45-54	55-64	65-74	> 75
Oesophagus	C15	131	19	32	40	25	15	21.3	10.9	11.9	10.5	12.6
Stomach	C16	129	18	22	43	33	13	23.5	25.7	27.6	15.8	
Colon	C18	57	9	11	13	15	9	12.8	21.0	37.0	31.9	0.0
Rectum	C19-20	67	13	12	22	12	8	25.7	12.0	10.6	64.9	71.0
Liver	C22	132	34	25	29	31	13	10.0		0.0	0.0	0.0
Larynx	C32	73	10	12	17	23	11	22.9	21.6	19.6	52.1	26.2
Lung	C33-34	116	14	21	35	37	9	8.3	16.5	12.9	7.7	19.4
Melanoma of skin	C43	101	29	26	24	13	9	93.0	69.2	82.5	54.3	104.9
Kaposi sarcoma	C46	151	147	4	0	0	0	5.2	0.0			
Breast	C50	258	70	69	51	37	31	51.2	62.2	52.8	66.9	122.8
Cervix	C53	264	109	67	52	27	9	41.5	40.5	24.8	49.2	76.5
Ovary	C56	63	27	12	14	7	3	30.4	39.4	56.5	0.0	64.4
Prostate	C61	64	0	2	11	31	20		0.0			
Urinary bladder	C67	130	22	22	37	28	21	34.0	15.7	22.7	61.4	88.7
Eye	C69	116	99	10	3	3	1	63.7	90.6		134.2	0.0
Hodgkin lymphoma	C81	39	35	3	1	0	0	50.4	73.9			
Non-Hodgkin lymphoma	C82-85+C96	99	63	19	12	3	2	17.7	19.8		42.1	246.1

** random sample of total incident cases*

Chapter 32

An overview of cancer survival in Africa, Asia, the Caribbean and Central America: the case for investment in cancer health services

Sankaranarayanan R, Swaminathan R, Jayant K and Brenner H

Abstract

Population-based cancer survival data, a key indicator for monitoring progress against cancer, are reported from 27 population-based cancer registries in 14 countries in Africa, Asia, the Caribbean and Central America. In China, Singapore, the Republic of Korea, and Turkey, the 5-year age-standardized relative survival ranged from 76–82% for breast, 63–79% for cervical, 71–78% for bladder, and 44–60% for large-bowel cancer. Survival did not exceed 22% for any cancer site in The Gambia, or 13% for any cancer site except breast (46%) in Uganda. For localized cancers of the breast, large bowel, larynx, ovary, urinary bladder and for regional diseases at all sites, higher survival rates were observed in countries with more rather than less developed health services. Inter- and intra-country variations in survival imply that the levels of development of health services and their efficiency to provide early diagnosis, treatment and clinical follow-up care have a profound impact on survival from cancer. These are reliable baseline summary estimates to evaluate improvements in cancer control and emphasise the need for urgent investment to improve awareness, population-based cancer registration, early detection programmes, health-services infrastructure, and human resources in these countries in the future.

Introduction

Population-based cancer survival data from 27 population-based cancer registries in 14 countries in Africa, Asia, the Caribbean and Central America are briefly described and discussed in this publication (Table 1). Survival data for 40 cancer sites are described in this chapter, although the number of registries reporting for each cancer site varied from 2 to 26 (Table 2). The countries contributing data in our study have variable levels of economic development, as indicated by the varying gross national income (GNI) per capita, and development of health services. The levels of development of health services and their efficiency in providing early diagnosis, treatments and clinical follow-up care have a profound impact on survival from cancer. Poorly developed and inaccessible health services obviously result in great disparity in early diagnosis, adequate treatment and follow-up care. We discuss the observed survival patterns and inter- as well as intra-country variations in this chapter, in the background of basic and effective early detection, diagnosis and treatment requirements for selected cancer sites, taking into account data quality issues, the wide differences in awareness, socio-economic development, human resources, health services investment, development and accessibility in the countries included in this study.

Case-finding and follow-up

The methods used by each cancer registry to identify and register all diagnosed cases from the various data sources in their geographical regions have been described in the individual chapters. In brief, the registries used a mix of both passive notification of cases and active registration by visiting and abstracting data on cases from different data sources to register all incident cancer cases in the populations they covered. They used quality assurance procedures as advocated by the International Agency for Research on Cancer (IARC) to validate the quality and completion of cancer registration in their target populations [1]. Uniform criteria [2] described in detail in Chapter 4 were adopted for inclusion of

with well-developed health services, such as Singapore and Turkey, than in other countries, underlining the importance of both early diagnosis and appropriate treatment (Figure 3a). Survival rates for the above cancer sites were lower in rural compared to urban areas of India and China, whereas the survival differences were minimal across Republic of Korea and Thailand.

The poor survival outcomes for most patients with head and neck cancer in our study and elsewhere [2,9] underscore the importance of primary prevention and early detection of these cancers. Most head and neck cancers are caused by tobacco use in any form [10,11] and alcohol drinking [12], and avoiding these risk factors has a substantial impact on preventing these cancers. A 35% reduction in oral cancer mortality following three rounds of oral visual screening among tobacco and/or alcohol users was documented in a randomized trial in Southern India [13]. Routine visual screening of such high-risk populations will improve survival and reduce oral cancer mortality.

Digestive tract cancers (Tables 3, 4d, 4e; Figures 1f–1j, 2e–2h and 4a–4b)

Five-year survival prospects of patients with liver, pancreas, gall bladder, oesophagus and stomach cancers were generally poor, not exceeding 15% in most populations studied, indicating the poor prognosis of cancers in these organs and the importance of primary prevention in controlling these tumours. Most of the cancers arising in these sites are rarely curable. The overall 5-year survival rate in patients amenable for radical definitive treatment by surgery or radiotherapy for oesophageal cancer ranges from 5% to 30%. Cytological and endoscopic screening have been evaluated in countries with a high incidence of oesophageal cancer. Although these efforts have shown that it is possible to detect cancers in an early asymptomatic stage, and those with very early disease have a better chance of survival, screening is unlikely to reduce mortality from oesophageal cancer and may result in some serious side-effects associated with endoscopy such as aspiration, perforation, bleeding and cardiopulmonary events. Improving general nutrition and controlling tobacco and alcohol consumption are important in the context of preventing oesophageal cancer. Symptomatic gastroesophageal reflux disease (GERD) has been identified as a risk factor of oesophageal adenocarcinoma.

The survival outcome of patients with stomach cancer is related to tumour extension beyond the gastric wall, regional lymph node involvement, and to a lesser extent on tumour grade [14,15]. Screening is unlikely to reduce mortality from stomach cancer. Overall stomach cancer incidence and mortality are declining across the world due to better food preservation using refrigerators, reduced consumption of salted, smoked and pickled food products, and wide availability of fruits and vegetables the year round. Risk factors for gastric cancer include the presence of precursor conditions such as chronic atrophic gastritis, intestinal metaplasia and pernicious anaemia. There is increasing evidence that Helicobacter pylori infection of the stomach is associated with both the initiation and promotion of gastric carcinoma.

Most patients with stomach cancer present with metastatic disease, either regional or in distant sites such as the liver. The curative treatment option for stomach cancer is radical surgery; however, the frequency of local failure in the tumour bed and regional lymph nodes and distant failures via haematogenous or peritoneal routes remains high. Although 30–50% of patients with localized distal stomach cancer can be cured, such disease accounts for less than 10% of cases. On the other hand, the 5-year survival rate of patients with localized proximal stomach cancer is less than 15%. None with disseminated disease survive at 5 years.

Survival for colorectal (large bowel) cancer varied from 4% in The Gambia to 64% in Seoul, Republic of Korea. The survival figures were less than 8% in the sub-Saharan African countries of The Gambia and Uganda and less than 30% in Harare, Zimbabwe, all of which have poorly-developed cancer health care infrastructure and limited availability of and accessibility to curative treatments for most patients. The survival prospects of patients with large bowel cancer is clearly related to the degree of penetration of the tumour through the intestinal wall, the presence or absence of regional lymph nodal involvement, and the presence or absence of distant metastases; these three characteristics form the basis for staging and treatment options for this cancer [16].

It is well established that screening with faecal occult blood testing reduces colorectal cancer mortality, and flexible sigmoidoscopy and colonoscopy leads to earlier detection of polyps and colorectal cancer. The standard treatment for patients with colon cancer has been open surgical resection of the primary and regional lymph nodes for localized disease. Patients with advanced disease may require combined modality therapy with chemotherapy with or without radiation therapy. The survival outcomes for colorectal cancer depend on the clinical stage at presentation and the ability of the health services to provide prompt standard care with radical surgery and other adjuvant therapies as indicated. Survival rates exceeding 50% reported from Hong Kong, Republic of Korea, Singapore, regions in Thailand and mainland China seem to reflect the wide availability of screening, endoscopy and treatment in their well- or moderately-developed health services. The flexible sigmoidoscope permits a more complete examination of the distal colon with more acceptable patient tolerance than the rigid sigmoidoscope. Virtually all the screening studies using these types of sigmoidoscopes have demonstrated an increase in the proportion of early cases and survival compared with cases diagnosed in a routine environment. It is quite likely that the early recognition of the clinical importance of flat lesions detected in colonoscopy by the endoscopy practices in east Asian countries has also led to earlier detection of colorectal cancers there [17]. The survival experience of large bowel cancer patients in Hong Kong and the Republic of Korea are similar to that reported for white patients in the United States Surveillance Epidemiology and End Results (US-SEER) [9].

The 5-year survival rates of localized and regional large bowel cancer were 64% and 46%, respectively in Singapore and Izmir, Turkey, as compared to 50% and 32%, respectively in countries with less-developed health services such as Thailand, India and the Philippines (Figure 4a). It is interesting to note that the survival experience of localized colorectal cancer patients in countries with less-developed health services and that of patients with regional disease in countries such as Singapore and Turkey with well-developed health services were almost similar (Figure 4b). The higher survival in Singapore and Turkey seems to be a reflection of both earlier stages of clinical presentation and the capability of the health services to promptly respond with early diagnosis and comprehensive management. On the other hand, the wide difference in the outcome between localized and regional cancers (18 percentage points) indicates the potential for early detection to prevent more deaths from colorectal cancer (Figure 4a).

The vast majority of patients with liver cancer die within a year, although a small fraction of those with localized cancers can be potentially cured by surgical resection. However, screening for liver cancer with ultrasonography and/or alpha fetoprotein (AFP) estimation does not reduce liver cancer mortality [18,19]. A vast majority of liver cancers are caused by chronic infection with Hepatitis B (HBV) or C (HCV) viruses, ingestion of foods contaminated with aflatoxins and alcohol consumption. Controlling these risk factors has a major impact on liver cancer prevention. A 69% reduction in the incidence of liver cancer among the vaccinated cohort has been recently demonstrated after the introduction of HBV vaccination in the national immunization programme of Taiwan [20].

Cancer of the pancreas is rarely curable, although complete surgical excision in patients with localized disease and small cancers (<2 cm) with no lymph node metastases and no extension beyond the capsule of the pancreas can result in 5-year survival rates around 20%. It is quite likely that survival rates exceeding 15–20% for these poor-prognosis cancers in our series suffer from over-estimation due to under-ascertainment of death events in many patients who might have been misclassified as alive at the closing date.

Lung cancer (Table 3; Figures 1l and 2j)

The 5-year survival from lung cancer was less than 15% in most countries and populations in our study (Table 3). Surgery is the most potentially curative therapeutic option for most localized non-small cell lung cancers (NSCLC). Radiation therapy, combined with chemotherapy, can produce a cure in a small number of patients and can provide palliation in most patients. Regardless of clinical stage and improvements in diagnosis and therapy made during the past 25 years, treatment outcomes are not satisfactory for most patients with lung cancer. Although a small proportion of NSCLC patients with surgically resectable disease may be cured, the majority of patients with lung cancer die of their tumour even with the best available therapy.

Small-cell lung cancer (SCLC) accounts for approximately 15–20% of lung cancers; without treatment, SCLC has the most aggressive clinical course of any type of lung cancer, with median survival less than 4 months. Although SCLC is more responsive to chemotherapy and radiotherapy, long-term survival and cure are difficult to achieve due to its tendency to disseminate early and widely. However, for patients with limited stage SCLC (confined to the hemithorax of origin), a median survival up to 24 months and 5-year survivals around 15–20% can be achieved [21]. Comparatively, a higher 5-year survival rates around 20% observed in Hong Kong and Republic of Korea may be a reflection of the wider accessibility to curative treatments in their health services, although some over-estimation cannot be ruled out.

The single most important risk factor for the development of lung cancer is tobacco smoking, as reflected by the fact that the risk for lung cancer is on an average tenfold higher than in lifetime non-smokers (defined as a person who has smoked <100 cigarettes in their lifetime). The risk increases with the quantity of cigarettes or smoking products (such as bidis or cigars), duration of smoking, and starting age. Smoking cessation results in a decrease in precancerous lesions and a reduction in the risk of developing lung cancer. However, former smokers continue to have an elevated risk for lung cancer for years after quitting.

Screening does not reduce mortality from lung cancer and would lead to false-positive tests and unnecessary invasive diagnostic procedures and treatments. Given the poor prospects for screening, early diagnosis and treatment to cure lung cancers, tobacco control offers the most cost-effective way of controlling it. Significant reductions in lung cancer mortality in developed countries such as the US, UK and Nordic countries have been due to their success in reducing consumption of tobacco by a variety of tobacco control measures including education, ban on tobacco advertisements, legislation, taxation and pricing. The incidence of and mortality from lung cancer is showing an increasing trend in many low- and medium-resourced countries due to failure to control tobacco use, and this trend should be reversed. Every effort should be taken to keep lung cancer incidence rates as low as possible in developing countries.

Breast cancer (Tables 3, 4f; Figures 1n, 2k, 5a–5b)

Five year survival rates exceeded 75% in Hong Kong SAR, Shanghai and Tianjin in mainland China, Singapore, the Republic of Korea, and Izmir in Turkey, indicating better care in terms of early diagnosis as well as availability and accessibility to surgery, radiotherapy and systemic hormone and chemotherapeutic treatments (Table 3). The survival experience in Hong Kong was similar to that reported for US-SEER White patients [9] and that of Singapore and the Republic of Korea are similar to figures reported from Europe [2]. There is considerable diagnostic mammography and ultrasonography activity in the health services in the Republic of Korea, Hong Kong, Singapore and Turkey, which would have led to much earlier detection of breast cancers in these health services. Screening mammography in women aged 40 to 70 years decreases breast cancer mortality, although to a higher extent in women aged 50–70 years [22]. The value of mass screening programmes using clinical and breast self-examination remain unclear.

Survival ranged between 65% and 70% in Costa Rica, Cuba, Saudi Arabia and in some regions of Thailand. The lowest survival, around 13%, was reported from The Gambia, which has no cancer-directed treatment available in the health services. The five-year survival observed in the capital cities of Uganda (46%) and Zimbabwe (58%), even with the limited cancer surgery, radiotherapy and chemotherapy available there, indicates the good prognosis from breast cancer that can be achieved with basic local (primary tumour directed) and systemic treatment. Survival rates ranged between 31% and 54% in different regions of India and 57% and 65% in Thailand (Table 3).

The 5-year survival for localized breast cancer was 90% in the more-developed health services of Singapore and Turkey, whereas it was 76% in the less-developed health services in Thailand, India and Costa Rica, among other countries (Figure 5a). However there was a wide difference (29 percentage points) between the survival outcomes for regional disease (indicating larger tumours or local spread to skin or chest wall or lymph nodes) between the two health care settings. In fact, the survival experience of patients with regional disease in Singapore and Turkey are similar to that of localized breast cancer patients in India and Thailand among other countries, and the two survival curves superimpose on each other (Figure 5b). Although some misclassification between localized and regional disease cannot be ruled out, inter-country differences in the availability and accessibility to early detection and appropriate treatment are predominantly responsible for this observation.

Breast cancer incidence rates are increasing steadily in all low- and medium-resource countries, and it is the most common cancer among women in many countries. The cause of breast cancer is not known, although risk factors such as family history of breast or ovarian cancer (particularly first-degree relatives on either the mother's or father's side); early age at menarche and late age at first childbirth, menopausal hormone use, obesity, and alcohol intake have been identified to increase the risk. Early detection and appropriate treatment are the currently available methods of preventing breast cancer deaths. The prognostic factors affecting survival outcome include the clinical stage of disease, menopausal status of the patient, histology and grade of the tumour, oestrogen (ER) and progesterone receptor (PR) status, and human epidermal growth factor receptor (HER2/neu) gene amplification status, all of which influence the choice of treatments.

Patients with breast cancer require a multimodal approach to curative treatment. Surgery is central to its management, and surgical options for breast cancer include breast-conserving surgery plus radiation therapy or mastectomy plus reconstruction or mastectomy alone. The axillary lymph nodes should be explored and histologically studied to aid in determining treatment and prognosis. Axillary node dissection, in the presence of clinically negative nodes, is a necessary staging procedure; controversy exists as to the extent of the procedure because of long-term morbidity (e.g., arm discomfort and swelling) associated with it. Lymphatic mapping and sentinel lymph node biopsy may be used in women with invasive breast cancer to decrease the morbidity of axillary lymphadenectomy while maintaining accurate staging. Radiation therapy is regularly employed after breast-conservation surgery. Adjuvant radiotherapy for post-mastectomy patients may be used to eradicate residual disease, thus reducing local recurrence. Approximately 5 years of adjuvant hormone therapy with tamoxifen is indicated in patients with ER positive cancers, and reduces the annual breast cancer death rate by 31%, irrespective of the use of chemotherapy and of age, progesterone receptor status, or other characteristics [23]. Ovarian ablation is another useful and feasible adjuvant systemic treatment option in premenopausal women. Adjuvant combination chemotherapy reduces annual risk of relapse and death by 37% and 30%, respectively, which translates into a 10% absolute improvement in 15-year survival (hazard ratio = 42% vs. 32%) in women under 50 years; for women over of 50 years, these values were 19%, 12% and 3%, respectively [23]. The 15-year cumulative reduction in mortality from 6 months of an anthracycline-based regimen (e.g. fluorouracil, doxorubicin, cyclophosphamide [FAC] or fluorouracil, epirubicin, cyclophosphamide [FEC]) was 38% in women younger than 50 years, and 20% in those aged 50 to 60 years.

The wide variation in breast cancer survival (from 13% to 90%) in our study indicates the vast potential for improving survival outcomes by ensuring early detection, resulting in the diagnosis of very small tumours (<2 cms) without axillary node metastasis, adequate staging and combined modality treatment and follow-up care. We believe that the higher survival rates in countries with well-developed health services are direct consequences of the above factors. Investing in improving breast awareness as well as the infrastructure and efficiency of health services is vital to achieve such cure rates as high as 90% 5-year survival.

Genital tract cancers in women (Tables 3, 4g-4h; Figures 1o-1p, 2l, 2m and 6a–7b)

Five-year survival rates exceeded 75% for cervical cancer in Hong Kong and the Republic of Korea, and 65% in Singapore. On the other hand, survival was less than 25% in The Gambia and Uganda (Table 3). The prognosis for patients with cervical cancer depends on the clinical extent of disease at the time of diagnosis. Early stage (stage I) cervical cancers may be treated by radical surgery or radical radiotherapy combining external beam therapy and intracavitary radiation. Surgery and radiation therapy are equally effective for early-stage small-volume disease, whereas locally advanced disease (stages II and III) are treated by a concurrent combination of radiotherapy and chemotherapy with cisplatinum containing combinations. Although clinical trials demonstrate significant survival benefit and reduced risk of death from cervical cancer for the concurrent chemoradiation therapy in regional disease, radiotherapy alone is still used for treating locally advanced regional disease due to the cost and limited availability of chemotherapeutic agents in many low-resource countries.

The 5-year survival for localized cervix cancer patients in our study was 70% in countries with well-developed health services and 73% in those less-developed services (Figure 6a). The lack of variation in the survival outcome of localized cervix cancer patients and the minimal difference in the outcome for locally advanced regional disease in these two groups of countries is interesting (Figure 6b). This probably indicates that facilities for cervical cancer treatment were not found wanting in these countries. Cervical cancer screening with Pap smear is widespread in Hong Kong, Singapore, the Republic of Korea and Costa Rica. Cervical cancer cases in these countries are more likely to be diagnosed in those who did not participate in screening and such cases may have a poor prognosis.

Cervical cancers are caused by persistent infection with one of the oncogenic human papilloma virus (HPV) types, and HPV vaccination is an emerging prevention option. While Pap smear screening has already reduced cervical cancer mortality in developed countries, new screening approaches such as HPV testing seem to be a more effective way of preventing cervical cancer [24,25] particularly in low-resource settings, with the eventual availability of affordable and rapid HPV tests [26] and when HPV vaccination becoming widespread, thereby reducing the prevalence of cervical precancerous lesions. In countries where HPV testing is not feasible due to costs and infrastructure, visual screening may provide an alternative screening option [27], but the subjective nature of the test, variations in test positivity and sensitivity, quality assurance and low specificity may pose challenges to obtaining optimum cost-effectiveness in routine health care settings. The commercial availability of affordable HPV tests such as the careHPV test [26] may make HPV testing feasible as a primary screening approach for cervical cancer in low- and medium-resource settings.

Five-year survival of ovarian cancer patients was less than 30% in India and Uganda and was above 60% in Hong Kong, Singapore and the Republic of Korea with well-developed health services (Table 3). The case mix between epithelial, germ cell and borderline ovarian malignancies, as well as the diagnostic practices, should be taken into account when interpreting overall survival from ovarian cancer. There was 20 percentage points difference in the 5-year survival outcome for localized ovarian cancer between countries with well developed health services and others with less developed services (Figure 7a). On the other hand, there were no major survival differences between these countries for locally advanced regional disease (Figure 7b).

Most patients with ovarian cancer have widespread disease at presentation due to early spread of tumour and symptoms such as abdominal pain and swelling, gastrointestinal symptoms, and pelvic pain often going unrecognized, leading to diagnostic delays. The most favourable prognostic factors for epithelial ovarian cancer include early stage (stage I), young age, cell types other than mucinous and clear cell, well-differentiated tumour, smaller disease volume prior to surgical debulking, absence of ascites and smaller disease volume following cytoreductive surgery.

Stages IA and IB ovarian cancer patients are treated with total abdominal hysterectomy and bilateral salpingo-oophorectomy with omentectomy. However, those with high-grade or adherent stage I or IC tumours will require systemic chemotherapy based on platinum compounds or in combination with alkylating agents. Patients with locally advanced ovarian cancer are treated with debulking cytoreductive surgery and platinum containing chemotherapy regimes. Surgery should include total abdominal hysterectomy and bilateral salpingo-oophorectomy with omentectomy and debulking of as much gross tumour as can be safely performed.

Germ cell tumours of the ovary are diagnosed most often in young women or adolescent girls. They are mostly unilateral and are highly curable if found and treated early. Use of combination chemotherapy after initial surgery has dramatically improved the prognosis for most ovarian germ cell tumours.

Urinary tract cancers (Table 3, Figures 1r, 2o and 8a–8b)

The 5-year survival exceeded 55% for kidney cancer in Hong Kong, Singapore, the Republic of Korea, and urban mainland China while it was less than 40% in India, Thailand and rural China (Qidong) which might be related to the ability of the health services to provide prompt diagnostic and surgical services (Table 3). This is again reflected by survival rates exceeding 70% observed for bladder cancer in Hong Kong, Singapore, the Republic of Korea, and urban mainland China as compared to less than 50% survival in other countries (Table 3). There was a 17 percentage point difference in the 5-year survival rate of localized bladder cancer and a 10 percentage point difference for regional disease between countries with highly developed and less developed health services (Figure 8a). Radical surgery is the mainstay of curative treatment for both kidney and bladder cancers. Five-year survival exceeded 85% for testicular cancer in Hong Kong, Singapore and the Republic of Korea (Table 3). Testicular cancers are treated by both surgery and chemotherapy, and the sustained availability of such services ensure high cure rates. The survival outcome for testicular cancer in countries such as India, Thailand and mainland China are highly encouraging and reflect the good prognosis for testicular cancer using currently available treatment options.

Lymphomas (Table 3; Figures 1t, 1u, 2p-2q and 9a–10b)

The 5-year survival rate exceeded 75% for Hodgkin lymphoma (HL) in Hong Kong, urban mainland China, Singapore and Republic of Korea, whereas it ranged between 37% and 58% in Cuba, India and half of the regions in Thailand (Table 3). HL is predominantly treated with radiotherapy (in early stages: non-bulky IA or IIA disease) and/or combination chemotherapy (in advanced stages: stages III and IV, bulky disease, presence of B-symptoms). These high survival figures reinforce the fact that more than 75% of all newly diagnosed patients with adult HL can be cured with combination chemotherapy and/or radiation therapy. The prognosis depends upon the stage of disease, presence or absence of symptoms, presence or absence of large masses, absolute sites of nodal involvement, extent of abdominal involvement and the quality of treatment.

There are 27-29 percentage points difference in the 5-year survival of HL between countries categorized as "High" with well-developed and as "Low" with less-developed health services (Figure 9a). On the other hand, the survival difference between countries classified as "Intermediate" with moderately-developed health services in India, mainland China, Thailand, and Cuba and less-developed services in sub-Saharan Africa are minimal, possibly indicating that sub-optimal treatments may have similar outcomes given the generally good prognosis for HL (Figure 9b).

The non-Hodgkin lymphomas (NHL) are characterized by a heterogeneous group of lymphoproliferative malignancies with variable clinical behaviour and responses to treatment. The clinical course of NHL is much less predictable than HL, and has high tendency to disseminate to extra nodal sites. The prognosis depends on the histologic type, stage, and treatment. The 5-year survival for NHL is much lower than for HL. The overall survival from NHL depends upon the case mix between indolent and aggressive NHL. Indolent NHL types have a relatively good prognosis, with a median survival as long as 10 years. Early-stage (stages I and II) indolent NHL can be effectively treated with radiation therapy alone, but NHL is usually not curable in advanced clinical stages. The aggressive type of NHL has a shorter natural history, but a significant number of these patients can be cured with intensive combination chemotherapy regimens. Aggressive lymphomas are common in HIV-positive patients, and treatment of these patients requires special consideration. Thus NHL assumes a special significance in regions with high prevalence of HIV infection such as sub-Saharan Africa. In general, with modern treatment of patients with NHL, overall survival at 5-years is approximately 50% to 60%. The survival for NHL ranges between 49% to 65% in Hong Kong, Singapore and the Republic of Korea, is lower than 50% in other Asian countries and less than 25% in the Gambia, Uganda and Zimbabwe (Table 3). The differences in outcome for NHL between these countries are striking (Figures 10a-b), and are possibly explained by the capacity of the health services to provide diagnosis, histological typing, accurate staging and appropriate treatment.

Conclusion

In summary, our results imply that the levels of development of health services and their efficiency in providing early diagnosis, treatment and clinical follow-up care have a profound impact on survival from cancer. Survival outcomes were higher in countries with highly-developed health services than in countries with less-developed services. The critical concentration of trained human resources for cancer control is definitely higher in developed health care services.

The large variation in survival observed within populations in different regions of China, India and Thailand reflects the varying levels of development of cancer health services and the availability of trained personnel within these countries, particularly in urban vs. rural areas. All three regions in the Republic of Korea showed no major differences in survival for any cancer, possibly reflecting equitably developed and accessible health care services across the country. The poor survival rates observed in The Gambia, Uganda and Zimbabwe emphasize the importance and urgent need for direct vertical investments to improve health services and to generate sufficient trained human resources by national governments of sub-Saharan African and other developing countries. It is quite likely that the survival rates in many low- and medium-resourced countries that were not included in this study, particularly those from sub-Saharan Africa, would be lower than those reported in our study.

This study would not have been possible without the availability of reliable population-based cancer registries. It is important to organize such information systems in the regions/countries that lack them. However, the registries must collect more reliable information on clinical stages, particularly in terms of composite clinical stages and Tumour, Node, Metastasis (TNM) categories according to internationally-accepted stage classifications and summary treatment data to explain the observed survival patterns and differences between different populations in a convincing manner. The staging information in terms of composite stages and/or TNM categories should be collected at least for treatable forms of cancers such as oral cavity, larynx, breast, cervix, ovary, lymphomas and childhood cancers. Treatment information in terms of proportions of patients completing prescribed treatment will be an important measure of health service efficiency and will be useful to describe observed survival variations.

Striking differences in cancer survival between countries reflect the large inequality in accessible and available cancer health services for populations across the world, and such inequality is clearly unacceptable. Health services need to be upgraded for cancers where there exist marked differences in survival for localized cancer between well-developed and less-developed countries. Urgent and adequate investment by countries in comprehensive cancer control, including improving public and professional awareness, early detection, prompt treatment using locally feasible yet effective regimens, health services infrastructure, human resources development and referral pathways, will reduce such inequality and ensure improved and equitable accessibility to health services. The current data can serve as a baseline to evaluate improvements in cancer control and cancer health services in the future.

References

1. Jensen OM, Parkin DM, Maclennan R, Muir CS, Skeet RG. *Cancer Registration Principles and Methods: IARC Scientific Publications No. 95.* IARCPress, Lyon, 1999.

2. Sant M, Allemani C, Santaquilani M, Knijn A, Marchesi F, Capocaccia R; EUROCARE Working Group. EUROCARE-4. Survival of cancer patients diagnosed in 1995-1999. Results and commentary. *Eur J Cancer*. 2009;45:

931–991.

3. World Health Organization. *International Statistical Classification of Diseases and Related Health Problems, Tenth Revision (ICD-10), Volume 1.* World Health Organization, Geneva, 1992.

4. Swaminathan R, Rama R, Shanta V. Lack of active follow-up of cancer patients in Chennai, India: implications for population based survival estimates. *Bull World Health Organ.* 2008;86:509–515.

5. Sriamporn S, Swaminathan R, Parkin DM, Kamsa-Ard S, Hakama M. Loss-adjusted survival of cervix cancer in Khon Kaen, Northeast Thailand. *Br J Cancer.* 2004; 91:106–110.

6. Swaminathan R, Sankaranarayanan R, Hakama M, Shanta V. Effect of loss to follow-up on population based cancer survival rates in developing countries. *Int J Cancer Suppl.* 2002; 13:172 (18th UICC Cancer Congress, 30 June - 5 July 2002, Oslo - Norway - abstract book).

7. Harrison LB, Sessions RB, Hong WK, eds. *Head and Neck Cancer: A Multidisciplinary Approach.* Lippincott-Raven, Philadelphia, 1999.

8. Cummings CW, Fredrickson JM, Harker LA, Krause CJ, Schuller DE, eds. *Otolaryngology - Head and Neck Surgery.* Mosby-Year Book, Inc., Saint Louis, 1998.

9. Ries LAG, Harkins D, Krapcho M, Mariotto A, Miller BA, Feuer EJ, Clegg L, Eisner MP, Horner MJ, Howlader N, Hayat M, Hankey BF and Edwards BK (eds). *SEER Cancer Statistics Review, 1975-2003.* National Cancer Institute. Bethesda, MD, 2006. http://seer.cancer.gov/csr/1975_2003/

10. World Health Organization. International Agency for Research on Cancer. *IARC Monographs on the Evaluation of Carcinogenic Risks to Human. IARC Monographs, Volume 83. Tobacco Smoke and Involuntary Smoking.* IARCPress, Lyon, 2004.

11. World Health Organization. International Agency for Research on Cancer. *IARC Monographs on the Evaluation of Carcinogenic Risks to Human. IARC Monographs, Volume 85. Betel-quid and Areca-nut Chewing and Some Areca-nut derived Nitrosamines.* IARCPress, Lyon, 2004.

12. World Health Organization. International Agency for Research on Cancer. *IARC Monographs on the Evaluation of Carcinogenic Risks to Humans. IARC Monographs Vol. 44. Alcohol Drinking.* IARCPress, Lyon, 1988.

13. Sankaranarayanan R, Ramadas K, Thomas G, Muwonge R, Thara S, Mathew B, Rajan B Trivandrum Oral Cancer Screening Study Group. Effect of screening on oral cancer mortality in Kerala, India: a cluster-randomised controlled trial. *Lancet.* 2005;365:1927–1933.

14. Siewert JR, Böttcher K, Stein HJ, Roder JD. Relevant prognostic factors in gastric cancer: ten-year results of the German Gastric Cancer Study. *Ann Surg.* 1998;228:449–461.

15. Nakamura K, Ueyama T, Yao T, Xuan ZX, Ambe K, Adachi Y, Yakeishi Y, Matsukuma A, Enjoji M. Pathology and prognosis of gastric carcinoma. Findings in 10,000 patients who underwent primary gastrectomy. *Cancer.* 1992;70:1030–1037.

16. Compton CC, Greene FL. The staging of colorectal cancer: 2004 and beyond. *CA Cancer J Clin.* 2004;54: 295–308.

17. Soetikno RM, Kaltenbach T, Rouse RV, Park W, Maheshwari A, Sato T, Matsui S, Friedland S. Prevalence of nonpolypoid (flat and depressed) colorectal neoplasms in asymptomatic and symptomatic adults. *JAMA.* 2008;299:1027–1035.

18. Zhang BH, Yang BH, Tang ZY. Randomized controlled trial of screening for hepatocellular carcinoma. *J Cancer Res Clin Oncol.* 2004;130:417–422.

19. Chen JG, Parkin DM, Chen QG, Lu JH, Shen QJ, Zhang BC, Zhu YR. Screening for liver cancer: results of a randomised controlled trial in Qidong, China. *J Med Screen.* 2003;10:204–209.

20. Chang MH, You SL, Chen CJ, Liu CJ, Lee CM, Lin SM, Chu HC, Wu TC, Yang SS, Kuo HS, Chen DS; Taiwan Hepatoma Study Group. Decreased incidence of hepatocellular carcinoma in hepatitis B vaccinees: a 20-year follow-up study. *J Natl Cancer Inst.* 2009;101: 1348–1355.

21. Jänne PA, Freidlin B, Saxman S, Johnson DH, Livingston RB, Shepherd FA, Johnson BE. Twenty-five years of clinical research for patients with limited-stage small cell lung carcinoma in North America. *Cancer.* 2002;95:1528–1538.

22. World Health Organization. International Agency for Research on Cancer. *IARC Handbook of Cancer Prevention, Volume 7. Breast Cancer Screening.* IARCPress, Lyon, 2002.

23. Early Breast Cancer Trialists' Collaborative Group (EBCTCG). Effects of chemotherapy and hormonal ther-

apy for early breast cancer on recurrence and 15-year survival: an overview of the randomised trials. *Lancet*. 2005;365:1687–1717.

24. Denny L, Kuhn L, De Souza M, Pollack AE, Dupree W, Wright TC Jr. Screen-and-treat approaches for cervical cancer prevention in low-resource settings: a randomized controlled trial. *JAMA*. 2005;294:2173–2181.

25. Sankaranarayanan R, Nene BM, Shastri SS, Jayant K, Muwonge R, Budukh AM, Hingmire S, Malvi SG, Thorat R, Kothari A, Chinoy R, Kelkar R, Kane S, Desai S, Keskar VR, Rajeshwarkar R, Panse N, Dinshaw KA. HPV screening for cervical cancer in rural India. *N Engl J Med*. 2009;360:1385–1394.

26. Qiao YL, Sellors JW, Eder PS, Bao YP, Lim JM, Zhao FH, Weigl B, Zhang WH, Peck RB, Li L, Chen F, Pan QJ, Lorincz AT. A new HPV-DNA test for cervical-cancer screening in developing regions: a cross-sectional study of clinical accuracy in rural China. *Lancet Oncol*. 2008;9:929–936.

27. Sankaranarayanan R, Esmy PO, Rajkumar R, Muwonge R, Swaminathan R, Shanthakumari S, Fayette JM, Cherian J. Effect of visual screening on cervical cancer incidence and mortality in Tamil Nadu, India: a cluster-randomized trial. *Lancet*. 2007;370:398–406.

Table 1. An overview of follow-up methods practised by the registries and countries

Follow-up of incident cancer cases carried out by			
Active method only	**Predominantly active method**	**Predominantly passive method**	**Passive method only**
The Gambia	**China**	**China**	**China**
India	Qidong	Shanghai	Hong Kong SAR
Barshi	**Philippines**	Tianjin	**Singapore**
Bhopal	Manila	**Costa Rica**	
Chennai	Rizal	**Cuba**	
Karunagappally	**Thailand**	**Saudi Arabia**	
Mumbai	Khon Kaen	Riyadh	
Pakistan		**Republic of Korea**	
South Karachi		Busan	
Thailand		Incheon	
Chiang Mai		Seoul	
Songkhla		**Thailand**	
Turkey		Lampang	
Izmir			
Uganda			
Kampala			
Zimbabwe			
Harare			

Table 2. Major cancer sites/types by number of registries and countries reported

Major cancer site/type	ICD-10 code	Number of registries	Number of countries
Tongue	C01-02	18	7
Oral cavity	C03-06	19	7
Tonsil	C09-10	14	7
Nasopharynx	C11	14	6
Hypopharynx	C12-13	15	5
Oesophagus	C15	18	7
Stomach	C16	19	8
Colon	C18	19	10
Rectum	C19-20	22	11
Liver	C22	15	7
Gall bladder	C23-24	11	4
Pancreas	C25	14	5
Nose/Sinuses	C30-31	11	4
Larynx	C32	20	8
Lung	C33-34	19	8
Bone	C40-41	11	4
Skin melanoma	C43	12	5
Skin others	C44	13	5
Mesothelioma	C45	5	3
Kaposi sarcoma	C46	2	2
Connective tissue	C47; C49	11	4
Breast	C50	26	13
Cervix uteri	C51	24	12
Corpus uteri	C54	11	4
Ovary	C56	19	8
Penis	C60	11	5
Prostate	C61	14	6
Testis	C62	9	5
Kidney/Renal pelvis	C64-66	12	5
Bladder	C67	19	8
Eye	C69	7	4
Brain & nervous	C70-72	12	5
Thyroid	C73	13	6
Adrenal/Other endocrine	C74	7	3
Hodgkin lymphoma	C81	16	8
Non-Hodgkin lymphoma	C82-85; C96	22	10
Multiple myeloma	C90	11	6
Lymphoid leukaemia	C91	16	6
Myeloid leukaemia	C92-94	17	6

Table 3. Comparison of 5-year age-standardized relative survival of major cancer sites/types between all registries

Cancer site/type	5-year age-standardized relative survival (0-74 years), %						
	China				Costa Rica	Cuba	The Gambia
	Hong Kong SAR	Qidong	Shanghai	Tianjin			
	1996–2001	1992–2000	1992–1995	1991–1999	1995–2000	1994–1995	1993–1997
Tongue	64.0		66.9	68.2		38.9	
Oral cavity	64.5	43.8	70.9	69.2		43.7	
Tonsil	47.8[$]		62.1	68.3		51.2	
Oropharynx						55.8	
Nasopharynx	74.0	36.4	57.6	57.6			
Hypopharynx	24.1		31.0	82.3			
Oesophagus	26.4	6.1	20.6	40.3			
Stomach	41.5	20.1	36.0	44.2			2.8
Colon	63.2	42.1	54.0	61.9		46.4	
Rectum	63.4[#]	34.5	51.0	58.1		50.7	
Liver	24.6	5.4	9.8	25.8			3.2
Gall bladder	29.7	17.5	21.0	50.3			
Pancreas	19.9	6.7	9.5	31.0			
Nose/Sinuses	70.2	22.3	52.4	61.6			
Larynx	73.4	48.7	67.2	69.7		58.1	
Lung	25.1	6.4	18.0	32.3			19.7
Bone	70.1	15.2	34.0	29.8			
Skin melanoma	61.7	26.6	61.7	62.8			
Skin others	100.1	37.3	85.9	86.7			
Mesothelioma	38.1			58.1			
Kaposi sarcoma							
Connective tissue	66.5	36.2	62.9	78.7			
Breast	89.6	58.3	79.4	85.6	69.6	70.4	12.5
Cervix uteri	79.5	47.9	63.5	70.5	53.5	56.3	21.8
Corpus uteri	85.1	62.2	86.9	91.3			
Ovary	67.3	35.1	47.9	64.4			
Penis	86.8		90.7	79.0			
Prostate	78.2	36.3	54.2	68.4			
Testis	92.1		81.7	76.4			
Kidney	70.5[@]	26.7	60.3	65.7			
Renal pelvis			71.2	93.9			
Ureter			73.0	77.9			
Bladder	81.2	47.3	74.5	81.1		68.8	
Eye	51.9		79.1	100.3			
Brain & nervous	48.7	11.1	51.1	49.5			
Thyroid	95.1	76.8	91.2	89.1			
Adrenal gland	71.2[+]		69.5	69.2			
Hodgkin lymphoma	87.4		77.6	81.9		57.5	
Non-Hodgkin lymphoma	64.7	13.4	45.6	53.2		50.3	25.5
Multiple myeloma	37.8	10.9	28.1	46.1			
Lymphoid leukaemia	59.1	5.4	30.4	64.9			
Myeloid leukaemia	42.3	6.0	30.0	68.0			
Unspecified leukaemia	36.8	7.1	14.6	22.0			

[$] includes oropharynx; [#] includes anus; [@] includes renal pelvis; [+] includes other endocrine

Table 3 (Continued).

Cancer site/type	5-year age-standardized relative survival (0-74 years), %									
	India					Pakistan	Philippines		Saudi Arabia	Singapore
	Barshi	Bhopal	Chennai	Karuna-gappally	Mumbai	South Karachi	Manila	Rizal	Riyadh	
	1993-00	1991-95	1990-99	1991-97	1992-99	1995-99	1994-95	1996-97	1994-96	1993-97
Tongue	11.8	13.1	23.4	29.6	29.7	39.3				44.3
Oral cavity	26.1	37.5	36.7	45.3	36.0	40.9				49.2
Tonsil			15.6		16.6	32.3				44.7
Oropharynx			20.7		20.4					
Nasopharynx					24.7					59.2
Hypopharynx	10.0	2.0	15.0	15.5	23.1					11.9
Oesophagus	5.3	3.6	8.6	18.5	16.2					12.1
Stomach	6.0	3.8	10.3	4.1	15.2					27.4
Colon		5.2			30.3		43.5			52.5
Rectum	14.7	6.5		32.6	31.1		30.6			52.1
Liver	0.0			4.5						6.5
Gall bladder										18.3
Pancreas			8.7	4.3	15.2					4.8
Nose/Sinuses										50.4
Larynx	15.7	15.7		28.3	36.0					65.7
Lung	5.3	1.0		7.8	13.4					9.3
Bone										38.5
Skin melanoma			38.0							44.5
Skin others	75.3		7.1	83.7						95.2
Mesothelioma										11.4
Kaposi sarcoma										
Soft tissue sarcoma										57.1
Breast	52.7	30.6	47.7	54.4	51.6		55.0	39.7	64.5	76.4
Cervix uteri	35.7	34.5	59.6	57.8	46.4		37.4			65.7
Corpus uteri										79.6
Ovary		18.9	28.5	27.8	22.9					62.4
Penis	64.1				53.3					74.8
Prostate				32.6	42.3					64.3
Testis					56.2					88.2
Kidney					35.2					55.0
Renal pelvis										43.9
Ureter										
Bladder		9.7	32.0	48.4	45.6					71.9
Eye										
Brain & nervous				16.2						29.6
Thyroid				90.0						91.2
Adrenal gland										32.1
Hodgkin lymphoma			37.8		52.2					75.4
Non-Hodgkin lymphoma	25.9	9.9	23.2	39.8	37.1					52.0
Multiple myeloma				13.4						26.0
Lymphoid leukaemia		12.6	16.4	45.6	15.5					42.9
Myeloid leukaemia	19.5	14.2	14.9	8.2	15.2					22.6
Unspecified leukaemia			11.2		7.1					12.9

Table 3 (Continued).

Cancer site/type	5-year age-standardized relative survival (0-74 years), %									
	Republic of Korea			Thailand				Turkey	Uganda	Zimbabwe
	Busan	Incheon	Seoul	Chiang Mai	Khon Kaen	Lampang	Songkhla	Izmir	Kampala	Harare[$]
	1996-01	1997-01	1993-97	1993-97	1993-97	1990-00	1990-99	1995-97	1993-97	1993-97
Tongue	52.8	52.0	59.6	24.3	32.4	33.2	31.4			
Oral cavity	48.4	54.4	51.6	22.0	41.9	37.2	35.3			
Tonsil	57.9	48.4	58.3	30.6		43.4	13.5			
Oropharynx	20.9		42.8							
Nasopharynx	53.2	53.6	47.1	41.5	34.6	39.9	47.4		0.0	
Hypopharynx	23.5	38.3	31.3	30.0		32.8	24.0			
Oesophagus	20.5	25.9	22.8	6.4		26.8	9.9		3.0	12.3
Stomach	46.5	50.0	49.2	12.1		20.4	8.8		0.0	22.8
Colon	57.0	57.4	65.7	32.5	44.3	39.4	52.8	52.2	8.2	28.6
Rectum	57.3	57.6	61.5	30.4	42.8	36.8	31.9	52.0	10.1	30.3
Liver	10.0	16.8	20.3	3.3		11.9	2.5		1.4	3.7
Gall bladder	21.8	25.3	30.3	6.4		18.5	14.4			
Pancreas	7.4	14.2	17.1	10.6		15.0	15.9			
Nose/Sinuses	39.3	63.4	50.9	30.8		50.7	25.9			
Larynx	58.9	61.6	75.6	28.0	26.5	49.1	44.6	71.4		29.7
Lung	13.7	20.6	19.7	4.8		12.1	8.6		0.0	11.4
Bone	39.7	46.9	39.8	8.5		19.9	27.5			
Skin melanoma	48.1	71.5	49.5	23.3		46.2	53.8			77.4
Skin others	89.4	85.4	92.6	59.2		85.4	76.6			
Mesothelioma	17.0		40.8							
Kaposi sarcoma									35.6	4.4
Connective tissue	40.8	55.6	55.7	44.6		52.6	32.0			
Breast	80.6	78.5	78.6	57.3	65.6	63.3	62.4	77.2	45.8	57.8
Cervix uteri	75.8	79.5	79.2	60.0	53.9	63.3	61.3	63.5	13.1	39.1
Corpus uteri	74.3	72.3	81.7	64.4		74.4	72.5			
Ovary	54.5	58.7	62.2	44.7	58.1	46.3	48.7	59.7	8.6	34.0
Penis	73.0		77.5	36.7		73.1	64.6			
Prostate	59.5	69.4	70.2	35.0		58.3	32.7		47.2	
Testis	72.2	98.3	93.9			61.1				
Kidney	64.1	67.9	70.3	23.1		29.0	37.0			
Renal pelvis	54.6	72.3	71.1			28.0				
Ureter	68.1	91.0	57.5							
Bladder	72.8	76.1	79.5	33.2	59.7	49.5	45.9	70.7		37.2
Eye	59.3		58.1						35.7	69.9
Brain & nervous	37.5	41.0	38.9	16.4		43.4	31.1			
Thyroid	93.0	92.6	94.4	65.4		73.1	86.9		10.8	
Adrenal gland	32.3[+]	78.4	31.6							
Hodgkin lymphoma	76.9	82.8	76.3	73.1	67.7	56.4	55.9	65.8		46.5
Non-Hodgkin lymphoma	49.0	57.4	58.0	28.1	39.3	44.3	47.7	50.6	25.1	26.0
Multiple myeloma	14.5	29.0	32.0				32.3	31.1		
Lymphoid leukaemia	32.7	40.3	38.5	15.4		44.1	36.5	50.1		
Myeloid leukaemia	27.5	36.0	26.3	10.9		35.0	15.4	34.2		
Unspecified leukaemia	6.1		16.8	11.0		12.9	17.0			

[$] *all races together; + includes other endocrine glands*

Table 4a. Frequency and 5-year absolute survival by clinical extent of disease for all registries: cancer of the tongue

Country/ registry	Period of registration	Frequency (%) L	R	D	U	5-year absolute survival (%) L	R	D	U
Cuba	1994–1995	35.5	39.8	2.2	22.5	46.7	27.3	20.0	16.8
India									
Bhopal	1991–1995	39.4	55.9	0.0	4.7	16.0	5.6	-	0.0
Chennai	1990–1999	4.4	86.8	2.6	6.2	59.2	17.3	15.4	14.7
Karunagappally	1991–1997	30.2	47.7	10.5	11.6	48.7	15.4	0.0	47.4
Mumbai	1992–1999	30.5	58.4	7.1	4.1	58.4	12.0	0.0	29.1
Pakistan									
South Karachi	1995–1999	37.8	50.6	0.6	11.0	57.4	11.7	0.0	47.6
Singapore	1993–1997	25.8	25.0	4.2	45.0	48.4	23.3	20.0	33.1
Thailand									
Lampang	1990–2000	23.6	68.4	4.0	4.0	32.6	36.2	0.0	33.3
Songkhla	1990–1999	19.9	30.6	7.1	42.3	40.0	27.9	26.0	26.0

L: localized; R: regional; D: distant metastasis; U: unknown

Table 4b. Frequency and 5-year absolute survival by clinical extent of disease for all registries: cancer of the oral cavity

Country/ registry	Period of registration	Frequency (%) L	R	D	U	5-year absolute survival (%) L	R	D	U
Cuba	1994–1995	44.2	34.6	0.4	20.8	52.6	22.2	0.0	24.4
India									
Bhopal	1991–1995	40.7	55.8	0.6	2.9	45.7	17.7	0.0	20.0
Chennai	1990–1999	3.5	88.7	2.7	5.0	54.9	30.0	10.0	30.9
Karunagappally	1991–1997	14.6	65.9	12.2	7.3	83.0	28.5	0.0	38.2
Mumbai	1992–1999	32.6	55.8	6.9	4.6	62.5	18.0	1.1	35.5
Pakistan									
South Karachi	1995–1999	36.3	53.0	0.5	10.2	58.3	18.6	-	18.3
Singapore	1993–1997	28.1	22.2	1.5	48.1	52.2	26.3	0.0	28.9
Thailand									
Lampang	1990–2000	21.2	66.1	4.2	8.5	35.6	30.7	0.0	40.0

L: localized; R: regional; D: distant metastasis; U: unknown

Table 4c. Frequency and 5-year absolute survival by clinical extent of disease for all registries: cancer of the larynx

Country/ registry	Period of registration	Frequency (%)				5-year absolute survival (%)			
		L	R	D	U	L	R	D	U
Cuba	1994–1995	51.3	23.0	1.3	24.5	65.5	34.5	10.0	22.2
India									
Chennai	1990–1999	6.6	85.5	3.6	4.3	44.3	30.3	-	34.1
Karunagappally	1991–1997	30.4	45.7	13.0	10.9	55.6	19.0	0.0	-
Mumbai	1992–1999	33.2	51.1	9.7	6.1	57.1	16.5	0.5	23.2
Singapore	1993–1997	35.7	12.2	2.3	49.8	63.6	28.6	14.3	41.8
Thailand									
Chiang Mai	1993–1997	11.8	82.4	3.8	2.0	52.4	21.4	16.7	0.0
Lampang	1990–2000	17.3	61.7	7.4	13.6	53.4	31.6	25.0	45.5
Songkhla	1990–1999	21.0	39.9	8.7	30.4	59.5	31.9	42.4	21.9
Turkey									
Izmir	1995–1997	32.1	23.0	7.5	37.4	74.8	45.1	47.6	65.8

L: localized; R: regional; D: distant metastasis; U: unknown

Table 4d. Frequency and 5-year absolute survival by clinical extent of disease for all registries: cancer of the colon

Country/ registry	Period of registration	Frequency (%)				5-year absolute survival (%)			
		L	R	D	U	L	R	D	U
Cuba	1994–1995	28.0	20.3	9.6	42.1	64.7	45.0	20.5	14.6
India									
Bhopal	1991–1995	37.5	27.1	18.8	16.7	11.1	7.7	0.0	0.0
Mumbai	1992–1999	38.7	26.7	25.9	8.7	51.8	19.1	1.6	27.5
Philippines									
Manila	1994–1995	33.8	33.1	17.9	15.2	68.9	34.3	0.0	29.2
Singapore	1993–1997	27.0	22.4	18.8	31.9	66.5	43.2	6.6	40.6
Thailand									
Chiang Mai	1993–1997	1.3	65.8	31.6	1.3	66.7	40.8	6.0	0.0
Lampang	1990–2000	8.4	44.2	33.7	13.7	60.0	56.8	2.1	37.5
Turkey									
Izmir	1995–1997	8.9	43.7	19.9	27.5	59.8	54.1	20.8	43.0

L: localized; R: regional; D: distant metastasis; U: unknown

Table 4e. Frequency and 5-year absolute survival by clinical extent of disease for all registries: cancer of the rectum

Country/ registry	Period of registration	Frequency (%)				5-year absolute survival (%)			
		L	R	D	U	L	R	D	U
Cuba	1994–1995	38.8	25.4	7.2	28.6	58.5	38.0	25.0	27.7
India									
Bhopal	1991–1995	41.0	33.3	15.4	10.3	12.5	7.7	0.0	0.0
Mumbai	1992–1999	46.2	26.0	20.3	7.5	46.5	19.8	1.6	32.4
Philippines									
Manila	1994–1995	34.0	27.2	15.5	23.3	56.0	26.4	-	23.1
Singapore	1993–1997	30.2	27.0	16.8	25.9	61.6	44.9	6.6	41.9
Thailand									
Chiang Mai	1993–1997	3.7	74.2	20.0	2.1	71.4	31.2	5.9	..
Lampang	1990–2000	9.2	59.8	17.7	13.3	42.3	41.8	4.5	48.5
Turkey									
Izmir	1995–1997	14.2	40.8	21.2	23.8	51.8	50.3	20.4	49.2

L: localized; R: regional; D: distant metastasis; U: unknown

Table 4f. Frequency and 5-year absolute survival by clinical extent of disease for all registries: cancer of the breast

Country/ registry	Period of registration	Frequency (%)				5-year absolute survival (%)			
		L	R	D	U	L	R	D	U
China									
Hong Kong SAR	1996–2001	12.2	34.6	1.5	51.7	94.9	79.1	31.8	82.7
Costa Rica	1995–2000	31.2	34.0	20.3	14.5	89.9	77.1	31.0	29.9
Cuba	1994–1995	43.5	33.3	4.9	18.3	81.6	58.9	30.2	43.3
India									
Bhopal	1991–1995	42.9	44.1	5.7	7.3	41.1	22.6	0.0	42.1
Chennai	1990–1999	1.7	67.9	13.0	17.5	70.8	48.9	12.3	46.6
Karunagappally	1991–1997	18.4	53.2	12.1	16.3	78.6	43.1	7.8	53.4
Mumbai	1992–1999	39.6	41.5	12.8	6.2	74.2	32.8	3.8	48.1
Philippines									
Manila	1994–1995	31.6	46.5	12.8	9.2	73.5	42.0	3.2	42.2
Rizal	1996–1997	17.5	43.7	9.9	28.9	65.3	35.0	11.9	34.8
Saudi Arabia									
Riyadh	1994–1996	30.9	32.6	20.8	15.7	70.4	55.7	56.7	62.3
Singapore	1993–1997	30.6	22.5	4.8	42.1	85.9	66.3	18.8	71.2
Thailand									
Chiang Mai	1993–1997	14.3	70.0	11.9	3.8	79.3	63.7	24.8	49.4
Khon Kaen	1993–1997	5.3	41.6	21.1	32.0	82.3	66.9	32.8	67.9
Lampang	1990–2000	22.5	52.9	14.2	10.4	84.1	65.2	8.2	82.5
Songkhla	1990–1999	17.1	34.7	14.4	33.8	82.8	66.2	27.0	59.6
Turkey									
Izmir	1995–1997	20.5	34.3	4.7	40.5	85.5	65.4	35.1	72.3

L: localized; R: regional; D: distant metastasis; U: unknown

Table 4g. Frequency and 5-year absolute survival by clinical extent of disease for all registries: cancer of the cervix

Country/ registry	Period of registration	Frequency (%)				5-year absolute survival (%)			
		L	R	D	U	L	R	D	U
Costa Rica	1995–2000	22.4	40.5	4.0	33.1	89.5	43.1	11.3	43.2
Cuba	1994–1995	41.3	34.3	1.7	22.7	73.9	41.5	33.3	45.0
India									
Bhopal	1991–1995	28.3	70.5	0.3	0.9	60.6	22.7	0.0	0.0
Chennai	1990–1999	6.4	86.0	3.7	3.9	69.1	55.3	12.4	43.4
Karunagappally	1991–1997	15.3	60.6	8.8	15.3	72.1	43.5	23.1	44.3
Mumbai	1992–1999	27.9	56.8	8.6	6.7	68.3	35.7	3.4	40.7
Philippines									
Manila	1994–1995	21.5	30.5	10.3	37.7	63.1	29.9	7.1	28.2
Singapore	1993–1997	45.5	5.7	5.0	43.8	69.7	48.0	20.4	55.7
Thailand									
Chiang Mai	1993–1997	26.1	69.7	3.7	0.5	81.2	52.7	12.2	75.0
Khon Kaen	1993–1997	17.3	53.8	6.3	22.6	65.1	48.7	30.6	57.0
Lampang	1990–2000	31.2	53.9	5.8	9.2	78.7	57.9	6.5	70.6
Songkhla	1990–1999	22.3	54.6	5.8	17.3	81.2	56.3	15.4	61.3
Turkey									
Izmir	1995–1997	41.8	41.8	6.1	23.2	67.7	54.6	9.3	69.1

L: localized; R: regional; D: distant metastasis; U: unknown

Table 4h. Frequency and 5-year absolute survival by clinical extent of disease for all registries: cancer of the ovary

Country/ registry	Period of registration	Frequency (%)				5-year absolute survival (%)			
		L	R	D	U	L	R	D	U
India									
Bhopal	1991–1995	66.7	8.7	13.0	11.6	21.7	33.3	0.0	12.5
Chennai	1990–1999	1.5	62.5	19.4	16.6	73.4	30.8	6.0	38.1
Karunagappally	1991–1997	17.1	11.4	54.3	17.1	100.0	0.0	8.8	44.4
Mumbai	1992–1999	28.6	11.4	49.9	10.1	59.7	27.5	3.0	26.4
Singapore	1993–1997	45.7	3.9	19.8	30.6	83.3	35.4	24.5	55.2
Thailand									
Chiang Mai	1993–1997	24.1	43.8	30.2	1.9	88.2	48.3	16.9	0.0
Khon Kaen	1993–1997	29.6	21.4	29.6	19.4	88.8	60.6	17.5	66.6
Lampang	1990–2000	22.8	34.7	30.1	12.4	86.2	56.6	0.0	75.0
Songkhla	1990–1999	24.3	28.9	12.7	34.1	92.1	30.0	19.8	43.0
Turkey									
Izmir	1995–1997	22.6	5.2	47.4	24.8	89.4	51.1	33.6	62.3

L: localized; R: regional; D: distant metastasis; U: unknown

Table 5. Classification of health services development based on a few indicators

Overall grading of health services development - Countries/ regions	GNI* (in USD)	Population* (millions)	Adult literacy[$] (%)	Diagnostic services		Treatment services			Population-based screening services	Palliative services
				Imaging	Pathology	Radiation (MeV)[a-c]	Surgery	Chemo		
A. Well developed	*9220-34 760*		*87-99*	*Extensively available and widely distributed*		*Extensively or adequately available and widely distributed*			*Routinely available*	*Adequate*
Hong Kong SAR	31 420	7.0	95	Extensively available; widely distributed		Adequately available; widely distributed *MeV: 9*	Extensively available; widely distributed	Adequately available; widely distributed	Exist	Adequate
Saudi Arabia	15 500	24.6	78	Adequate and widely distributed		Adequate and widely distributed *MeV: 27*			No	Adequate
Singapore	34 760	4.8	94	Extensively available; widely distributed *MeV: 10*					Exist	Adequate
Republic of Korea	21 530	48.6	99	Extensively available; widely distributed *MeV: 69*					Exist	Adequate
Turkey	9340	73.9	87	Extensively available; widely distributed		Adequately available; widely distributed	Extensively available; widely distributed	Adequately available; widely distributed	Exist	Adequate

* *GNI: Gross National Income per capita 2008, Atlas method. World Development Indicators Database, World Bank, 7, 2009. http://web.worldbank.org/WBSITE/EXTERNAL/DATASTATISTICS/0,,contentMDK:20535285~menuPK:1192694~pagePK:64133150~piPK:64133175~theSitePK:239419,00.html*

$ *World Health Statistics 2008 (WHO); UNDP Report 2009, Pg 171; MeV: Megavolt machines total*

Source:

a Tatsuzaki and Levin (2001). Radiotherapy and Oncology; 60: 81–89

b Zubizarreta, Poitevin and Levin (2004). Radiotherapy and Oncology; 73: 97–100

c Levin, Gueddari and Meghzifene (1999). Radiotherapy and Oncology; 52: 79–84.

Table 5. Classification of health services development based on a few indicators (continued)

Overall grading of health services development - Countries/ regions	GNI* (in USD)	Population* (millions)	Adult literacy[$] (%)	Diagnostic services		Treatment services			Population-based screening services	Palliative services
				Imaging	Pathology	Radiation (MeV)[a-c]	Surgery	Chemo		
B. Moderately developed	*980-6060*		*50-99*	*Adequate in urban; inadequate in rural*		*Variably developed even between urban areas; inadequate in rural*			*Not routinely available*	*Variably developed*
China (Mainland)	2940	1325.6	91	Adequate in urban; inadequate in rural		Adequate in urban; inadequate in rural *MeV: 667*	Adequate	Adequate in urban; inadequate in rural	Available in selected metropolitan areas	Adequate in urban; inadequate in rural
Costa Rica	6060	4.5	95	Adequately available; widely distributed		Adequately available; *MeV: 6*	Adequately available;	Adequately available;		
Cuba	>3856	11.2	99	Adequate	Adequate	Adequate *MeV: 12*	Extensive	Adequate	Available	Adequate
India	1070	1140.0	61	Adequate in urban; inadequate in rural	Adequate in metropolitan areas; not in others	Adequate in metropolitan areas; not in others *MeV: 291*	Adequate in urban; inadequate in rural	Adequate in metropolitan areas; not in others	No	Adequate in urban; inadequate in rural
Pakistan	980	166.0	50	Adequate in urban; inadequate in rural *MeV: 34*					No	Adequate in urban; inadequate in rural
Philippines	1890	90.3	93	Adequate in urban; inadequate in rural *MeV: 17*					No	Adequate
Thailand	2840	67.4	93	Adequate in urban; inadequate in rural *MeV: 50*					Available	Adequate

** GNI: Gross National Income per capita 2008, Atlas method. World Development Indicators Database, World Bank, 7, 2009. http://web.worldbank.org/WBSITE/EXTERNAL/DATASTATISTICS/0,,contentMDK:20535285~menuPK:1192694~pagePK:64133150~piPK:64133175~theSitePK:239419,00.html*

$ World Health Statistics 2008 (WHO); UNDP Report 2009, Pg 171; MeV: Megavolt machines total

a Tatsuzaki and Levin (2001). Radiotherapy and Oncology; 60: 81–89; b Zubizarreta, Poitevin and Levin (2004). Radiotherapy and Oncology; 73: 97–100

c Levin, Gueddari and Meghzifene (1999). Radiotherapy and Oncology; 52: 79–84.

Table 5. Classification of health services development based on a few indicators

Overall grading of health services development - Countries/ regions	GNI* (in USD)	Population* (millions)	Adult literacy[$] (%)	Diagnostic services		Treatment services			Screening services	Palliative services
				Imaging	Pathology	Radiation (MeV)[a-c]	Surgery	Chemo		
C. Least developed	*390-975*		*69-89*	*Inadequately developed*		*Inadequately developed and not widely distributed*			*No*	*Inadequate*
The Gambia	390	1.7	n.a.	Inadequate and not widely distributed	Not available	Not available	Available in capital city	Not widely distributed	No	Inadequate
Uganda	420	31.7	67	Inadequate	Available in capital city	Available in capital city *MeV: 2*	Adequate in capital city	Inadequate	No	Inadequate
Zimbabwe	<975	12.5	89	Adequate in capital; inadequate in others	Adequate in capital; inadequate in others	Adequate in capital; inadequate in others MeV: 5	Adequate in capital; inadequate in others	Adequate in capital; inadequate in others	No	Inadequate

** GNI: Gross National Income per capita 2008, Atlas method. World Development Indicators Database, World Bank, 7, 2009. http://web.worldbank.org/WBSITE/EXTERNAL/DATASTATISTICS/0,,contentMDK:20535285~menuPK:1192694~pagePK:64133150~piPK:64133175~theSitePK:239419,00.html*
[$] World Health Statistics 2008 (WHO); UNDP Report 2009, Pg 171; MeV: Megavolt machines total

Source:
a Tatsuzaki and Levin (2001). Radiotherapy and Oncology; 60: 81–89
b Zubizarreta, Poitevin and Levin (2004). Radiotherapy and Oncology; 73: 97–100
c Levin, Gueddari and Meghzifene (1999). Radiotherapy and Oncology; 52: 79–84.

Figure 1. 5-year age-standardized relative survival (ASRS%; 0-74 years) by country and cancer site/type *(median {minimum-maximum} of values if more than one registry is contributing)*

Figure 1a. Tongue

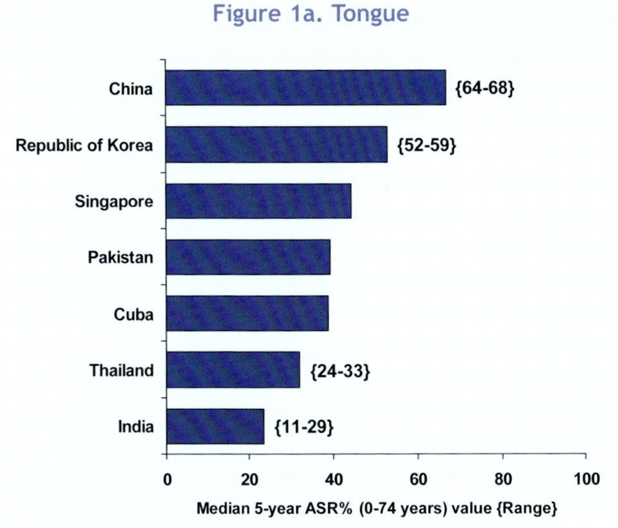

Figure 1d. Nasopharynx

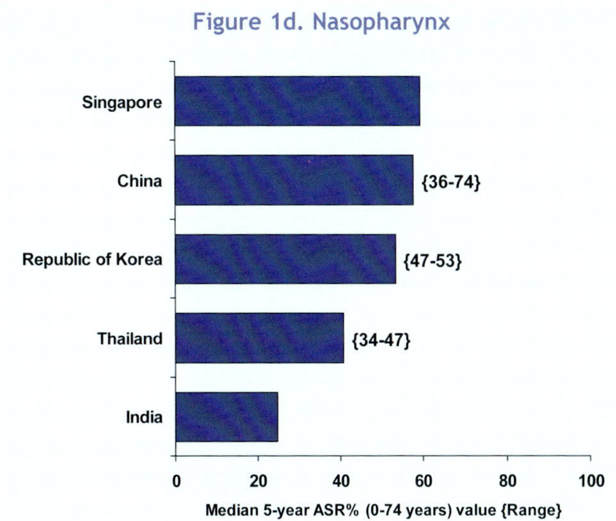

Figure 1b. Oral cavity

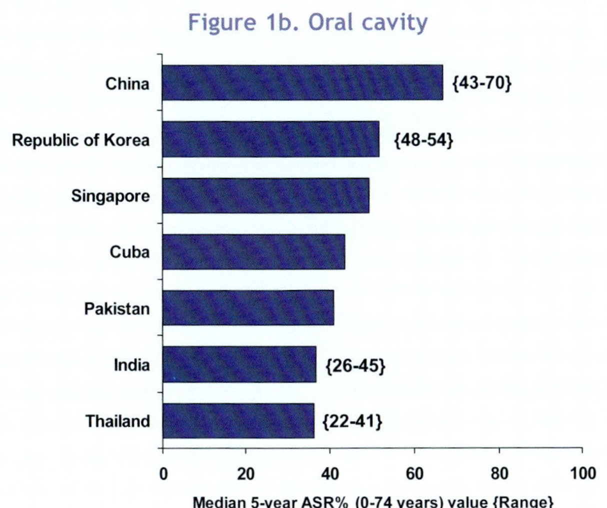

Figure 1e. Hypopharynx

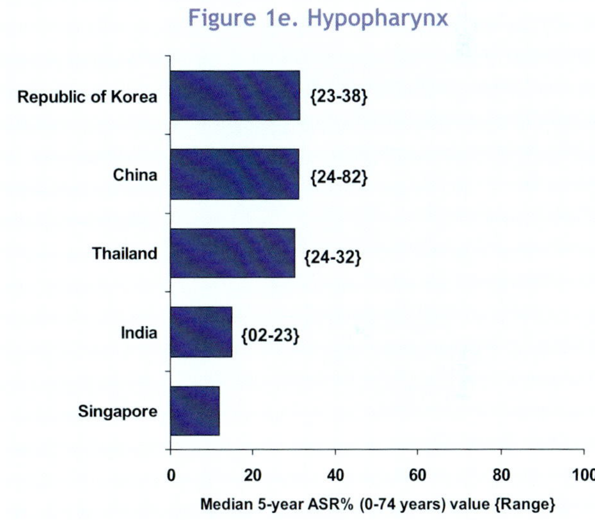

Figure 1c. Tonsil

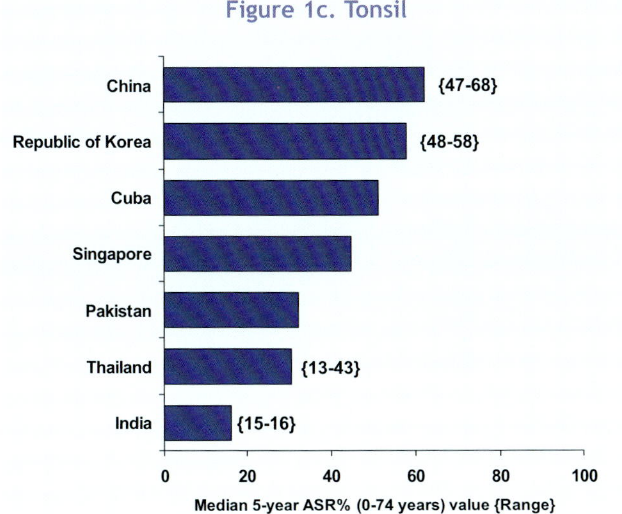

Figure 1f. Oesophagus

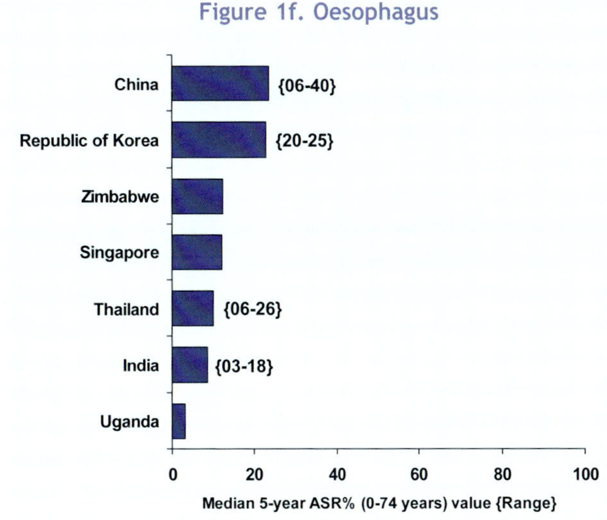

Figure 1 (Continued).

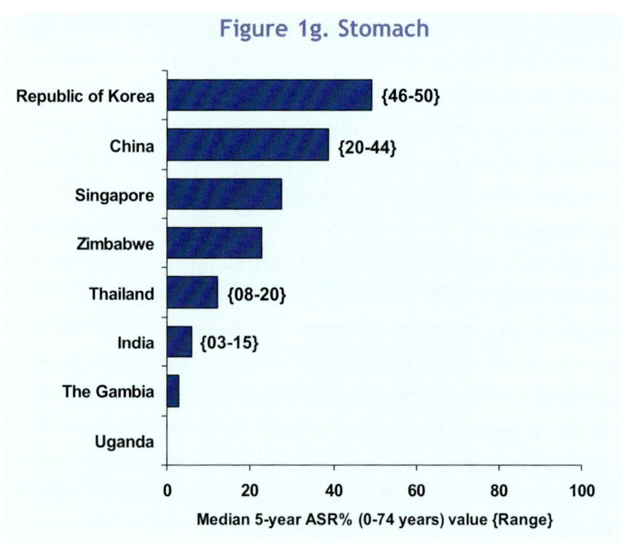

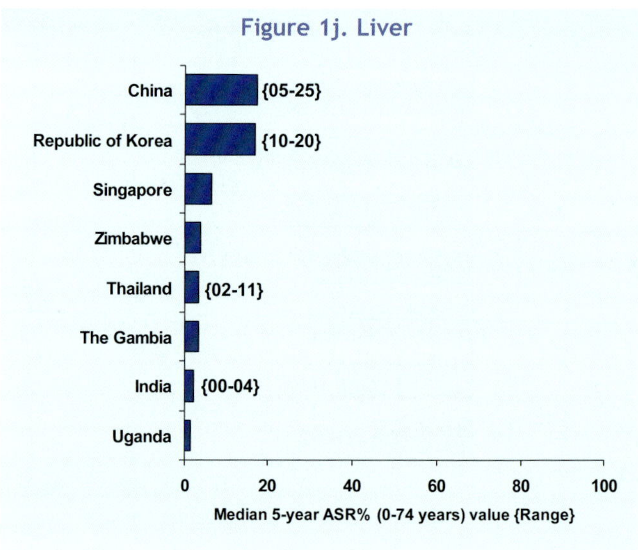

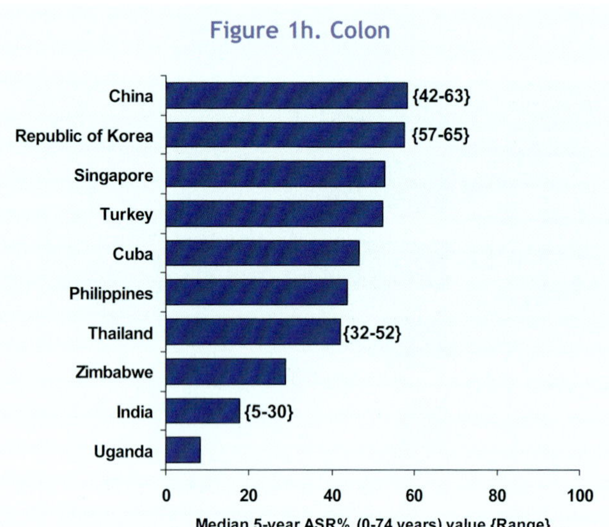

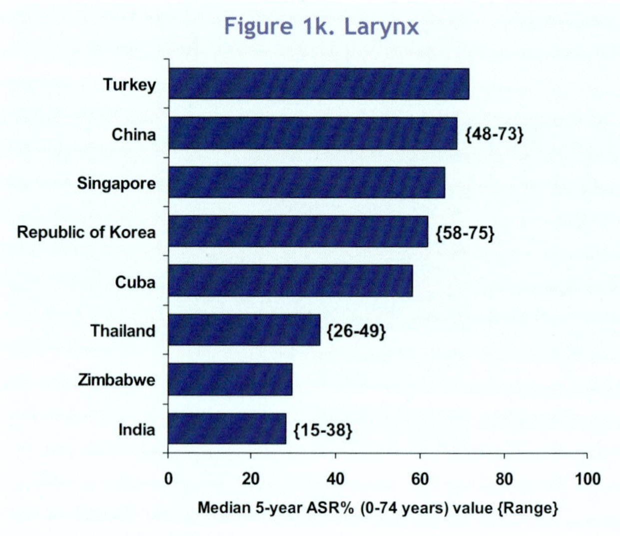

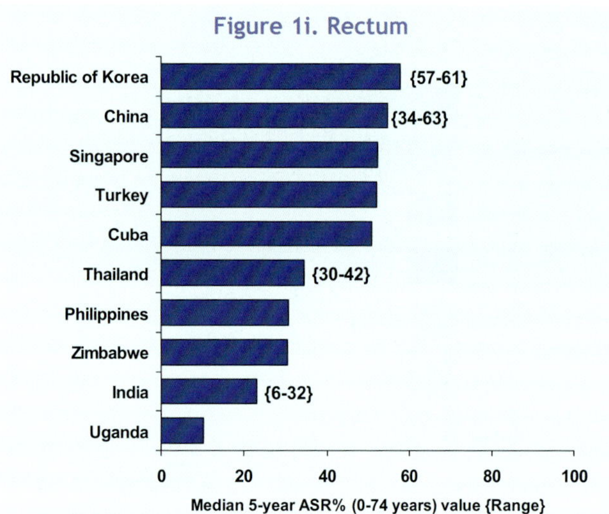

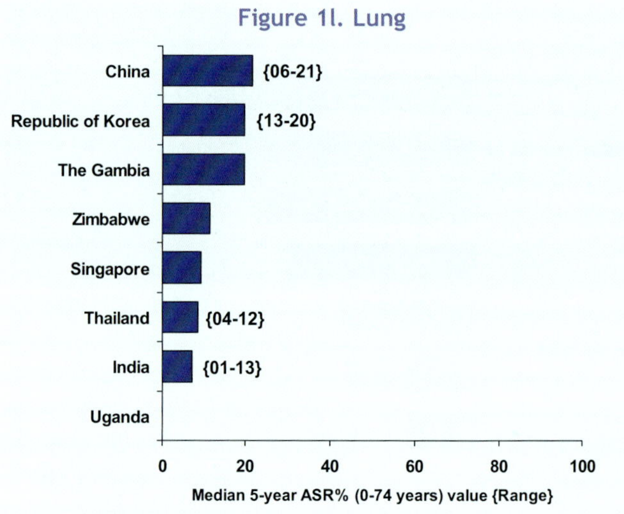

Figure 1 (Continued).

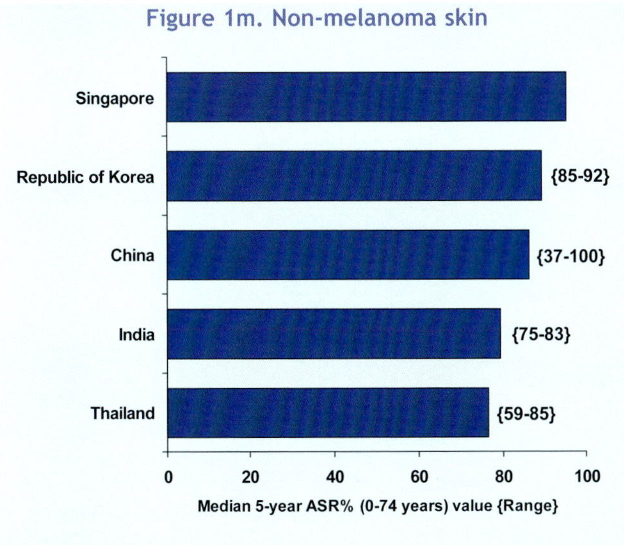

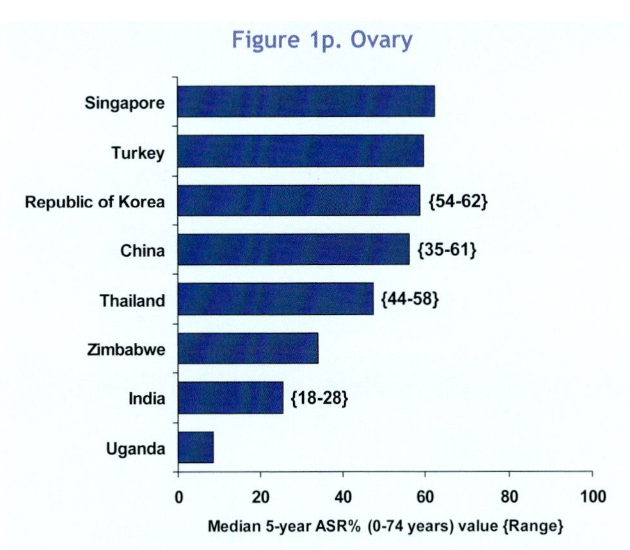

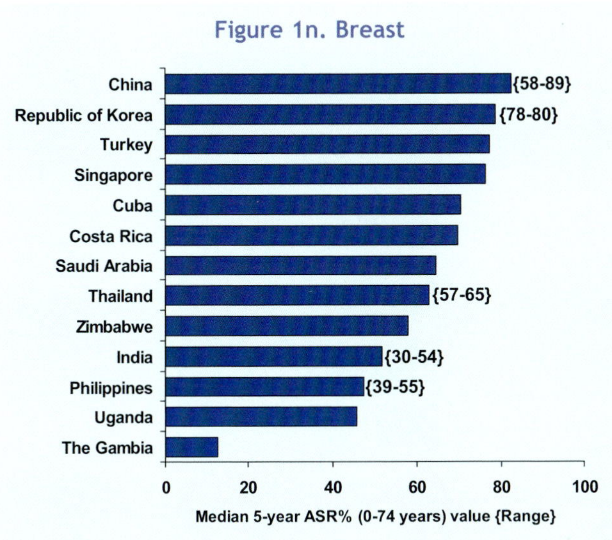

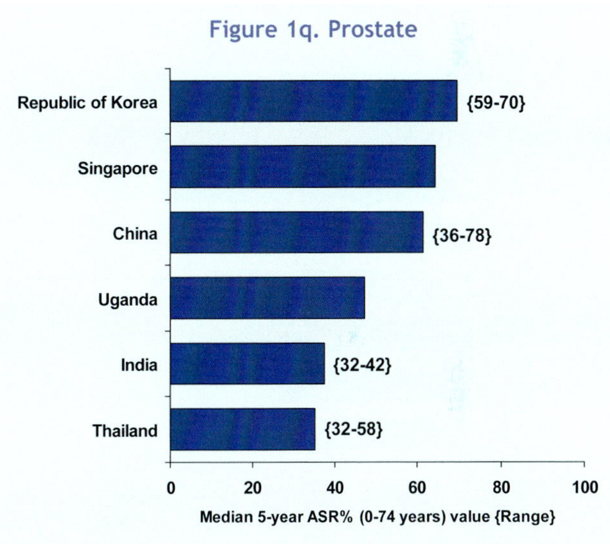

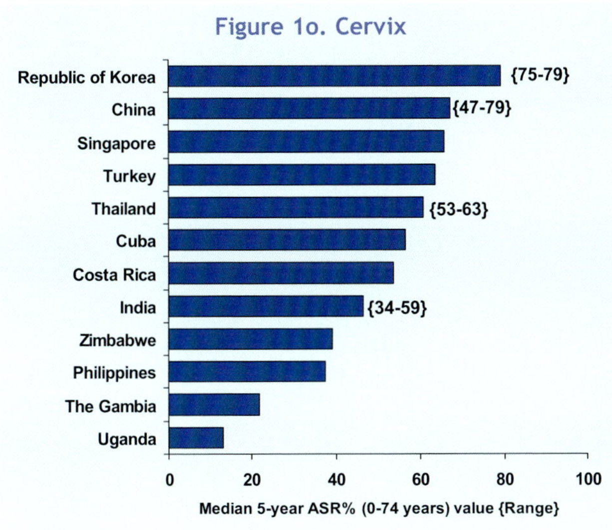

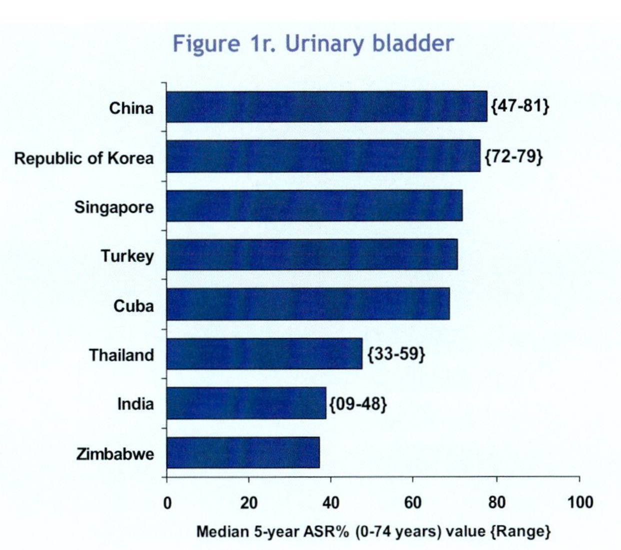

Figure 1 (Continued).

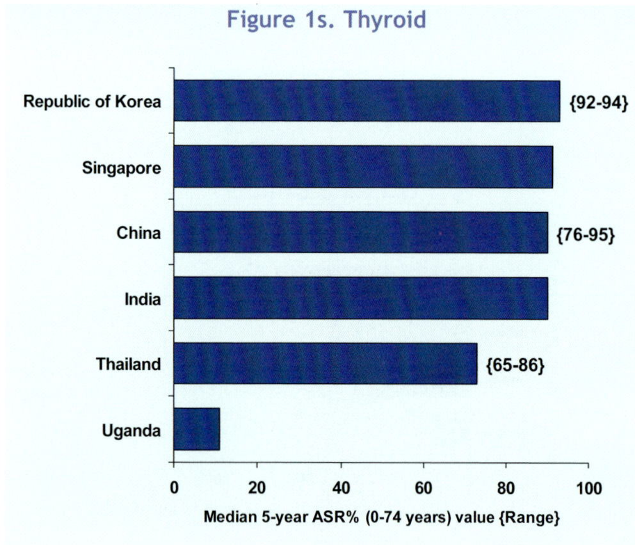

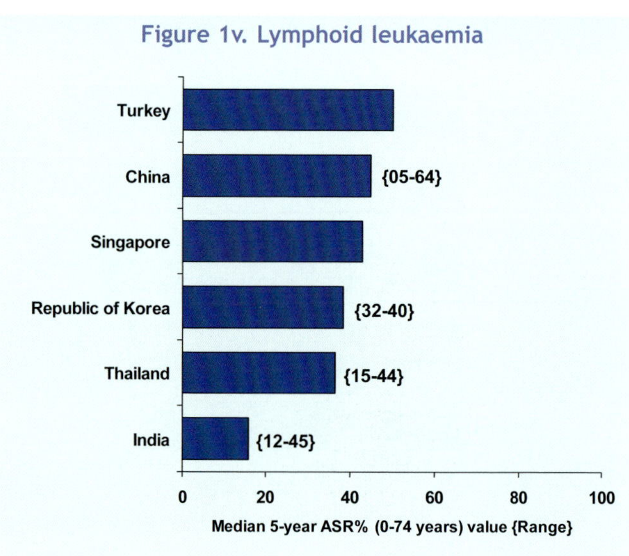

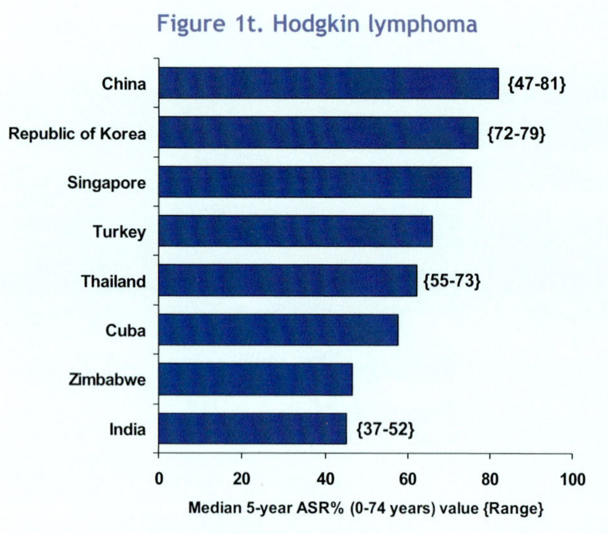

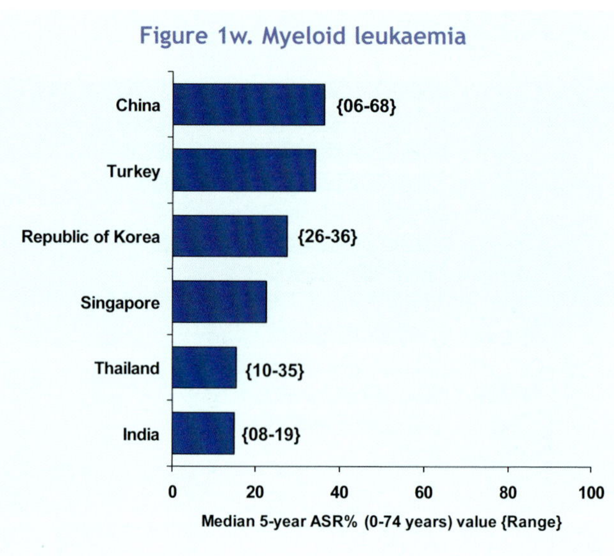

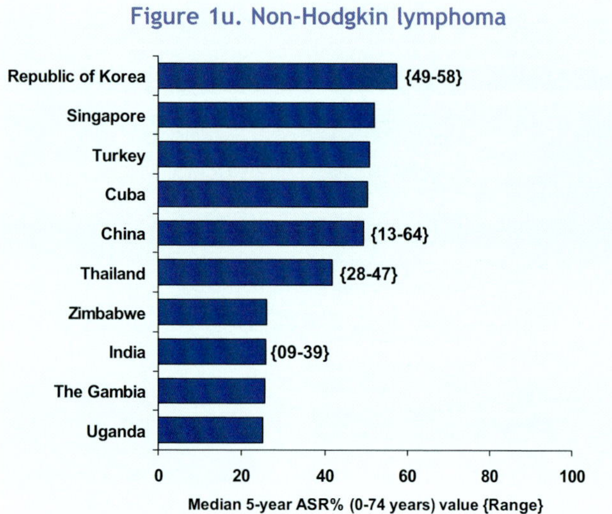

Figure 2. 5-year age-standardized relative survival (ASRS%; 0-74 years) of selected cancers by all registries (ranked on ASRS)

Figure 2a. Tongue (ICD-10: C01-C02)

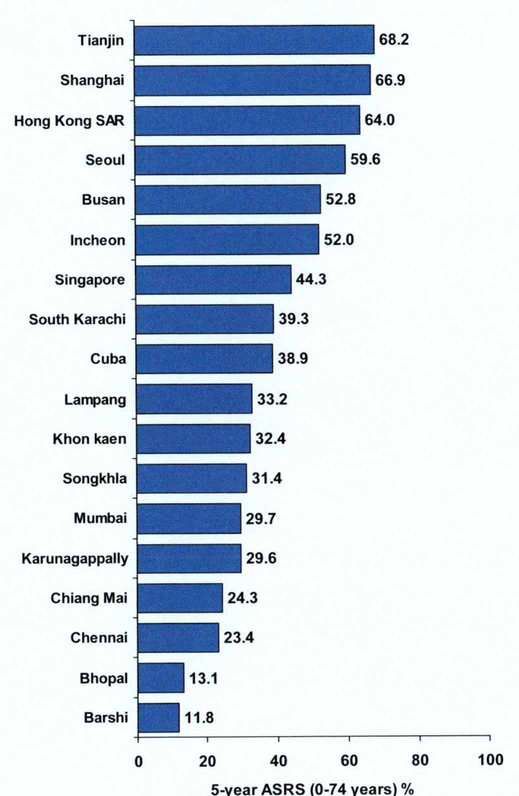

Figure 2c. Nasopharynx (ICD-10: C11)

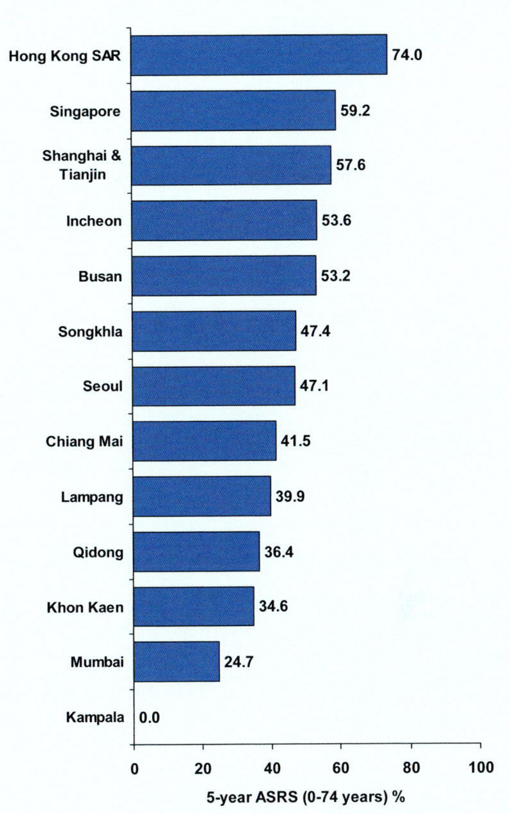

Figure 2b. Oral cavity (ICD-10: C03-06)

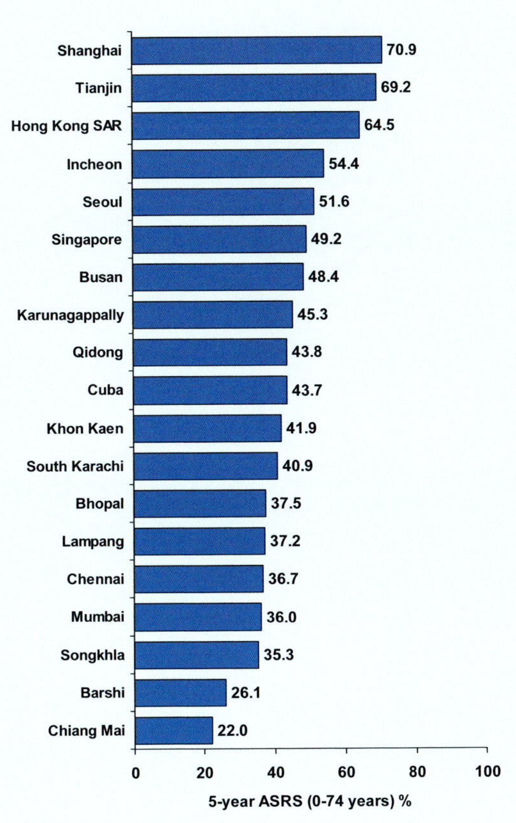

Figure 2d. Hypopharynx (ICD-10: C12-13)

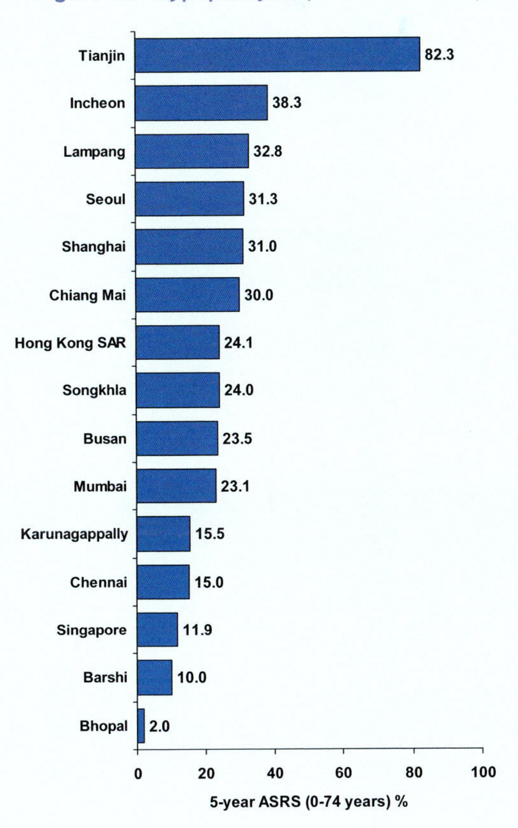

Figure 2 (Continued).

Figure 2e. Oesophagus (ICD-10: C15)

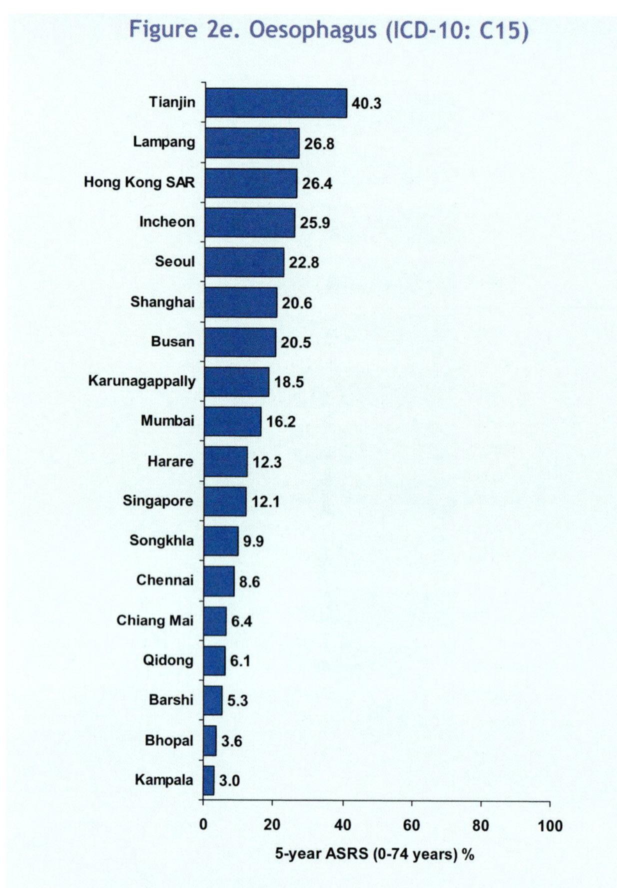

Figure 2g. Colon (ICD-10: C18)

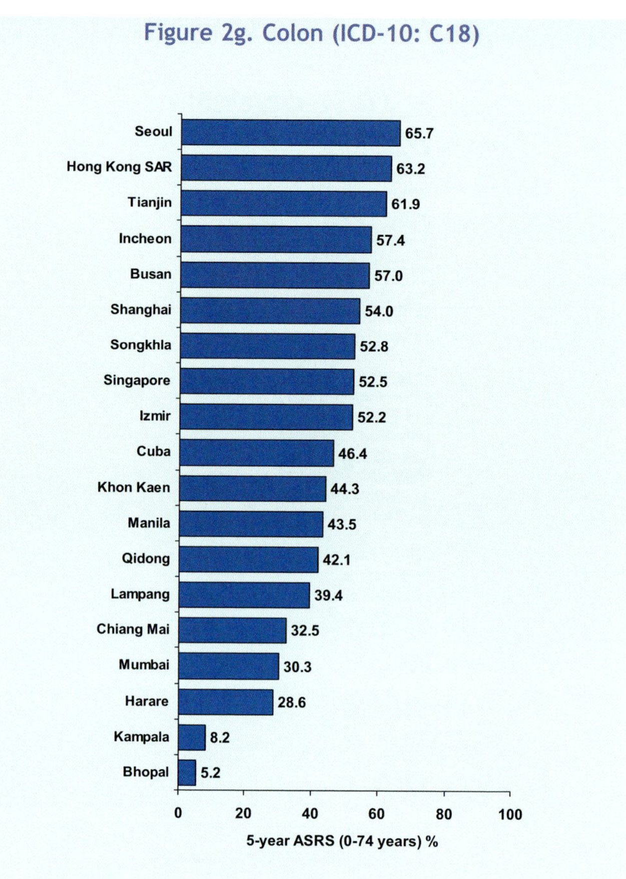

Figure 2f. Stomach (ICD-10: C16)

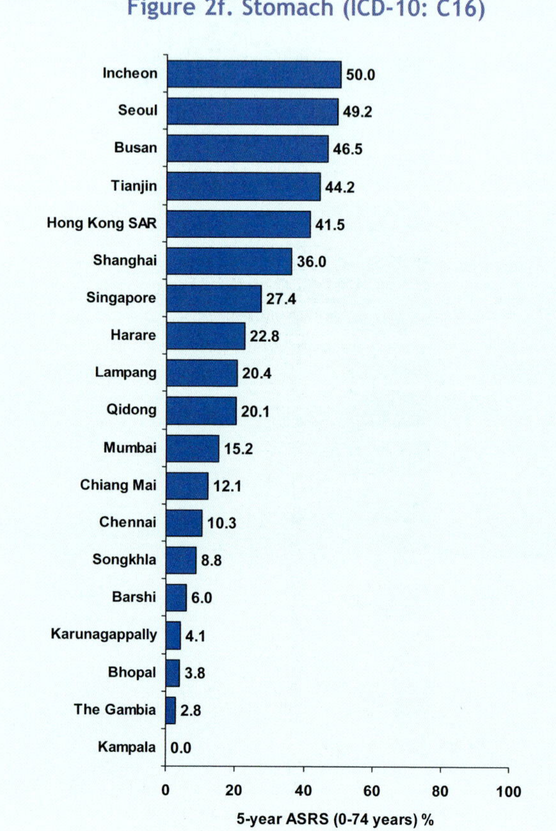

Figure 2h. Rectum (ICD-10: C19-20)

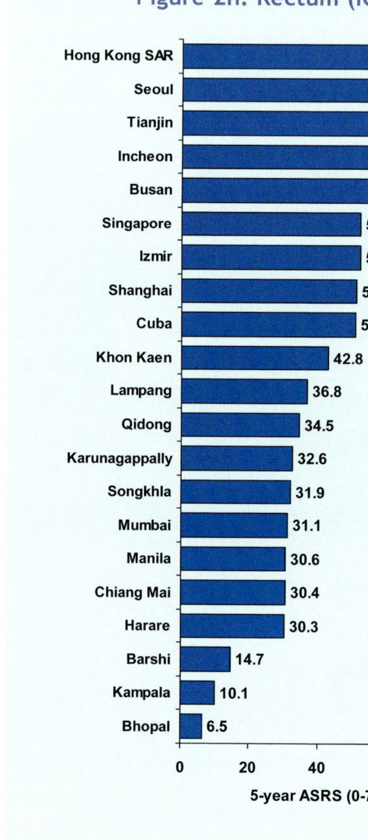

Figure 2 (Continued).

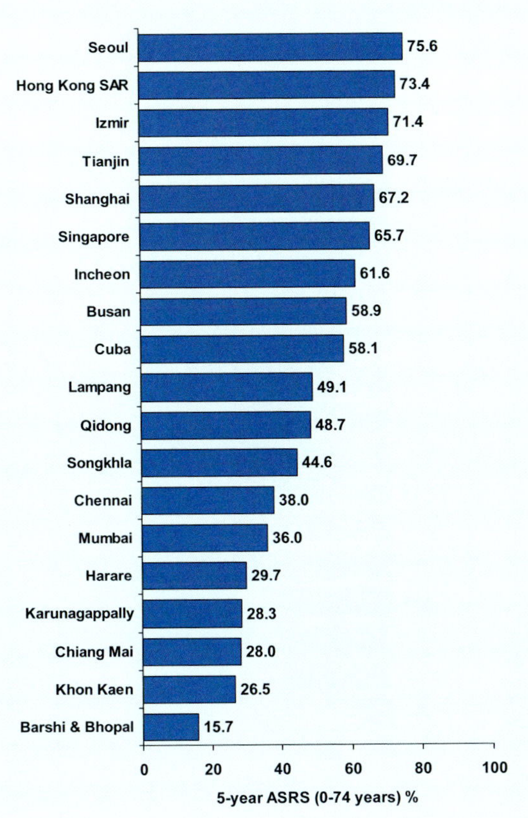

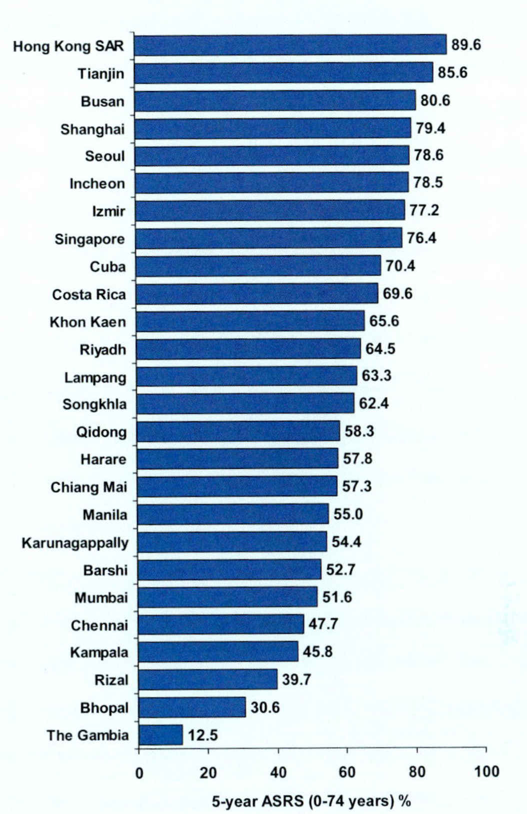

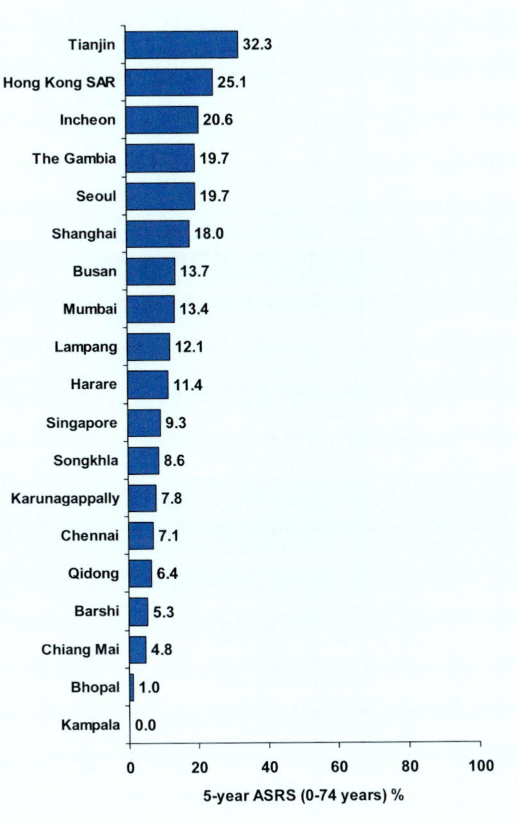

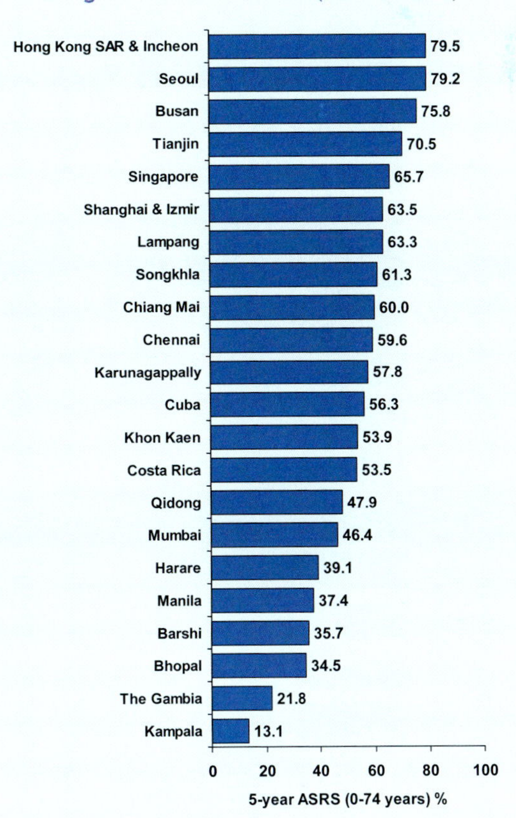

Figure 2 (Continued).

Figure 2m. Ovary (ICD-10: C56)

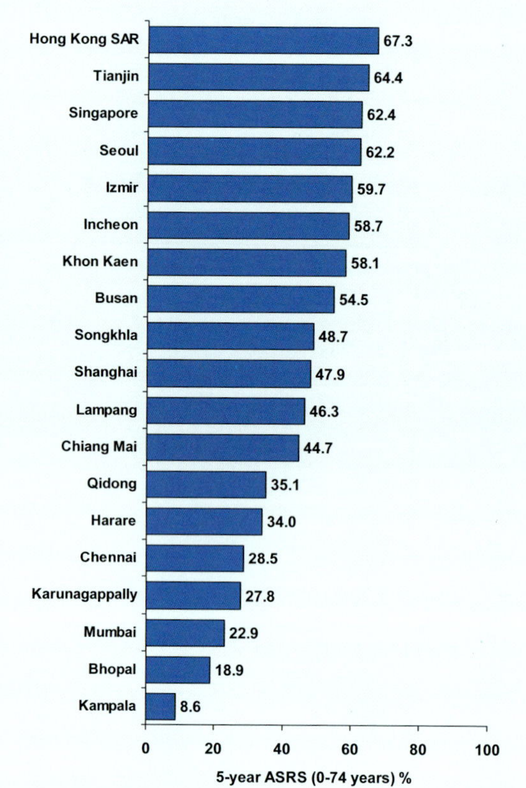

Figure 2n. Prostate (ICD-10: C61)

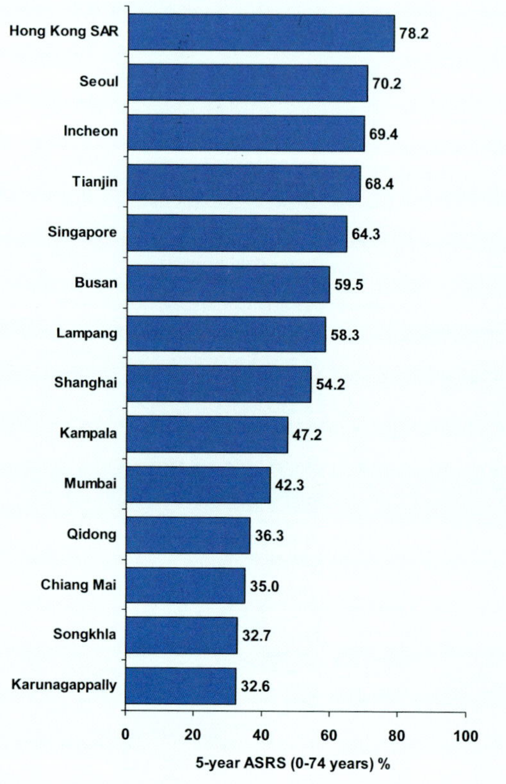

Figure 2o. Urinary bladder (ICD-10: C67)

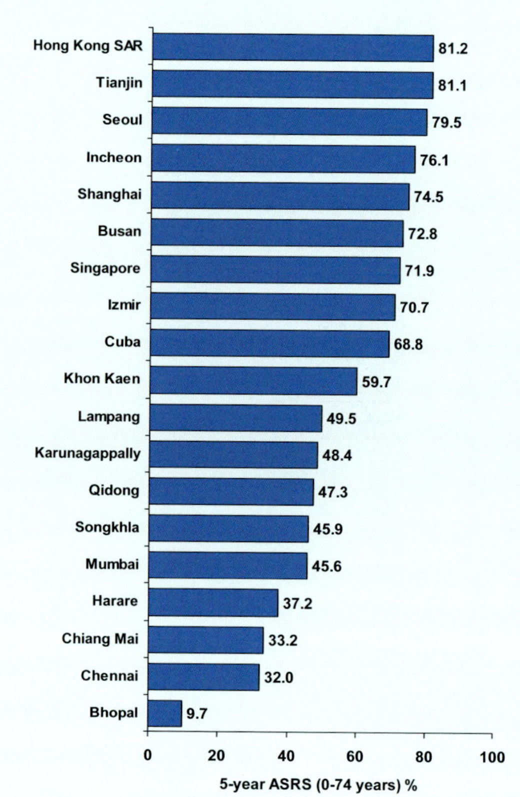

Figure 2p. Hodgkin lymphoma (ICD-10: C81)

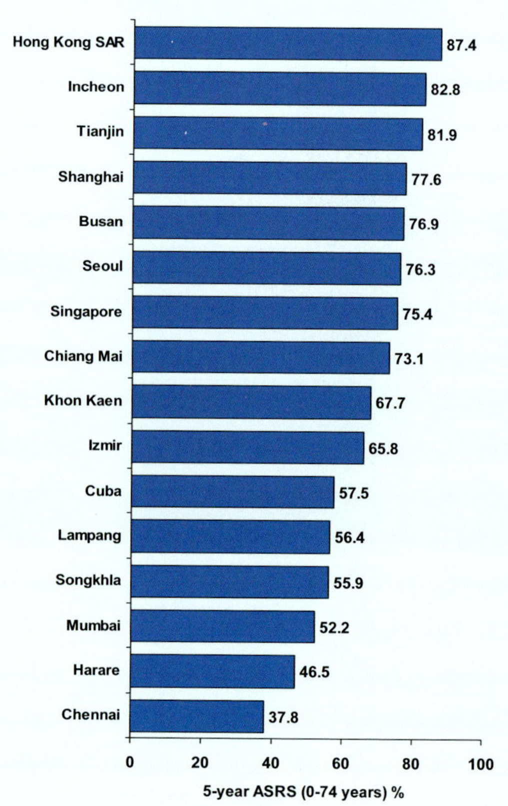

Figure 2 (Continued).

Figure 2q. Non-Hodgkin lymphoma (ICD-10: C82-85; C96)

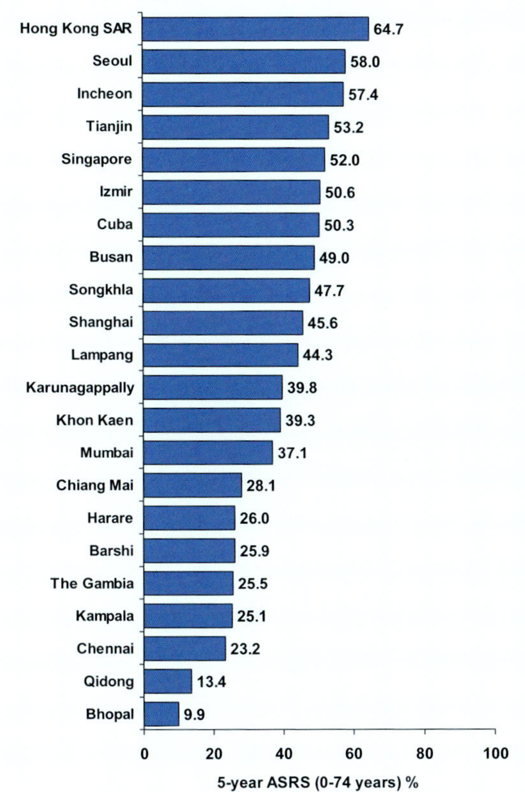

Figure 2r. Lymphoid leukaemia (ICD-10: C91)

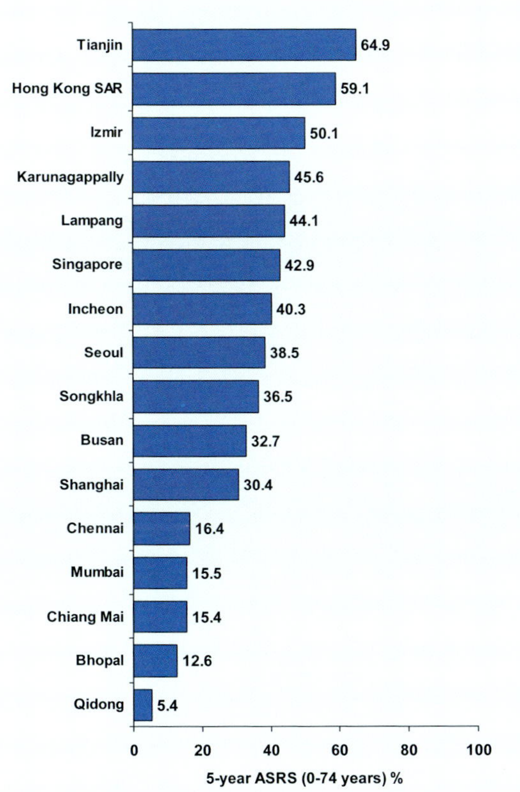

Figure 2s. Myeloid leukaemia (ICD-10: C92-94)

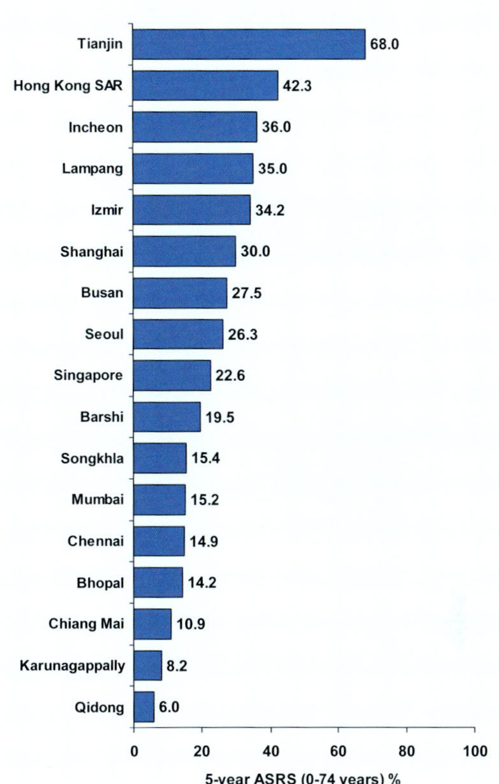

Figure 3. Localized and regional extent of disease among more and less developed health services, larynx cancer

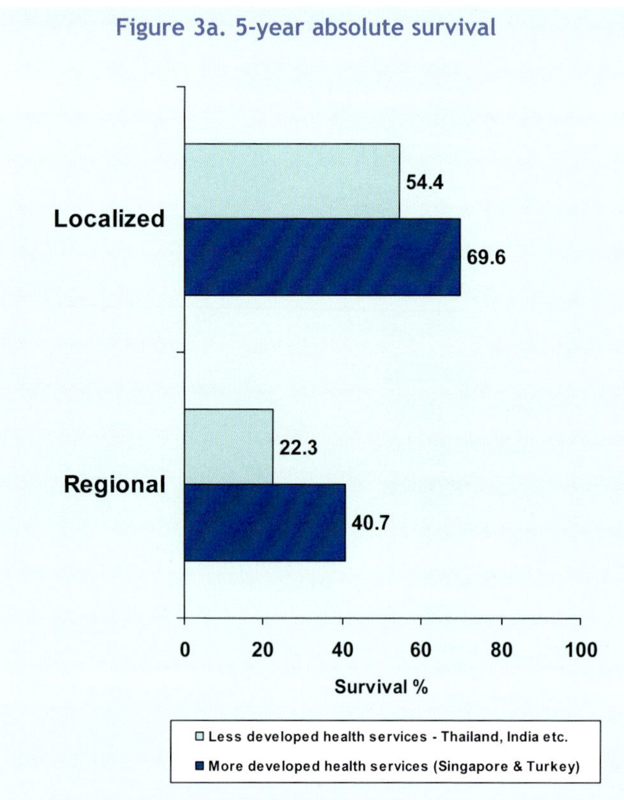

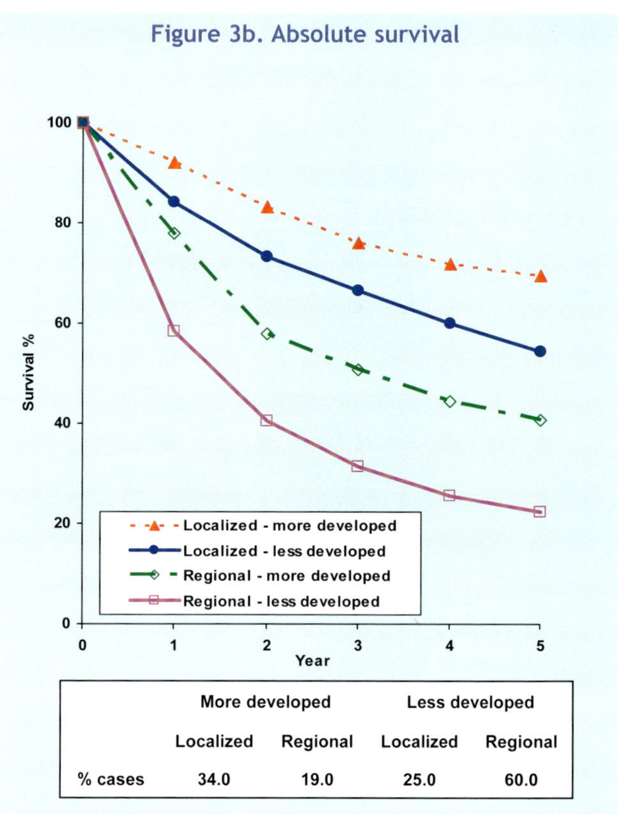

	More developed		Less developed	
	Localized	Regional	Localized	Regional
% cases	34.0	19.0	25.0	60.0

Figure 4. Localized and regional extent of disease among more and less developed health services, large bowel cancer

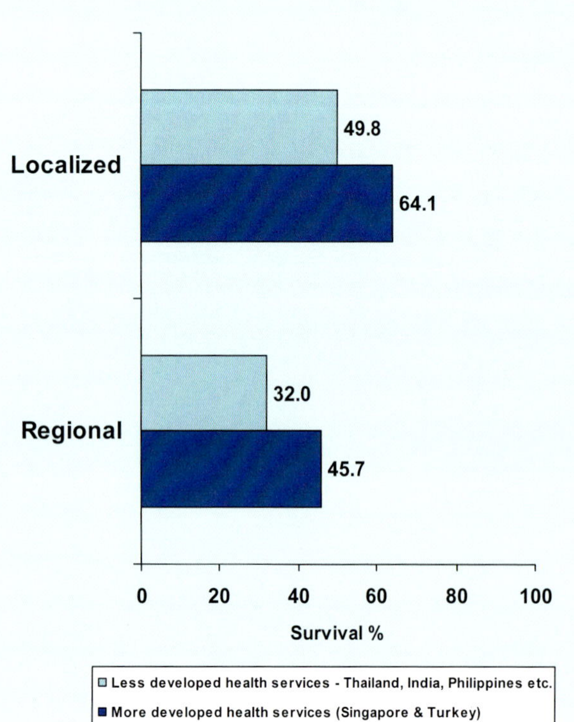

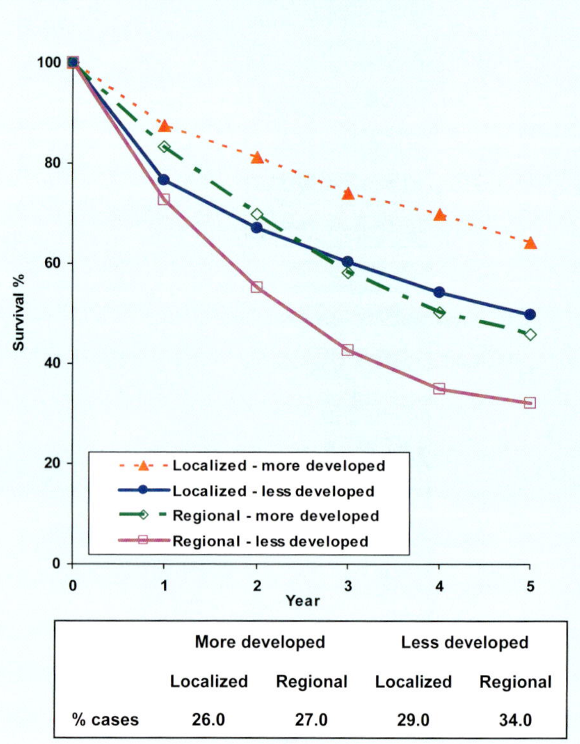

	More developed		Less developed	
	Localized	Regional	Localized	Regional
% cases	26.0	27.0	29.0	34.0

Figure 5. Localized and regional extent of disease among more and less developed health services, breast cancer

Figure 5a. 5-year absolute survival

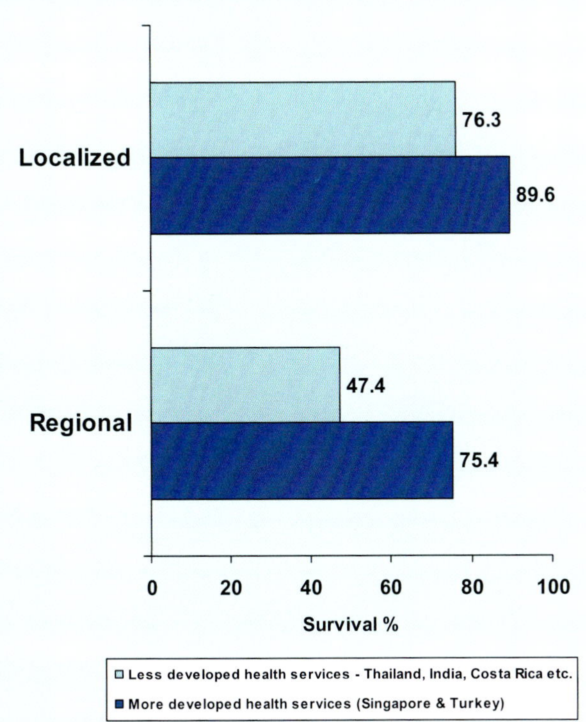

Figure 5b. Absolute survival

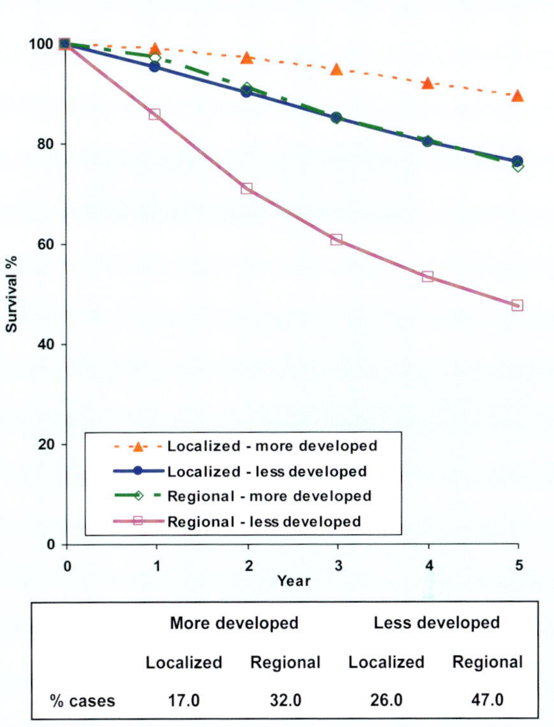

	More developed		Less developed	
	Localized	Regional	Localized	Regional
% cases	17.0	32.0	26.0	47.0

Figure 6. Localized and regional extent of disease among more and less developed health services, cervix cancer

Figure 6a. 5-year absolute survival

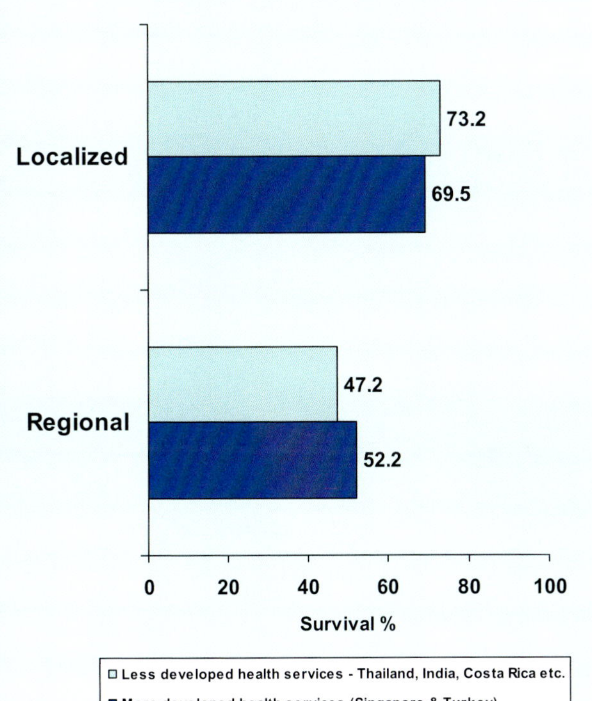

Figure 6b. Absolute survival

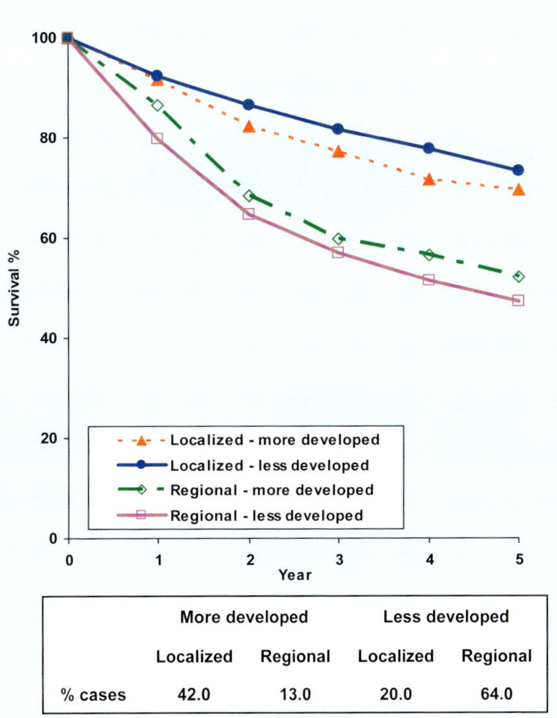

	More developed		Less developed	
	Localized	Regional	Localized	Regional
% cases	42.0	13.0	20.0	64.0

Figure 7. Localized and regional extent of disease among more and less developed health services, ovary cancer

Figure 7a. 5-year absolute survival

Localized
63.8
84.1
Regional
34.5
39.7
0 20 40 60 80 100
Survival %
Less developed health services - Thailand, India etc.
More developed health services (Singapore & Turkey)

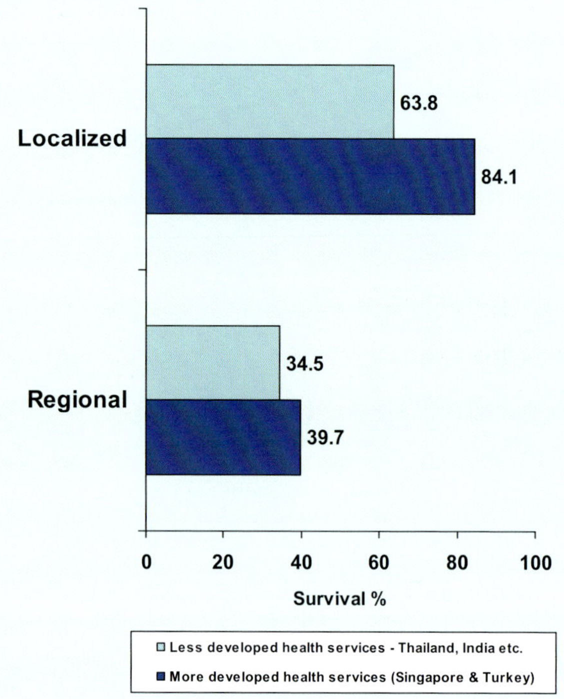

Figure 7b. Absolute survival

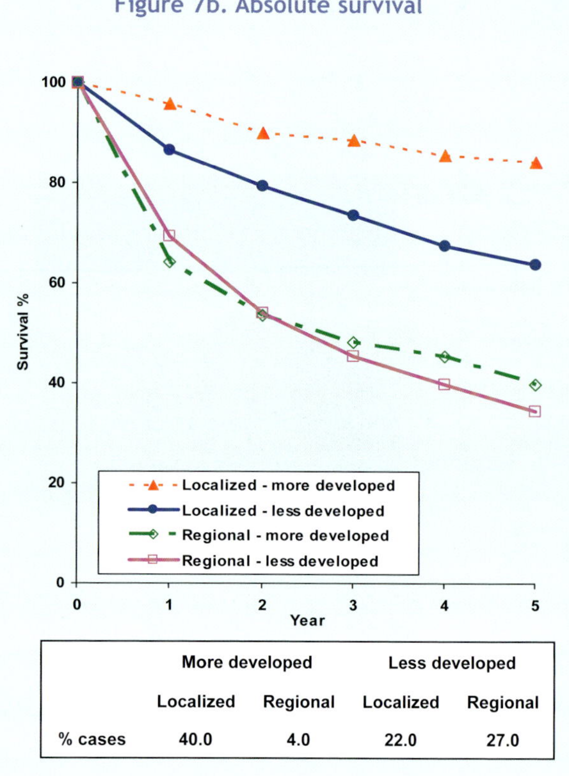

	More developed		Less developed	
	Localized	Regional	Localized	Regional
% cases	40.0	4.0	22.0	27.0

Figure 8. Localized and regional extent of disease among more and less developed health services, bladder cancer

Figure 8a. 5-year absolute survival

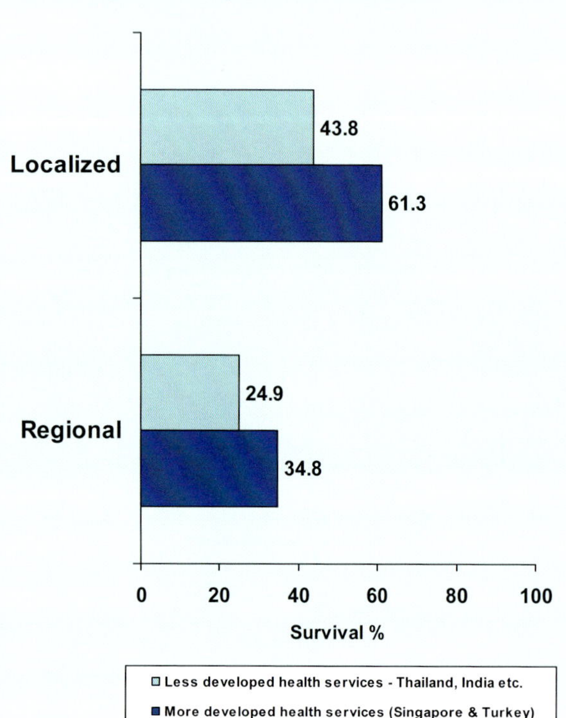

Figure 8b. Absolute survival

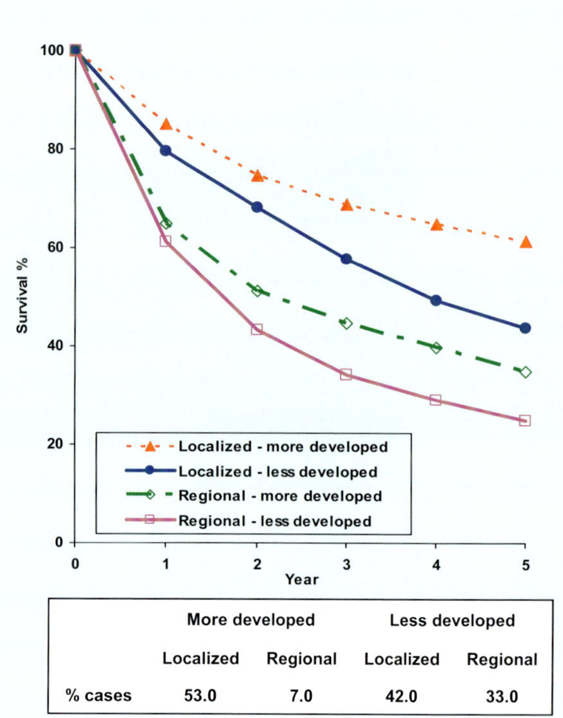

	More developed		Less developed	
	Localized	Regional	Localized	Regional
% cases	53.0	7.0	42.0	33.0

Figure 9. Survival among grouped countries with varied development of health services, Hodgkin lymphoma

Figure 9a. 5-year absolute survival

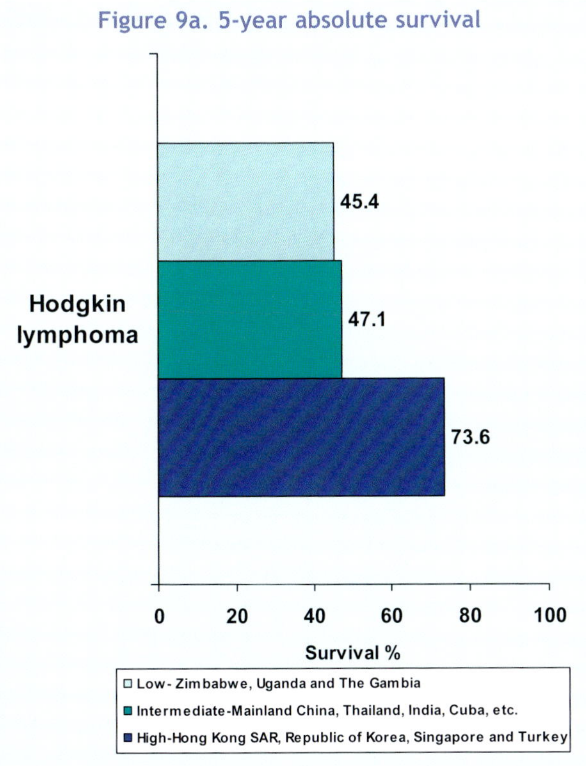

Figure 9b. Absolute survival

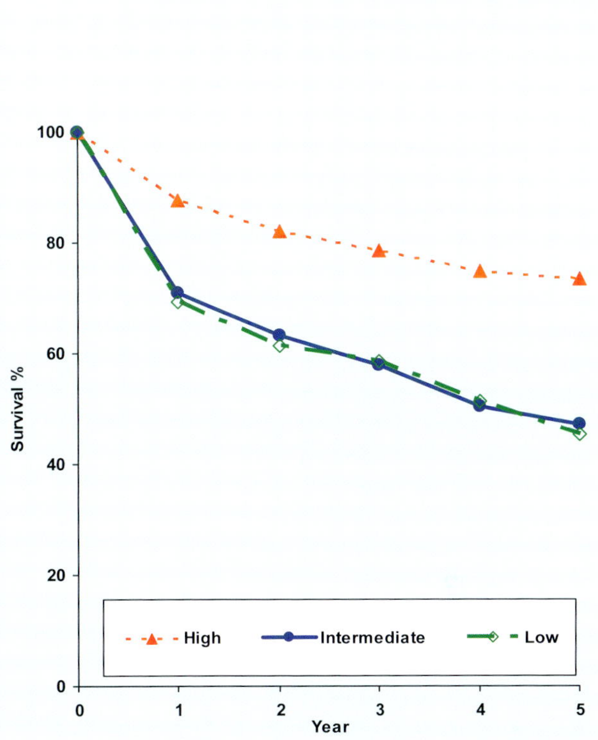

Figure 10. Survival among grouped countries with varied development of health services, non-Hodgkin lymphoma

Figure 10a. 5-year absolute survival

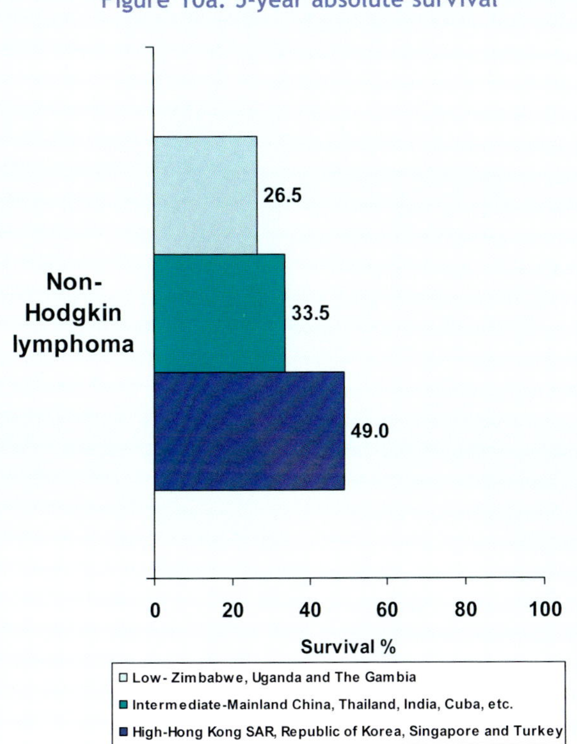

Figure 10b. Absolute survival

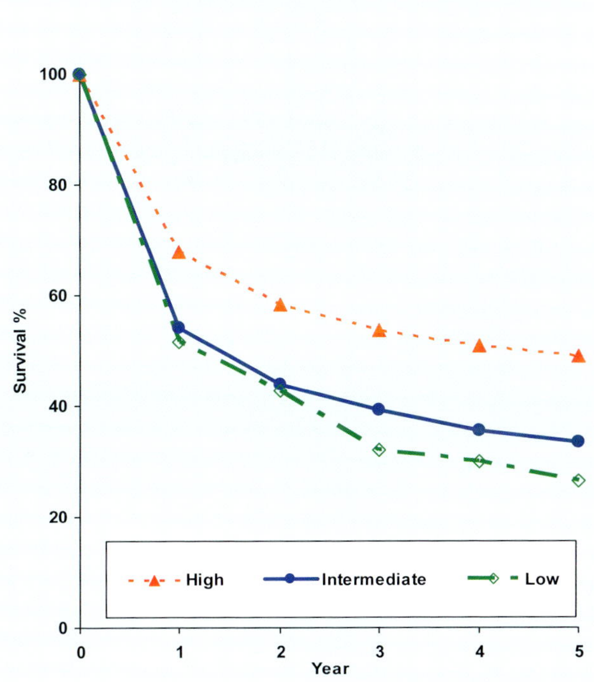

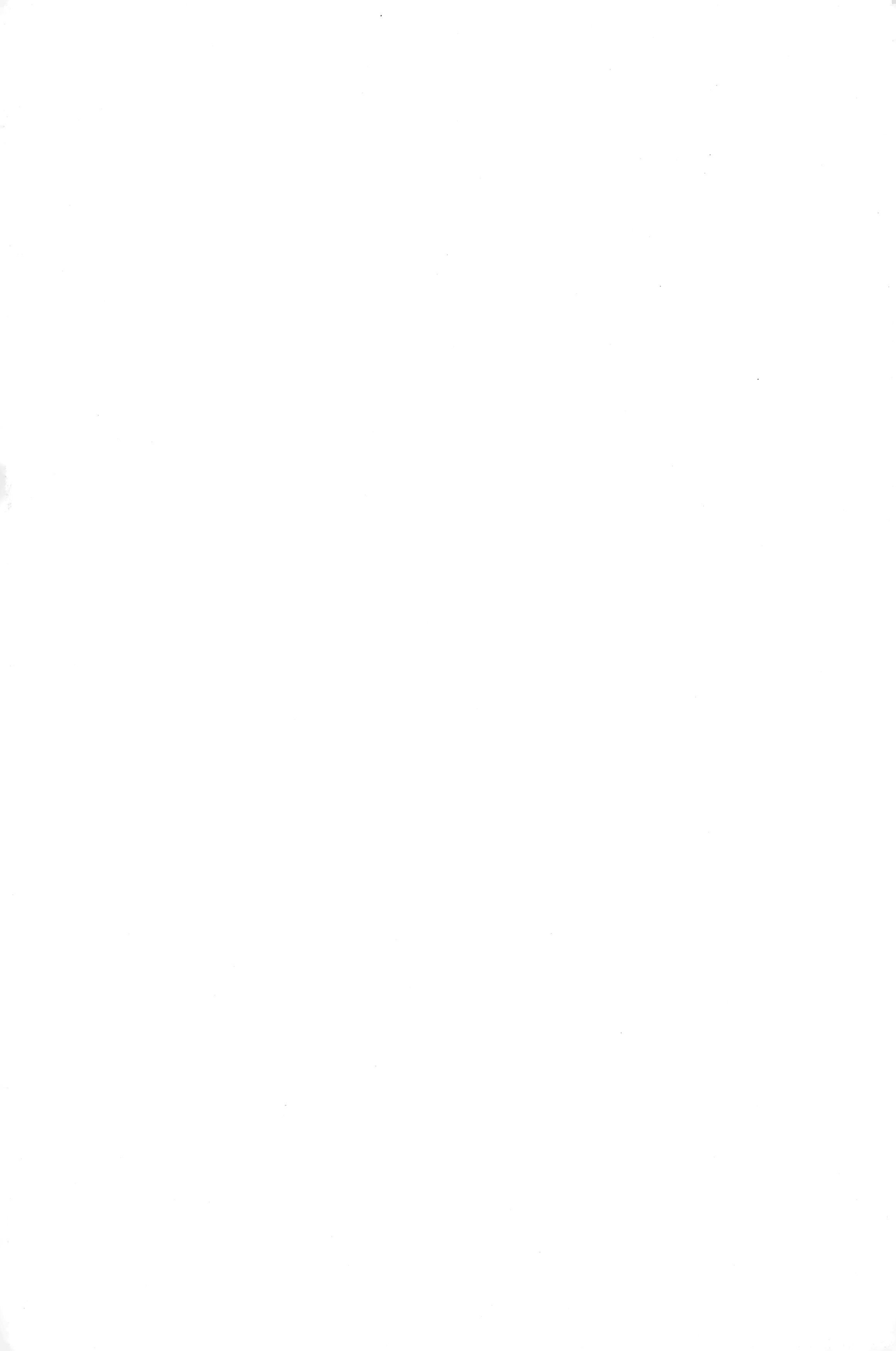